Optimum Health

Optimum Health

*A Natural
Lifesaving Prescription
for Your Body and Mind*

STEPHEN T. SINATRA, M.D.

BANTAM BOOKS
NEW YORK · TORONTO · LONDON · SYDNEY · AUCKLAND

Though this book represents the recommendations I make to my patients concerning a healthy diet and nutritional supplementation, it is not intended to provide medical advice or to substitute for the advice of your physician. The reader should regularly consult a physician in matters relating to his or her health and individual needs, particularly in respect to any symptoms that may require diagnosis or medical attention.

OPTIMUM HEALTH
A Bantam Book / published by arrangement with the author

Publishing History
Lincoln-Bradley Publishing Group edition published 1996
Bantam edition / July 1997

All rights reserved.
Copyright © 1996, 1997 by Stephen T. Sinatra, M.D.
Book design by Robert Bull Design.
No part of this book may be reproduced or transmitted in any form or by any means, electronic or mechanical, including photocopying, recording, or by any information storage and retrieval system, without permission in writing from the publisher.
For information address: Bantam Books.

Library of Congress Cataloging-in-Publication Data

Sinatra, Stephen T.
[Cardiologist's guide to optimum health]
Optimum health : a natural lifesaving prescription for your body
and mind / Stephen T. Sinatra
p.   cm.
Originally published: New York : Lincoln-Bradley Pub. Group, 1996
under the title: A cardiologist's guide to optimum health.
Includes bibliographical references and index.
ISBN 0-553-10613-9 (hardcover)
1. Nutrition.   2. Health.   3. Weight loss.   4. Dietary
supplements.   I. Title.
RA784.S56   1997
613.2—dc21   96-50340
CIP

Published simultaneously in the United States and Canada

Bantam Books are published by Bantam Books, a division of Bantam Doubleday Dell Publishing Group, Inc. Its trademark, consisting of the words "Bantam Books" and the portrayal of a rooster, is Registered in U.S. Patent and Trademark Office and in other countries. Marca Registrada. Bantam Books, 1540 Broadway, New York, New York 10036.

PRINTED IN THE UNITED STATES OF AMERICA

BVG   10 9 8 7 6 5 4 3 2 1

For my deceased father, Salvatore Charles Sinatra, who not only took me to church as a young boy and who taught me how to cook and dance in my adolescence, but also gave me the gift of unconditional love. For my mother, Elizabeth Patricia Sinatra, who loved and supported me through all my endeavors. She taught me more about health and illness than any professor, colleague, or patient. Her unfortunate lifelong struggle with diabetes, glaucoma, blindness, osteoporosis, fractures, and chronic pain has made me look deeper into myself to become a physician who truly cares and heals from his heart.

TABLE OF CONTENTS

ACKNOWLEDGMENTS ix

INTRODUCTION An Allopathic Physician in Recovery xiii

ONE Eight Nutritional Rules for Optimum
Health 1

TWO Fat in America 17

THREE Basic Nutrition: Back to School 25

FOUR Fiber Can Be Fun 35

FIVE Cholesterol: Myth, Fact, and Fiction 43

SIX Fat, Good Fat, and Bad Fat 53

SEVEN The Good, the Bad, and the Ugly:
Water, Salt, Alcohol, and Caffeine 71

EIGHT The Truth about Free Radicals,
Vitamins, and Antioxidants 81

NINE Minerals, Botanicals, and Enzymes 113

TEN Women and Children First 137

ELEVEN Emotional Healing 153

TWELVE Move! 169

THIRTEEN Foods That Heal 185

FOURTEEN Nutritional Healing for the Year 2001 199

FIFTEEN Recipes for Preventive Medicine 215

SIXTEEN The Agony and Ecstasy of Change 239

SEVENTEEN The Search for the Fountain of Youth 247

EIGHTEEN Optimum Health 263

APPENDIX 267

GLOSSARY 285

SELECTED REFERENCES 291

INDEX 309

ACKNOWLEDGMENTS

The research, writing, and editing of this book, as well as an earlier book of mine entitled *Lose to Win*, have consumed considerable energies over the last seven years. There are several people whose contributions have assisted me in taking these books from a vision to a reality.

Steve Williford, who worked on the first edition of this book, has been especially important in making this project a reality. His calming influence, professional direction, and commitment have helped to make the book better. His willingness to travel to my home in Manchester, Connecticut, and work for endless hours is truly appreciated. My predominantly vegetarian household was surely a shock to his meat-and-potatoes diet. Fortunately, an organic turkey was an amazing grace to his soul.

Julia Molino and *Ellen Lieberman* were instrumental in developing the contents of *Lose to Win*. Their writing and editing were most helpful, particularly regarding the issues of love and sexuality as they relate to weight loss. My editor at Bantam, *Brian Tart,* helped me bring my message to a wider audience.

A special thank-you goes to *Jo-Anne Piazza* for her friendship, assistance, and guidance in my mission. As president of Optimum Health International (OHI), LLC, she has endured many hours of hard work and has totally invested her heart in our mission. I appreciate her assistant,

Jo-Anne Renna, who is truly a jack-of-all-trades. I wish to thank *Susan Graham*, LPN and massage therapist, for her creativity and editing. I also could not have completed this project without the continued support of my office staff, *Rosemary Pontillo, Carol Gustamachio, Rebecca Rossick*, and *Caron Maker*. To *Sun King Wan, MD*, and *Laurel Gay, PAC*, my cardiological associates who have endured long hours of clinical work as I was preparing this book, I offer my gratitude. To *Donna Chaput*, who assisted with the typing, to *Genevieve Slomski, PhD*, who assisted in editing the second edition, and to *Peggy Johnson* and *Pat Morolt*, who participated in preparing the first edition of this book, I say thank you.

Additional and significant thanks go to *Brendan Montano, MD*, my good friend, colleague, and an expert in depression and weight management. Your friendship and support have been instrumental in my growth. To *Jose Mullen, MD*, a homeopathic physician who treated my son with homeopathy and love. To *Nicholas Palermo, DO, Anthony Posteraro, MD, Lester Kritzer, MD, Michael Kovalchik, MD*, and *Robert Galvin, MD*, outstanding traditional physicians with open attitudes regarding alternative care. To *Bruce Sobin, MD*, an internist and co-owner of my health food store, Natural Rhythms, for your assistance in editing the first book. To *Ronald Buckman, MD, Joseph Guardino, MD, Daniel Tardiff, MD*, and *Gio Hoang, MD*, who believe in nutritional healing and contributed to the development of my health food store. To *Richard Delany, MD, FACC, Harvey Zarren, MD, FACC, Bruno Cortis, MD, FACC, Peter Langsjoen, MD, FACC*, and *Steven Kunkes, MD, FACC*, cardiological colleagues with parallel belief systems in healing the heart.

To *Arthur B. Landry Jr., MD, FACC*, my former partner and perhaps the best clinical-traditional cardiologist I ever had the opportunity to work with. Your continued friendship, trust, and sincerity I have always treasured.

To *Alexander Lowen, MD*, who touched my heart and life, and to *Philip Helfaer, MD*, my bioenergetic trainer and mentor. To *Frank Hladky, MD*, and *Virginia Wink-Hilton, PhD, Joyce Bellis, John Pierrakos, MD*, and the late *John Bellis, MD*, all inspirational teachers and psychotherapists whom I admire and respect.

To *Hazel Stanley*, my present spiritual guide and adviser—a wise woman with whom I can consult on matters pertaining to the spirit and soul. To *Ann Dahlberg*, my Rolfer, who has worked with my lower back discomfort for the past five years and continues to do so. To my physical therapist, *David Cameron*, on whom I can always count when I am in trouble. To my chiropractors, *David Van Hoeyck, DC,* and *Sharon Vallone, DC,* who give me much physical comfort.

To *Holly Hatch, CSW,* and *Marilyn Anderson, MA,* two therapists who heal from their hearts.

To my men's support group, *Bud Harris Stone, PhD, John Bustelos, Jerry Ainsworth, PhD, Rod Lane, PhD, Paul Nussbaum, MD,* and *Doug Gibson, MD.* Thanks for all of your listening and the feedback from your hearts.

To *Sean Truman* and *George Allen, PhD,* my coinvestigators at the University of Connecticut studying the impact of nutritional supplementation on mind and body.

To pharmacists *Mel Rich* and *Raj Chopra,* two GMP (Good Manufacturers Procedures) manufacturers who have helped me realize my goal of developing my own antioxidant and nutritional formulas. Thanks to *Stanley Jankowitz* for pointing me in the direction of these knowledgeable men. You have been extremely supportive and helpful, especially with your knowledge of nutrition. To *Gordon Stagg,* who participated in the development of OHI. To *Fred Mendelsohn* of Environmental Lighting Concepts, Inc., who introduced me to the world of television. To *Tony Little,* a man whose mission to promote exercise is enhancing the lives of literally millions of people. To *Karen Berney, Kate Fiedler, Bobbie Lieberman, Amy Painter, Julia Noble, Karen Phillips, Dan Kagan, Donna Engelgau, Lisa Goldman,* and *Lorna Newman* of Phillips Publishing Company, for helping me in my educational mission for the *HeartSense* newsletter.

To my former wrestling coaches, *Donald Jackson* and the late *Ken Hunte.* Through their warrior activities, I experienced the gift of discipline with the agony and ecstasy of intensive training, hard work, and winning.

To my attorneys, *Michael Darby* and *Dominic Squatrito.* Thanks for the endless hours of difficult negotiations and for protecting me in the pursuit of my vision.

Thanks to *Jeannine Cyr-Gluck* and *Elizabeth Marx,* the librarians at Manchester Memorial Hospital, who provided me with vital information. To *Anna Salo,* my secretary in the Department of Medical Education.

To *Bev Grady, RN, Mo Criascia, RN,* and *Lisa Holmes, RN,* for taking the risks in teaching alternative care.

To *Barbara Palmer,* who manages my health food store, and *Kye*

Cohen, a former employee. Thanks to you and all my employees for the great food prepared with love.

To *Roberta Ruland, RD,* my nutritional consultant, who integrates the dynamics of eating and behavior.

To my special friends, *Bill* and *Ursula Niarakis, Tony* and *Roberta Visconti, Dr. John* and *Mary Puskas, John* and *Jean Fleet,* and *Drs. Bob* and *Kathy Lang.* Your continued support of me and my work has been so greatly appreciated.

To *Fran Kovarik, PhD,* and *Steve Novil, PhD,* of the Academy of Antiaging Medicine, and *Ruth Buczynski, PhD,* of the National Institute for the Clinical Application of Behavioral Medicine, for supporting my mission in preventive medicine at the national conference level. Your commitment to high-quality education is truly admirable. To *Stanley Cheslock, Louis Zemsky, MD,* and *Richard Johnson, CPA,* my college wrestling teammates and fraternity brothers at Lambda Alpha fraternity.

To my ex-wife, *Suzy Sinatra,* my lifelong friend and mother of my children, who gave me tremendous support through my early clinical years. To my brother, *Richard,* and my sisters, *Pam* and *Maria.* Your love and encouragement have touched my heart. To my children, *March, Step,* and *Drew,* who are such tremendous treasures in my life. You are all lovable "messengers" in your very own unique ways. To *Jan DeMarco, RN,* who has been truly helpful in the writing and editing of both editions of this book. Your continued love and support have been valued and appreciated.

There are many other individuals who contributed to this work, particularly the patients I have treated for years. I have grown to love them as we all age through what, sometimes, are difficult and treacherous times. They undoubtedly have been my best teachers. Their struggles in battling disease have touched my heart on so many occasions.

An Allopathic Physician in Recovery

W̶e in the very late twentieth century are on the verge of witnessing a total transformation of health care in the United States. Skyrocketing health care costs are bankrupting the individual, the family, and the entire country. In today's disease-oriented society, most physicians wait until symptoms occur and then treat their patients with hospitalization, surgery, and expensive drugs. The cost of this type of care is high. According to recent statistics, Americans spend over eighteen billion dollars on coronary artery bypass surgery annually. But what is the alternative?

The alternative, quite simply, involves a paradigm shift from disease to health and prevention. This shift is not only necessary; it is inevitable. But it would mean that disease would no longer be big business. And it would mean that instead of rushing to make quotas, we would have to do it the old-fashioned way—we would have to care for patients' minds and spirits as well as their bodies.

Our era of high-tech medicine stands in direct contrast to the 1920s, when Dr. Francis W. Peabody stated in the *Journal of the American Medical Association* that the most important aspect of medicine is "caring for the patient." Our government and our politicians have failed to assist the medical profession in adopting a health care system that is both affordable and humane. Gone are the days of empathy, nurturing, and true healing.

As a clinical cardiologist, I have worked with many cases of heart disease, but my introduction to true healing emerged during my training as a psychoanalyst. After twelve years of study in both Gestalt and bioenergetic psychotherapy, it became clear to me that pathology (becoming ill) is often a form of dis-ease that emerges from the chaotic imbalance of mind, body, and spirit.

My interest in writing this book has been a slowly evolving and growing passion. Over the past twenty years I have cared for patients struggling with heart-related disease and have come to understand some of the processes that lead to this illness.

When considering illness, diagnosis, and treatment, I began to focus not only on the disease and the physical dysfunction it caused, but also on all the human operational planes. I soon developed a new appreciation for conscious as well as unconscious drives. I realized that to be on such a journey, I needed to be more in touch with the body's energy systems.

The healthy operation of the human energy system involves both generative and maintenance phases. Adequate formation of energy depends on the intake of sufficient oxygen and essential nutrients. But maintaining balance is based on a more complex set of variables. A deficiency or an imbalance in any part of the system may contribute, over time, to the impaired functioning of our cells, tissues, organs, and eventually our entire bodies. Thus the concept of energy is both quantitative and qualitative. A proper balance of oxygen and nutritional components, such as vitamins, minerals, enzymes, and cofactors, is required for cells to function properly.

The realization that true healing takes place only when this balance is restored ignited my interest in exploring the energetic/metabolic/nutritional constituents that make up the whole process of optimum health. Just how important is this process?

FACT   Coronary artery disease is the leading cause of death in the industrialized world.

FACT   Cancer is the second-leading cause of death.

FACT   Coronary artery disease and cancer may be preventable by risk factor modification.

FACT   Obesity is a risk factor for both heart disease and cancer.

FACT   The way to good health is a balanced diet, proper weight maintenance, exercise, and appropriate nutritional supplementation.

FACT Prevention is easier than cure.

FACT A study recently published in *The Lancet* reported that elderly people taking multivitamins with minerals had improved immune function and had 50 percent fewer sick days.

FACT Increased intakes of antioxidant vitamins (beta carotene, vitamin C, vitamin E) could potentially prevent or postpone 50 to 70 percent of cataracts.

FACT Two studies recently conducted at the Harvard University School of Public Health and Harvard Medical School showed that taking 100 IU per day of vitamin E supplements for more than two years reduced the risk of heart disease by 26 percent in a group of more than 45,000 men, and by 41 percent in a group of more than 85,000 women.

FACT Environmental toxins such as polluted air, radiation, chemical poisons, heavy metals, auto emissions, and cigarette smoke boost our need for supplemental nutrients.

FACT The common degenerative diseases of the twentieth century, such as atherosclerotic cardiovascular disease, cancer, osteoporosis, diabetes, arthritis, and Alzheimer's disease, have been associated with premature aging due to free-radical oxidative stress. Many of these diseases can be largely prevented by lifestyle modification.

FACT A California study suggested that vitamin C greater than 300 to 500 mg per day may increase life expectancy due to a decrease in heart attacks and various forms of cancer.

FACT In a Chinese study of 29,000 people, the ingestion of beta carotene, vitamin E, and selenium produced a 13 percent reduction in esophageal and gastric cancer and a 9 percent reduction in death from these diseases as compared to the population not taking supplements.

FACT Clinical research has shown that meditation and/or silent prayer have resulted in reduced blood pressure.

FACT Nutrition is still a great unexplored area in science, medicine, and health and plays a major role in optimum health.

I'm convinced that life can be healthier for most people than it presently is. I think the message of how to achieve optimum health and enhance the quality of life needs to be shared with as many people as possible.

In this book, I focus on how you can nurture your body with nutritional, emotional, and spiritual healing. I try to provide simple answers to complex questions on how to achieve optimum health. Although healing is truly a multifaceted process, this book offers clear and concise information about vitamins, minerals, fat, fiber, and cholesterol. It includes valuable facts about exercise and healing foods as well as the latest information about antiaging strategies. It also explains how nutritional supplements can make a difference in your life.

One more thing. I realize that I provide a *lot* of information—maybe more information than you want. I guess because I'm a researcher as well as a clinical cardiologist, I want to share as much information as possible with my peers, patients, and friends. Let me suggest that you use this book as a handy health reference. Even though you might not be immediately interested in every topic I cover, chances are that one day you'll need some information in this book for yourself or someone close to you.

HEALING THE HEART

Like me, many physicians have experienced a gradual shift in their approach to illness. We have become interested in the philosophy and psychology of healing and in complementary and alternative care techniques. Still, we need to ask ourselves the question, What is it that makes some people ill? For example, why do some people catch the flu and others don't? Are there certain constitutional weaknesses in some individuals that make them more vulnerable?

I applied this question to the phenomenon of sudden cardiac death. Clinically, this unexpected event occurs as the first symptom of heart disease in up to 40 percent of cases. This is a somber statistic for a cardiologist to deal with. As I gained more experience in treating heart disease, it became evident that heart disease is usually a slow process that evolves over time. However, a heart attack may occur at any time and may or may not lead to sudden death.

Your vulnerability to heart attack arises from a combination of traditional risk factors, including stress, emotional arousal, unaccustomed physical activity, intense psychological and emotional needs, depression, and dissatisfaction with life. For many, the pathological condition of heart disease involves both controllable and uncontrollable risk factors.

The uncontrollable risk factors include family history, gender, and age. Controllable risk factors include cigarette smoking, high blood pressure, high cholesterol, sedentary living, obesity, psychological stress, and other variables. Many of these risk factors are actually extensions of our personality and character. For example, consider that high blood pressure may be related to repressed feelings, particularly anger and rage, and that cardiac arrhythmias may be related to fear, anxiety, or panic.

Over the years I have come to appreciate firsthand that illness has strong emotional and psychological components. It is true that for many, coronary artery disease arises from years of self-destructive behavior. For others, however, the disease often reflects an unconscious, maladaptive search for one's true self. Many of my patients have testified that heart disease has offered them an opportunity to delve deeper into their emotional and spiritual being, thus changing the way they choose to live in the world. Let me explain.

In addition to treating heart attacks with the traditional medical approach, I am now more interested in and committed to looking for the reasons why a patient had a heart attack in the first place. I even inquire as to the specific time of the heart attack in order to look for contributing factors. After recovery, I attend to the patient's nutritional, emotional, psychological, and physical needs. We examine together the relationship between a maladaptive lifestyle and heart disease. My role as a physician has evolved from treating physical illness to seeing and treating the patient as a whole person.

Disease or catastrophic illness has the incredible potential to cause an emotional and psychological shift, bringing the individual to a new awareness of who he or she really is. For many of my patients, heart disease has enlightened them and led them to take what M. Scott Peck calls "the road less traveled." Simply put, this is the spiritual road to healing. I have spent many tender moments with my patients as they gain new insights into themselves. Some even begin to see their heart disease as a "gift," moving them to a higher level of growth.

STRESS AND ILLNESS

Is the heart just a pump that circulates blood throughout the body? Or is it a place for thoughts, emotions, passions, and feelings, as the poets say? Finding the answer has been my quest throughout my more than twenty years as a cardiologist and fifteen years of practicing bioenergetic analysis.

Early in my career, I noticed that many of my patients who suffered from heart disease also experienced high levels of stress. I began researching this correlation. Later I published some of my findings on the relationship between stress and disease, with particular application to the heart, in medical journals. Then I realized that I needed to pursue specialized training in the field of psychotherapy. The more I read, the more I wanted to know. The connection among mind, emotion, and heart became more clear to me, but I still needed to put it all together. The missing piece was the study of one's character, including my own.

My investigation further convinced me that the power of emotion is directly related to health and illness. The study of the relationship between the mind and body is so vast and intricate that the more I pursued these relationships, the more inadequate I felt. The subject was broad and, at the time, relatively unexplored.

Although there was some research into the relationship between stress and illness and between personality and heart disease, there was little data available on the development of character and its effect on subsequent cardiac illness. I wanted to know if there was something beyond type A behavior. Was type A behavior just a symptom of one's personality? Was there something more profound that was as yet undiscovered and worthy of further analysis? Might this be the missing link?

I had begun my search for causative factors that may have the potential to render one vulnerable to heart disease. The identification and modification of these character traits for enhancing and prolonging life became my purpose. This is why, as a traditionally trained cardiologist, I decided later to become a psychotherapist as well. (To my knowledge, I am the only certified cardiologist who is also a certified bioenergetic psychotherapist.)

Bioenergetic therapy is a psychoanalytically based therapy originating from the works of Wilhelm Reich. Reich, an Austrian psychiatrist and a student of Freud's, proposed that love and healthy sexuality could cure the ills of mankind. Reich was known for his writings on the relationship among disease, emotions, and the denial or absence of pleasure. He described cancer as a resignation from life and believed that cancer originates because of unreleased feelings of sadness and anger that cause depression.

Recently it has been verified that emotions do play a major role in cancer. Bernie Siegel, in his book *Love, Medicine, and Miracles,* discusses the "cancer personality" as being one who is stuck and willing to give up. Siegel says that fighting back through releasing anger and suppressed feeling, as well as forgiving and loving the self and visualizing the self overcoming the enemy cancer within, is the way to heal. You cannot rely on your physician to heal you, Siegel says; you must take a proactive role—and I agree.

Alexander Lowen has spent a lifetime expanding Reich's theory and developing his own. As a student of Reich's, Lowen created the therapy called bioenergetics, a body-oriented analytic therapy focusing on the muscular tensions in the body that are the physical counterparts of the emotional conflict in the personality.

In bioenergetic analysis, the therapist can determine where tension is located and where energy is blocked. By utilizing various techniques and exercises to charge and discharge the body, the bioenergetic therapist can release trapped energy, which allows for dissipation of tension.

Lowen's theory incorporating emotional conflict and physical expression in the disease model so appealed to me that I decided to study under him in a program of self-exploration and psychotherapy. I was particularly struck by Lowen's focus on breathing. It became more apparent to me that energy and breathing were related to heart disease. I have seen an "inability to breathe" and restricted breathing patterns in many of my coronary patients. For example, many of us have noticed aggressive, coronary-prone individuals suck in air during conversations (even while continuing to speak) and emit brief sighs and/or muffled grunts when breathing out. This disturbance in respiration becomes a charged, nonpulsating energetic cycle, which makes it hard to relax. Many of these patients also tend to hold their breath as well. Such respiratory motility problems cause rigidity and chest wall tension.

Thus, learning to breathe is an essential ingredient in obtaining optimum health. Why? Because deeper, fuller breathing not only increases the physical amount of oxygen needed to drive the body's metabolic processes, but also assuages tissue spasticities and releases tension. By freeing up blocked feelings and emotions, breathing gets the body in touch with feeling. As a psychotherapist, I have seen many patients perform deep-breathing exercises and as a result experience deep feelings, crying, and emotional release. This release in itself is healing. Breathing is thus the focus of any body-oriented therapy.

I learned the value of deep and fuller respirations, not just in my own bioenergetic therapy with Lowen but also in a Rolfing program, which I decided to enter to further my healing after my father died of a ruptured aorta. Rolfing is an intense body therapy aimed at loosening up deep tissue spasticities by direct myofascial massage. Rolfing, deep tissue work, and massage are all excellent therapies designed to get you in touch with your body and its feelings. I still continue to have monthly Rolfing sessions. In addition to loosening up the spasticities in my lower back and pelvis, Rolfing also assuages the sympathetic nervous system. Like meditation, yoga, tai chi, and qi gong, Rolfing is an alternative therapy with considerable potential for healing the body.

Alternative medical care is in direct contrast to allopathic care, or traditional care, which relies on acute crisis intervention, pharmacology, surgery, and various other "cookbook" approaches to treat underlying disorders. For example, the cardiologist treats an acute heart attack with a multitude of drugs and invasive interventions. In an emergency, such traditional therapies are lifesaving for the patient. However, in nonemergent situations, you have many options from which to choose.

THE ALLOPATHIC MEDICAL MODEL

The standard allopathic model is crisis-oriented or, in simple terms, a Band-Aid fix. Consider the use of aspirin for a headache. Although aspirin may give you some relief for the headache, in most cases we do not examine why the headache occurred or how to prevent it from recurring. The typical model of medicine in this country is based on fixing problems with pharmacological, surgical, and other external interventions.

For example, many heart patients rely on bypass surgery or angioplasty alone to prevent further attacks. Although these treatments may buy time for the patient to heal himself or herself, *bypass and angioplasty procedures are not cures.* They are only "aspirin for a headache." In heart disease, the real healing needs to take place after the bypass or angioplasty. Unfortunately, many patients do not understand preventive medicine and are not sufficiently educated by their physicians.

Even with a physician's advice, it is the patient who must assume personal responsibility for healing. Many of my patients put considerable pressure on me, requesting an instant cure. They rely on my knowledge and experience in the use of pharmacological agents and want a "magic bullet" to end their suffering. In these instances, my patients wish to relinquish their power to me. Although this is an adequate system for some, for many this medical model simply does not work.

I had my own family experience of how a straightforward medical model can be insufficient. Both of my sons have struggled with asthma since they were six years old. I noted that at times their asthmatic attacks were precipitated by emotional stress. The boys were often most vulnerable when there was no outlet for their frustration, hurt, or anger. At other times there were obvious infectious or environmental precipitants that triggered the abrupt inability to breathe, which was often an emotionally terrifying experience for them.

My oldest son, Step, had asthma from age six to age fourteen. His condition was treated with traditional medicine—that is, occasional antibiotics, steroids, and various sprays to open up his airways. Although his health care providers performed skin tests and gave him allergy shots, there was no investigation of nutritional, emotional, or psychological concerns. When he could not breathe, he became powerless. He was totally dependent on medications to get him over the crisis of not being able to breathe.

One day my son had a powerful realization while sitting in the doctor's office. He looked around, observing other children clinging to their parents' arms as they awaited their turn to see the physician. Step said he made a decision that day. He came to the realization that he did not want to be "like those other kids . . . victims, scared, weak, and dependent on everyone and everything else." I believe my son had a major "aha" that day in his own personal growth. He made a decision that he was not going to use his sprays or pills or even obtain any further allergy shots. When he discussed this with me, I offered him my wholehearted support. He decided to follow my advice and alter his diet, cut out junk food, and particularly restrict his dairy intake. However, giving him permission to vent his feelings—especially his anger and sadness—was just as important as altering his diet, since these emotions may precipitate asthma attacks.

Following this internal commitment to be well, Step had perhaps one or two minor flare-ups of his condition. To this day, he has been completely free of any asthmatic bronchitis. My son was able to cure himself by accessing his own inner healing ability. Recently Step discussed this experience with Drew, my younger son. Drew motivated his own inner healer in a similar way, using his own power to promote healing. He, like Step, found the courage to heal himself.

HEALING AND EMPOWERMENT

Getting well requires a mobilization of our intrinsic forces against disease. We must remember the great physicians of history: nature, time, and patience. Paracelsus, a physician during the Reformation, stated, "Nature cures; the doctor only nurses." Both the physician and the patient must participate in the healing process. Patients have the power to enhance healing, but it is the role of the physician to help stimulate and nurture the power that the patient possesses.

Just as a good coach can take an athlete to a higher level of self-confidence and achievement, a good physician can help a patient to regain balance and health. Like a coach, the physician has to believe in the patient and make the patient believe that the opponent, illness, can be defeated. You, and only you, can make it happen. My twenty years of experience in medicine have reinforced one thing more than anything else—it takes a combination of nature and the patient's inner healer to cure heart disease. A good physician will promote the power inherent in every patient to regain his or her own balance and health.

Unfortunately, the sick person may not share this view. The difficult reality for the physician is that patients often feel that the sickness and discomfort come only from external sources. The sicker they become, the more they believe the sickness is caused by forces outside of themselves. In this belief system, patients are vulnerable to becoming victims of the illness; stuck, fearful, confused, withdrawn, upset, and even despairing. They can't figure out why they cannot get "fixed." In desperation, patients unconsciously seek out physicians who share their point of view.

Sometimes a "magic bullet" such as penicillin works for a strep throat or pneumonia, and real healing does take place. Where this is possible, it is almost mandatory that the physician choose such a "bullet" to help ease the patient's suffering. If the patient has a positive expectation and faith in the physician's remedy, often more positive results will occur. This may be due to a combination of choosing the right agent and the optimistic attitude of both the patient and the doctor. Sometimes remedies also work because of the placebo effect. Regardless of how the healing takes place, both the patient and the physician are satisfied.

However, if the remedy fails, patients will often blame their health care providers for failing to cure. Sometimes patients will go to physician after physician, hoping that someone will find the solution and save them. Such recurrent failures set the stage for total dependence and powerlessness. The power of the patient to heal himself or herself is soon lost to the perceived power of others.

In this disturbed codependency, energy grows stagnant. Thinking becomes limited. A division occurs between thinking and feeling, mind and body. The natural pulsatile flow of energy is disrupted. Although the healer may have some influence over the disease the patient is confronting, it is the patient's willingness to take responsibility for his or her own healing that is crucial. The physician and the patient must share and collaborate in the healing process. Indeed, patients have within themselves the power to enhance healing. Once again, physicians must help patients find, stimulate, and nurture that power.

IMPORTANCE OF MULTIPLE HEALING TECHNIQUES

Physicians, in general, have large egos. It takes a strong ego to survive medical school and vigorous postgraduate training. But sometimes our greatest confidence can be our greatest weakness. The need for the physician to "be right" may get in the way of healing. I have a problem with doctors who tell their patients that "vitamins are worthless," "psychotherapy does not work," or "cardiac rehabilitation is a waste of time." I have heard these phrases over and over from my patients. I have even seen cardiologists "fire" their patients for taking nutritional supplements. On the other hand, it is genuinely touching when a physician approaches me to inquire about targeted nutritional supplements, supportive psychotherapy, and emotional release.

Many times my journey has been a lonely one. I often face rejection, antagonism, and even criticism from my peers for not adhering to the accepted standard of care. At times I have felt hurt, shamed, and even humiliated by these remarks. And yet I believe that I have offered my patients treatment that goes far beyond the traditional standard of care. When necessary, I recommend cardiac catheterization, angioplasty, and even bypass surgery for my patients. But I firmly believe that complementary therapies—vitamins, antioxidants, nutritional supplements, psychotherapy, mental imagery, Rolfing, martial arts, meditation, and other strategies—when combined with traditional medicine, offer the patient much more than what has been established as the standard of care.

When catastrophic illness becomes a major threat, mobilizing the patient's inner healer through whatever means possible is of critical importance. Consider, for example, the traditional treatment of cancer. Radiation and chemotherapy are not magical cures; the justification for their use is that they kill cancer cells. The physician must continually balance potential gain (death of cancer cells) with potential loss (killing of normal cells). The negative side of chemotherapy is that it damages our immune system, the body's own defense against cancer cells, infections, and other diseases. This additional burden on the body's own defense system can indirectly leave the patient vulnerable to secondary infections, illnesses, and rapidly multiplying cancer cells. Such a case comes to mind from my internship at Albany Medical Center in 1972.

I was treating a man in his early fifties who had been recently diagnosed with lung cancer. Previously a heavy smoker, he unfortunately had developed a large, inoperable tumor in his right lung. His prognosis was grim, to say the least. I remember the oncologist's instructions to give him a powerful but toxic chemotherapy agent called Cytoxan. After the administration of the anticancer drug, the patient died within thirty-six hours due to overwhelming infection and shock. Although this gentleman would have ultimately succumbed to the cancer, the fact remains that the drug used in this case hastened his death.

Many patients do live longer because of the use of chemotherapeutic agents and radiation—oftentimes with exhausting and debilitating side effects. This occurs because the body is given the monumental task of repairing healthy as well as diseased tissue. It is the wise physician who recognizes the need to counteract the negative impact of traditional medicines, chemotherapy, and radiation by strengthening the body and its immune system. This necessitates high-quality nutrition as well as freedom from stress, tension, and depression.

In addition, mobilizing the patient's will to live and inspiring hope are critical strategies in combating catastrophic illness. Techniques integrated in the field of alternative medicine offer the physician an array of tools to help engage the body's inner healer in a mind/body/spirit approach to illness.

Recent studies performed at Ohio State University found that severely depressed, nonpsychotic patients had a significantly poorer ability to repair DNA in immune cells exposed to radiation than their less depressed counterparts. Both depressed groups fared significantly less well in DNA repair than the psychologically healthy, nondepressed control group. These findings suggest that depression or emotional stress may contribute to the incidence of cancer by directly diminishing immune surveillance and integrity. Lifting the patient out of depression is not easy, but neither is it beyond reach. Again, healing requires a totally integrated approach to the mind, body, and spirit.

Researchers are now acknowledging that the mental processes that can cause disease can also be redirected to cause healing. Jeanne Achterberg, a pioneer in mental imagery, believes that nature has created few one-way processes. If we can become ill as a result of mental stress in our lives, we must also have the inherent power to improve health with the use of purposeful and positive mental processes. Positive imagery has been known to stimulate the body's production of lymphocytes, T cells (natural killer cells), and neutrophils, which help fight disease. According to research, imagery can also help reduce levels of adrenal corticosteroids in high-stress individuals. Excessive levels of cortisol can not only enhance premature coronary artery disease but also premature dementia, commonly referred to as Alzheimer's disease. Imagery also alleviates emotional strain and reduces physical pain while altering the course of disease and improving the individual's outlook on his or her illness.

As a cardiologist, I rarely treat cases of cancer. However, some cancer patients have approached me, requesting that I participate in their healing. In addition to the emotional support that I can give, I recommend a broad nutritional approach that includes the elimination from the diet of long-chain fatty acids, which are found in animal protein and dairy products. Long-chain fatty acids are great fuel for cancer cells. If you can eliminate the fuel, you may stifle the cancer growth. I also recommend vitamins, minerals, coenzyme Q_{10}, glutathione, phytonutrients, natural healing foods, and various forms of visualization and psychotherapy that I will discuss later.

For example, consider that L-arginine (an amino acid) stimulates the production of T cells that enhance the body's natural killing mechanisms.

This simple nutritional approach may be used as an additional therapy, especially in the treatment of breast cancer, along with traditional approaches. When the body's own responses are mobilized together with the cancer-fighting techniques of modern medicine, the combination can frequently bring about remarkable results.

Treating an illness or dysfunction is incomplete if it just addresses part of the body. In other types of healing, such as alternative, naturopathic, or homeopathic care, the healer takes a holistic approach to illness. For example, the healer may investigate not only the physical manifestation of the illness, but also its emotional, psychological, nutritional, metabolic, and in some cases spiritual ramifications. Thus a holistic approach provides an understanding of the patient and his or her illness in terms of the whole person.

Nowadays the treatment of dysfunction requires an investigation of mind, body, and spirit. But this has not always been the case. For example, consider my own medical school experience. In the 1970s a physician's training focused on pathology, illness, and treatment. Preventive medicine had no place in medical schools at that time. Interactions between the mind and the body were yet to be considered. Our course work on nutrition included minimal instruction on the role of fat, fiber, and cholesterol in heart disease and cancer. We also studied the harmful effects of alcohol on the body and the uses of B-vitamin supplementation.

However, there was no education about the health hazards posed by processed foods, polluted water, heavy metals, and radiation leaking into the environment. There was minimal education about the perils of vitamin and mineral deficiency. As a young physician, my own understanding of nutrition was very limited; the subject received no emphasis during medical school, internship, medical residency, or even my fellowship in cardiology. Not until the latter part of the 1970s, when the Framingham study data were released, was high cholesterol recognized as a major contributor to heart disease.

In the early 1970s there was also very little time to investigate why people became ill. I focused on comforting the sick and attempting to slow down or cure the diseases they already had. Pharmacological agents became my first line of treatment. After all, the medical profession became drug-oriented after the discovery of penicillin in the 1940s. My training emphasized disease models and treatment with the multitude of pharmacological agents that were available to me.

As a student of this traditional Western medical model of health and disease, I studied hard, worked long hours, and often played the "midnight hero" in many highly charged medical dramas. Although I enjoyed my work and felt highly competent in what I was doing, I was somehow not fulfilled. Something was missing in my role of physician and healer. As battling illness began to take its toll on me, I searched for missing links in the quest for healing. In my studies as a psychotherapist, I began to appreciate the deeper processes by which health is maintained, lost, regained, and often lost again. I began to direct my energies more toward preventive medicine, looking deeper into lifestyle, eating habits, emotional factors, nutritional needs, and relationship needs. Over time I began to realize that I was becoming an allopathic physician in recovery.

OBESITY AND HEART DISEASE

Obesity often has its roots in emotional issues. Eating disorders are critically linked to self-esteem, love, acceptance, and even sexuality. I was indeed fortunate to be the leader of a courageous group of men and women who entered the weight-loss program at Manchester Memorial Hospital in Connecticut. We spent six months together, working in three-hour sessions on a weekly basis. The members of this group taught me invaluable lessons about the emotional and psychological issues behind weight loss and weight gain. I also learned that obesity is a very common metabolic disturbance in humans.

There is absolutely no reason for people to develop heart disease or other illnesses as a result of being overweight. Unfortunately, obesity is still a primary contributor to major diseases such as high blood pressure, diabetes, heart disease, and even some cancers. Yet a healthy diet will not only reduce your weight but will also protect you from illness.

IMPROVING DAILY NUTRITION

High-quality nutrition can help prevent illness and improve your quality of life. As a sample of the things I'll be talking about later in the book, consider the following:

Onions contain quercetin, which prevents the harmful lipoprotein LDL from injuring our bodies. They are also an excellent natural antihistamine I've used in the treatment of my child's asthma.

Broccoli contains sulphoraphane, which helps prevent cancer.

Cabbage has isothiocyanates, which also help prevent cancer.

Mackerel, sardines, and salmon are abundant in coenzyme Q_{10}, a miracle nutrient for the heart.

Anchovies and other fish have DMAE, a substance known to improve one's memory. For years folklore has touted fish as a brain food. Now we learn that this folklore was fact rather than fiction.

Asparagus contains folic acid, a vital nutrient for women anticipating pregnancy. Folic acid has also been discovered to prevent heart disease, especially in the elderly.

Spinach has lutein, a bioflavonoid that is vital in healing advanced macular degeneration of the retina, which is the leading cause of blindness in the United States.

In addition to these, there are literally thousands of flavonoids and hundreds of carotenoids that will prevent and even cure illnesses and diseases.

It is so important for us to learn about the nutritional secrets hidden in common foods and become aware of the dangers of preservatives and additives in processed products. A diet rich in foods and nutrients that heal may well be our best line of defense against the country's leading degenerative killers, such as cancer, heart disease, and autoimmune disorders. Our diet is one of the most powerful weapons in our arsenal. As trite as it sounds, you *really* are what you eat!

NUTRITIONAL SUPPLEMENTATION

Consider that many of us cannot get enough of the essential natural nutrients, such as magnesium, vitamin E, coenzyme Q_{10}, B vitamins, and flavonoids, even in the best of diets. A deficiency of any of these components will impair the healthy functioning of our cells, ultimately resulting in disease.

The National Cancer Institute recommends consuming from five to nine servings of fresh fruits and vegetables a day. Although I try to do this on a daily basis, sometimes I find that eating this many fruits and vegetables is absolutely impossible. Therefore, I take a daily vitamin and mineral supplement as an insurance policy.

ANTIAGING STRATEGIES

Although for years I had been very comfortable taking vitamins, minerals, antioxidants, and coenzyme Q_{10}, I had never really investigated the antiaging supplements such as DHEA, melatonin, DMAE, and so on. But at a 1994 conference devoted to antiaging strategies, I was shocked to find that many university professors were not only taking vitamins and minerals, but also consuming these antiaging supplements. I also met researchers who presented well-substantiated data about antiaging technologies. I now know, for example, that heart disease, various forms of cancer and autoimmune diseases, and Alzheimer's are really a sort of premature aging. As I again began to reconsider the experiences of my patients in the light of my new understanding of aging, I realized anew that specific nutritional and dietary deficiencies are rampant in our population. Later I will detail some specific antiaging strategies that build upon these insights. By raising consciousness and initiating a healthy preventive lifestyle, individuals can prevent premature aging and the diseases that result from it.

HEARTSENSE

In 1994 I was recruited as an editor for a national newsletter, *HeartSense,* which incorporates traditional, complementary, and alternative methods for healing the heart. This book has evolved from my work on the newsletter and my more than twenty years as a healer. It focuses on nurturing the body with nutritional, emotional, and spiritual healing. This book will tell you the facts about vitamins, minerals, herbs, healthy fats, and other healing foods. It will address the tremendous confusion and controversy about high-carbohydrate, low-fat diets and say why I am convinced they are not the saviors we thought they were. It will also demonstrate to you how nutritional supplements can make a difference in our lives. It also includes a section devoted to the special needs of women and children. New antiaging strategies are discussed as well.

This book is intended to expand your consciousness. Today is a time of awareness, of taking responsibility for yourself, and of living in harmony with your body. I believe this book can lead you to a new consciousness and awareness that will make a difference in the quality and even longevity of your life. Take this journey with me to an exciting new plateau of awareness and health. The rest is up to you!

Optimum Health

CHAPTER One

Eight Nutritional Rules for Optimum Health

There are many comprehensive programs that tell you how to live a healthy lifestyle. You may have tried some of them. But if they haven't worked, read on. The eight rules for optimum health that I present in this chapter integrate the essential emotional, physical, and nutritional aspects of healing. They focus on nutrition because that is the most important first step you can take.

RULE NUMBER ONE: DENIAL OF PLEASURE CAN LEAD TO OBESITY AND EARLY DEATH

"Well," you might say, "I can understand how eating disorders can lead to early death, but how can denial of pleasure do that?" As a cardiologist and psychotherapist, it is easy for me to see that self-denial can cause extreme unhappiness that sets the scene for stress and heartbreak, which in turn can lead to heart disease and, frequently, death. Denial of love, denial of human contact, and denial of emotional outlets clog the system just as surely as do fats and cholesterol.

Always doing what we "think" is best, not acting on what we truly feel, stopping ourselves from doing what we always wanted because of fear of rejection or loss, denying ourselves the simple sensual pleasures of life that came so easily in childhood—all these things stop the natural flow of energy that is our very life force. Just as stagnant water can become poisonous and toxic, the blocking of our intentions, feelings, intuition, pleasures, and desires can be equally toxic, leading to frustration, unhappiness, and despair.

When we try to lose weight, one of two things usually happens:

1. We deny ourselves the pleasures of eating, and through a series of small victories (and perhaps one or two slipups) we lose weight. Great! But denial of pleasure breeds resentment, and resentment harbors self-contempt, fostering feelings of guilt and frustration.

2. Because food is often seen as either friend or enemy, small setbacks are seen as failures. We give up in defeat, vowing to start anew tomorrow, or we justify going off our diet by saying that we might as well be fat and fulfilled. Both attitudes are wrong. We might be physically full, but we are not emotionally fulfilled. We feel guilt and self-loathing, and these unforgiving feelings start the cycle of denial all over again.

Weight loss and healthy eating require a true commitment to awareness and the attainment of a level of consciousness that supports self-nurturance. This can be done without denial of pleasure. People who constantly gain weight and then lose it, only to gain it back again, are not doing themselves any favors. The best approach to weight loss is finding foods that not only taste good, but also nurture the body.

Recently my friends and I had a celebratory dinner that was healthy yet just as delicious as any Thanksgiving dinner I've ever had. The menu consisted of roasted turkey, fresh green and yellow beans, a tofu salad, and a salad of cucumbers and tomatoes sprinkled with extra-virgin olive oil. We ended the meal with fresh fruit pies. Because the rest of the meal contained the right kinds of fats, in reasonable quantities, and was high in fiber, I chose not to deprive myself and to have a small piece of pie, though I realized that the crust of the pie was probably made with lard, a pure animal fat frequently used in baking. A two-inch piece of pie contains 10 to 15 grams of fat, which was more than the fat content of the entire meal I just consumed. The American Heart Association recommends a daily intake of no more than 75 grams of fat a day for an average-sized man such as myself. Since the rest of the meal contained healthy fats, I was able not to deprive myself, knowing that the total fat content for this meal, including the "forbidden" pie, was only about 30 grams! This is eating with awareness. And this is healing.

On the other hand, a typical fast-food meal, including a double cheeseburger, french fries, a shake, and an apple pie, contains an alarming 70 to 80 grams of fat! And this is only one meal. If you ate like this at every meal, you could conceivably eat 200 to 225 grams of fat a day. This not only leads to weight gain, but also is dangerous.

RULE NUMBER TWO: FORGIVE YOURSELF

If we embark on a program of awareness and allow ourselves a little bit of what we are being denied, we can become masters of our own enjoyment and be fulfilled. (More on this later as we get into "how." For now, let's stick with "why.") If, on the other hand, we try to force ourselves to stick to an extremely rigid diet but fail, we often berate ourselves, thereby adding to our feelings of failure and self-doubt. But if we can allow some leeway for human frailty, we can begin anew.

Let's not kid ourselves, though. Allowing ourselves only a limited amount of our favorite foods isn't always easy. A taste of ice cream may lead to an entire bowl. But the key is forgiving yourself and getting support from others.

Frequently, overweight adults come from families in which achieving is more important than being oneself—where there is little acceptance of the children as they really are because they are not as their parents want them to be. Does this mean we should blame our parents for not giving us unconditional love? Not necessarily. They probably received similar treatment from their parents, or from a society that encouraged them to believe that this was the way to instill a success mentality in their children. On the contrary, too much pressure (even for adults) only tempts us to rebel or to loathe our shortcomings—what we have come to call failure.

RULE NUMBER THREE: GET SUPPORT

Aside from trying to lose weight, we may have work pressures, family pressures, and sexual issues begging to be resolved. Where does one "problem" stop and the others begin? We have had a bad day at work and so follow it up with a cocktail or two. This activates our libido, but rather than risk rejection, we try to satisfy our desires with ice cream instead. Of course, the cycle goes on and on. In an *aware* consciousness, however, we can direct our energies. We can call or meet with others who know our struggles and who can encourage us to come over for a glass of juice instead of a cocktail, or who can talk us through our work frustrations and then help us to plan dinner.

Social occasions can be extremely difficult as well. A friend of mine, Roger, gained so much weight that he approached the four-hundred-pound mark. Unfortunately, during this weight gain he lost friends—many not because they thought Roger was any less interesting or amusing than he was before, but because Roger felt too vulnerable to accept their invitations. He became more and more isolated, even from his wife, literally barricading himself with fat and cutting off the very support that is necessary for achieving any goal. Just as Roger was carrying nearly four hundred pounds of physical weight, he was also carrying about four hundred pounds of emotional baggage. His psychic pain was devastating—he thought of himself as an outcast and acted like one, becoming lonely and alone. How many of us, when in pain, turn away from those who love us, those who could help us most? And, as friends, how many of us refuse to support another in a similar situation? What is not needed are comments like "Are you eating again? You are just going to get fatter and fatter." Rather, we need to say to a friend confronting a weight problem, "Instead of eating that bag of potato chips, can I fix you a bowl of crunchy popcorn?"

RULE NUMBER FOUR: EAT HIGH-FIBER AND HEALTHY-FAT FOODS

High-fiber and healthy-fat food choices will allow you to lose weight without giving up naturally good-tasting food. This fact has been substantiated by many of my patients who started out using my dietary recommendations for a high-fiber diet in order to heal their hearts. Healthy foods that contain healthy (unsaturated omega-3) fats instead of unhealthy ones include fish, soybean products such as tofu, and some nuts. A diet low in saturated fats reduces blood levels of LDL, which contributes to hardening of the arteries and heart attacks. And a diet high in fiber keeps the body and appetite nourished while allowing most of the refuse of the digested food to be easily flushed away by the intestines. While my patients started on this diet to heal their hearts, they ended up losing weight! Why? The answer is simple. If my patients choose foods high in fiber and healthy fats, they tend to cut down on the number of carbohydrates they consume, which helps prevent a phenomenon called insulin resistance.

The effects of insulin resistance have become widely studied in recent years, as it appears to be a major cause of weight gain. Overweight people who eat lots of carbohydrates produce greater quantities of insulin. However, the insulin is used inefficiently; instead of "burning" carbohydrates, it encourages fat deposition. It is this elevation of insulin levels and subsequent high blood sugar levels that cause the accumulation of body fat as well as enhance the progression of coronary artery disease. I talk more about this later.

When Roger, my four-hundred-pound friend mentioned in the previous section, was trying to lose weight about fifteen years ago, many of the newly engineered diet foods were unavailable, but this is not what caused him to turn to a high-fiber/healthy-fat diet. First he tried every diet available: the Scarsdale Diet, the Grapefruit Diet, the Aviator's Diet, and protein drinks. With none of them, however, could he keep the weight off when he returned to "normal" eating. Obviously it was the "normal" eating that needed to be changed. Fifteen years ago the public was beginning to learn about the benefits of fiber. Roger took this information to heart. He would snack on high-fiber crackers that even he says did not have a good taste, and he would eat fruit, a source of natural sugar, when he felt his energy was low. Being a steak lover, Roger didn't eliminate red meat from his diet, but he did cut it back significantly, and he would always remove all the visible fat before taking even one bite. In this way he didn't feel deprived, yet his eating was *contained*. He was aware that if he ate the steak, he could not follow it with bread, butter, and french fries. Roger didn't know it, but with his omission of many carbohydrates, he was combating insulin resistance.

RULE NUMBER FIVE: AVOID SALT, SUGAR, AND CAFFEINE WHILE CONSUMING AS MUCH WATER AS POSSIBLE

Now, this may sound like denial, but let me explain. Salt, sugar, and caffeine do not need to be avoided altogether, but they should be used in moderation for both improved health and weight loss. Sugar quickly boosts the blood sugar and thus our energy level, but this effect quickly wears off, thereby causing a sugar craving in order to boost energy again. Caffeine works in a similar manner: It boosts our energy level, which quickly drops again, thus causing a craving for a sweet or another cup of coffee to keep us going. While increasing sugar or caffeine consumption increases energy temporarily, it creates a cycle of eating sugar and/or drinking coffee as often as every two hours! Such increased sugar intake can obviously lead to an increase in accumulated fat.

The way to prevent this cycle is to begin your day with a breakfast that includes some carbohydrates (while trying to limit breads as much as possible) and protein. A serving of salmon or trout, an omelet with vegetables, or even two poached eggs with Canadian bacon will be converted to blood sugar slowly. Instead of the quick boost that a sweet roll gives, a bowl of oatmeal, for example, will allow a more gradual increase and subsequent decrease in blood sugar and, therefore, will prolong the amount of time you feel full. Eating a combination of complex carbohydrates and fiber, such as shredded wheat with blueberries or strawberries, will control hunger even longer because fiber taken with water or another liquid will bulk up in the gastrointestinal tract, thus creating a longer-lasting feeling of fullness.

If you choose a breakfast that combines fiber, protein, and complex carbohydrates, you may safely have a cup of coffee (without added sugar) without beginning the sugar/caffeine cycle. While the caffeine may cause a food craving, it will be satisfied by the gradual release of energy caused by the slow burning of the complex carbohydrates. Remember, anything that is sugary-tasting or sticky-feeling is probably made with processed sugar, so *read labels!* The ingredients are listed in order of quantity. Remember that high-fructose corn syrup and dextrose are sugars too.

A good breakfast may begin or prevent a day of overeating, so choose wisely. Try to replace the tempting foods on the left with the tasty alternatives on the right in the following chart:

Avoid	*Replace With*
Sugared cereals	Whole-grain cereals
White bread	Whole-grain bread
Commercial pancakes with processed syrup	Buckwheat cakes with fresh kiwi fruit
Belgian waffles with whipped cream	Whole-grain waffles with spreadable fruit

Avoid	Replace With
Sweet rolls	Oatmeal
Blueberry muffins	Bran muffins

When making food choices, there's a general rule of thumb that is easy to remember: The closer the food is to its original form, the better. If you must have bread, whenever possible, buy whole-grain bread from your local baker instead of white bread from the grocery market. While you can still use convenience foods, choose frozen waffles from a health food store instead of the kind found in supermarkets. You can make a batch of buckwheat pancakes by merely adding water to a mix available at many health food stores, instead of using a processed biscuit or pancake mix.

Even my sixteen-year-old son prefers buckwheat pancakes (see recipe in chapter fifteen) to those he gets at his friends' homes, because my pancakes have a chewier texture and a fuller flavor. And I serve them to him with pure maple syrup tapped from the trees around a cabin I own in Vermont. Okay, okay. You don't have to tap your own trees, but if you can splurge on a jug of pure maple syrup instead of the ordinary supermarket varieties, which are mostly artificially flavored corn syrup, not only will the flavor be more robust, but it will be healthier as well. Another healthy choice is to spread a dollop of honey on the pancakes; while dousing them in either syrup or honey is not advised, a small amount of honey adds much flavor. Fresh fruit or spreadable fruit, of course, tastes great on pancakes or waffles and is an excellent choice.

I also recommend consuming generous quantities of fluids at breakfast, whether skim or soy milk, decaffeinated coffee or tea, or even just plain water. Water is a cardinal ingredient in health—it cleanses the organs of excess sodium that is often hidden in many of today's foods, especially commercially packaged convenience foods such as canned soups, boxed mixes and sauces, and even sweets. Foods especially high in sodium include pickles, ketchup, mustard, soy sauce, and pickled fish, to mention a few. Sodas can be one of the worst offenders—even some low-calorie carbonated soft drinks have sodium in them. So if you are in the habit of drinking a diet beverage instead of water with a meal or to quench thirst, check the label; too much sodium will not only prevent a good opportunity to cleanse the system, but will also add to its contamination.

Remember that a high sodium intake also contributes to high blood pressure and heart disease, so it's wise to replace all sodas with water, tap or bottled, and to drink as much water as possible throughout the day. In addition to sodium and sugar content, many soft drinks contain emulsifiers, artificial coloring, phosphoric acid, and antifoaming agents. These chemicals cause metabolic stress to our body, as do other additives, preservatives, and synthetic agents commonly used in processed foods.

RULE NUMBER SIX: READ LABELS AND EAT NATURAL

The Food and Drug Administration (FDA) has come to the aid of the label-reading consumer with new guidelines that help eliminate misleading label and advertising information. The FDA is tackling such questions as: How much fat is permitted in a product that calls itself low-fat? What does low-sodium mean? Or for that matter, what does low-calorie mean? Manufacturers in the past have boasted that a product is "cholesterol free," yet it may contain large amounts of saturated fat, which is eventually turned into cholesterol in the body. With the new definition, *cholesterol-free* is legally defined as a product with less than 2 mg of cholesterol per serving. Likewise, a *low-cholesterol* food must contain less than 20 mg of cholesterol.

High-fiber is another term that is frequently unregulated, but new legislation requires that a food contain a specific number of grams of fiber per serving in order to be labeled high-fiber. New FDA standardizations make it easier for consumers to rely on factual nutritional information. Not only are consumers now able to determine the amount of calories in a particular item, they also are given information about the number of calories from fat and the amount of saturated fat, cholesterol, fiber, protein, sodium, and vitamins and minerals in a given product.

Okay. Enough about the good news. What about the bad? What are the feds doing about the chemicals, preservatives, and other harmful ingredients that are added to many commercially packaged foods? Although the FDA has issued formal regulations on literally hundreds of food additives, there are many that are still listed as GRAS (generally regarded as safe). These food additives include artificial flavors, colors, bleaches, emulsifiers, softeners, thickeners, hydrogenators, deodorizers, conditioners, fortifiers, driers, alkalizers, firming agents, stabilizers, and buffers.

They add color and visual appeal to food that does not need refrigeration, but for all practical purposes, these agents are literally "dead"; that is, they do nothing useful but extend shelf life. And are they *really* safe?

Two commonly used GRAS additives, butylated hydroxyanisole and butylated hydroxytoluene, frequently referred to as BHA and BHT, are antioxidants made from petroleum. BHA and BHT are found in almost every processed food, including cereals, shortening, ice cream and other dairy foods, peanut butter, potato chips, meats, dressings, snacks, and so on. They do indeed give goods an extended shelf life and also prevent rancidity. However, these additives have been reported as having a causal relationship to allergies and nervous-system disorders.

Monosodium glutamate (MSG) is also considered a food enhancer and is in thousands of foods. Convenience foods such as TV dinners, processed meats, meat tenderizers, and salad dressings often contain considerable quantities of MSG. In fact, industry officials indicate that MSG is the most widely utilized chemical flavoring agent. MSG has been used in the United States since 1907 and has been closely scrutinized. It has been proven to cause side effects such as asthma, heart palpitations, chest pain, weakness, and heartburn in some people. In experimental animals, MSG has also been shown to cause permanent brain damage. Headache is probably the leading symptom of MSG intake, frequently sending patients to their doctors for unnecessary evaluations and interventions when a good nutritional history and diet change would suffice.

What does all this mean to the consumer? Unfortunately, the average consumer takes in numerous chemical additives in his or her food. But we cannot blame it all on the food industry. We really do want convenience, speedy preparation, and a longer shelf life. Major food companies take advantage of the consumer with advertising campaigns that are impressive but sometimes misleading. Although processed foods may be inexpensive, the consumer does pay a price in terms of physical symptoms and perhaps increased susceptibility to illness.

We need to become more discriminating shoppers. Read labels and look for items that say "no preservatives" and "free from additives." Look also to see if artificial flavorings or colorings have been added. Watch out for labels that list "natural flavoring," "hydrolyzed protein," "sodium caseinate," and "autolyzed yeast." These terms are used frequently to disguise MSG. We need to be suspicious of chemical names and ingredient abbreviations.

Avoid BHA, BHT, sodium nitrate, sodium nitrite, caffeine, sulfur dioxide, butyric acid, diethylene glycol, sodium benzoate, and amyl acetate. If you don't understand the language, or if you feel you need an advanced degree to figure out the contents, then you should avoid the product. Be aware of the toxic ingredient aluminum, and be particularly cognizant of the use of white flour additives such as ammonium chloride, potassium bromate, and propionic acid (sodium or calcium propionate); these are all unnatural to living organisms. Just as industrial chemicals can pollute the environment, these chemicals pollute the body. We need to realize that additives and chemicals actually add nothing to the nutritional value of foods. They are frequently added to make inferior substances taste better. The far better option is to consider natural and organically grown foods. Try to learn about and seek out organic foods, which are free of pesticides and chemical fertilizers.

Recent surveys have indicated that 55 percent of pesticide residues in the average American diet are supplied by meat. Dairy products provide 23 percent of the total intake of pesticides, and vegetables, fruits, and grains account for 11 percent. An alarming 94 percent of the chlorinated hydrocarbon pesticide residues in the American diet are attributable to meats, dairy products, fish, and eggs.

In the last few years, numerous studies have indicated that women on high-fat diets increase their risk of breast cancer. Although their diet may be a factor, new research indicates that it may not be the fat itself that causes the problem but rather the toxins and pesticides contained in the fats. Studies have determined that breast tissue from cancer patients had higher levels of the pesticide DDT and higher concentrations of PCBs (polychlorinated biphenyls), which are petroleum by-products. Man-made pollutants such as DDT and PCBs are chemicals that react with estrogen receptor cells in human breast tissue, are absorbed into the body, and are stored in human fat. DDT is the most notorious pesticide linked to breast cancer and is part of the class called organochlorides. Although DDT is banned in the United States, it is still produced in the third world, particularly in Latin America, China, and India. In a study involving Israeli women, the banning of organochloride pesticides resulted in a cancer decline of 20 percent. Prior to the ban of DDT in Israel, Israeli women had one of the highest breast cancer mortality rates in the world. But these two environmental toxins are just the tip of the iceberg.

Presently in the United States, there are over 75,000 different industrial chemicals used for agricultural and commercial purposes. Minimizing or eliminating pesticide use around the home, avoiding air pollution, and drinking purified water are some ways you can reduce your risk of exposure. I would also recommend eating as many organic foods as possible. The term *organic* indicates that the soil in which the food is raised has been free of any artificially produced fertilizers for several years or even decades. Natural foods are gradually becoming more and more popular with consumers. Although you may have to pay a few pennies more for organic foods and accept a shorter shelf life, the dividend can be a healthier body and mind. We have to be willing to give up precooked, instant, refined, and chemically treated foods. If you want good health, you need to compromise and take more responsibility for the ingredients you put into your body. Be a detective when it comes to food and guard your body, since this is the only one you will ever have.

RULE NUMBER SEVEN: MOVE!

A calorie is a unit for measuring energy. This means that for every calorie that we take in, we must expend an equal amount of energy in order to remain at a balanced weight. When we take in more calories than we expend, we gain weight. When we expend more energy than we take in, we lose weight. And when the two are balanced, we can remain at a constant weight.

Okay, so you know this already. You may even feel hopeless that you could ever expend more energy than you take in because you are not an athletic person. Don't believe it. Any amount of activity greater than what you are doing now will burn more calories. So even if you are consuming the same amount of food today as you were yesterday, but you add a bit more movement to your day, you will lose weight slowly. Now, substitute in today's diet some foods less dense in calories than what you ate yesterday, and you will lose weight even faster.

Notice that I say *movement,* not *exercise.* I think *exercise* can sometimes be a scary word. People visualize themselves running down the road in sweaty shorts and sneakers, or pumping iron. Professionally speaking, I must say I don't recommend either. Both put a tremendous amount of stress on the heart muscle and other muscles and tendons. Let's take it easy. Remember, this is a program of nondenial and enjoyment.

Let's start out *walking.* The evening breeze is cool, and spring or fall crispness might be in the air. Or perhaps there is a beautiful red August moon that you can see from your window. Get up. Walk outdoors. Enjoy nature. This is a holistic way of living. Mind and body are one. Human life and wildlife are on the same planet. Let's enjoy each other, as we are all part of the same universe. Even if you can't find time to walk every other day (though I think you might, once you get used to the beauty of the land- or cityscape), think of every little movement you make and take it one step beyond. Walk out to the driveway to get the mail instead of picking it up in your car on the way home. Walk around the bed to make up the other side rather than reaching over. While watching television, my daughter does leg lifts. Think of this not as strenuous exercise, but as an efficient use of exercise time!

When my friend Roger first started losing weight, he couldn't even reach over to tie his shoes. He couldn't walk more than a few yards. Four hundred pounds is a lot of weight to move around. So he started walking out for the newspaper each morning and taking out the trash. He even began cleaning out closets. Roger was a successful businessman who, if he so desired, could hire a housekeeper to clean closets. But Roger knew that each added movement would add to his successful weight loss. Every little movement counts. As with a savings account, Roger added more and more movement to his daily regimen until he accumulated the lifestyle he has today. Now he plays racquetball three times a week and even won his division in the North Carolina state championship. He was one of the oldest men to win this title—and to think that only six years before he could barely walk far enough to take the trash out!

RULE NUMBER EIGHT: ADD VITAMINS AND MINERALS TO YOUR DIET

Once you are on a balanced diet, you can decide if you want to take supplements or choose to get your vitamins and minerals through your food. I suggest a combination of fresh foods and nutritional supplements.

Some people question why they need to take vitamins and minerals in a supplemental form when they can get them in the foods they eat. Unfortunately, the "apple a day" principle does not hold as true today as it did a century ago. In this day and age, the need for vitamin and mineral supplementation is critical. Few adults (perhaps 9 percent) eat a balanced diet containing at least five to nine servings of fruits or vegetables per day. Even when eating such a balanced diet, most people are unlikely to get the larger amounts of certain vitamins (especially beta carotene, vitamin

C, and vitamin E) that have been shown effective in clinical trials. Although you may consider vitamins in foods the best way to stay healthy, the foods we eat today may not be as rich in nutrients as they were years ago. Also, food processing frequently strips our food of many of its most important nutrients.

We need a wide assortment of vitamins, minerals, and accessory nutrients to stay healthy and to help prevent disease. We also need to eat in a way that satisfies our hunger but will not make us fat. You may not be getting everything you need from the food you eat, even with my recommended menu. Why not?

Most food doesn't come with a label that specifies how much of each nutrient is in the portion you eat. Your brain tells you when you're hungry, but your brain can't tell you if it needs a particular vitamin or mineral. It can't say, "I need a magnesium fix today, and I'm running short on iron. Go out and buy some pumpkin seeds and add them to the menu." Your brain can only tell you, "Eat something," and it will continue to fuel your appetite until satisfaction is achieved.

Our need for supplemental nutrients is also increased by exposure to environmental toxins such as polluted air, radiation, chemical poisons, and heavy metals, as well as other man-made risk factors such as auto emissions, cigarette smoke, and the increasing usage of fats in our diets. These factors cause dangerous free radicals to form in our bodies, causing premature aging and disease.

OPPORTUNITIES FROM CRISIS

Roger tells the story of the time he and another four-hundred-pound friend got into Roger's Corvette in front of his luxury auto dealership. With much effort, they struggled into the low-slung car and, once seated, attempted to shut the doors simultaneously. But neither could. Between them, there was just too much man inside that little car. With his employees watching, Roger didn't want to risk further humiliation by getting out and admitting defeat, so he became determined to get the doors shut. First he leaned outward and told his friend to pull his door shut, then to reverse the action while Roger pulled his shut. Since their first attempts were unsuccessful, their repeated efforts created a rocking motion, and the two four-hundred-pound men swayed from side to side as they tried to physically reposition, and figuratively remold, their huge bodies into ones that would fit into a sleek Corvette. Roger admits that the car's rocking must have been a funny sight. His employees began gathering at the windows of the dealership and laughing hysterically. Roger waved to them, smiling and encouraging their fun while pushing down his true feelings of hurt and shame. Finally he and his friend got the doors shut and left the embarrassing situation behind.

It was with the same single-minded resolve that Roger finally decided to lose weight. Not long after becoming stuck in a chair in a shoe store and dumping an unsuspecting lady on the floor when he stood up and took a row of connected seats with him, he was rushed to the hospital. For some time before that, Roger had been feeling some discomfort sleeping and breathing; he was running a slight temperature and his head felt stuffy. His doctor had examined him and listened to his chest but could find nothing more, so he diagnosed a cold. After almost a month the symptoms got worse, so Roger saw another physician. Again the doctor could not hear congestion in Roger's chest when he listened with a stethoscope, and there was something more. He asked for a chest X ray. And when the doctor saw it, he suggested Roger be hospitalized immediately. Roger had a severe case of pneumonia that couldn't be detected with a stethoscope through the layers of fat around his sixty-inch chest.

When Roger was checked into the hospital, they took his vital signs and wanted to check his weight. However, the nurses feared he was too large even for medical scales, which went up only to three hundred pounds, and told him he might have to go to their laundry room to be weighed. His shame and humiliation were intense. Luckily, they brought in a special scale that saved him the further pain of being weighed as cargo. As he was waiting for the process to be over, he saw a cadaver being wheeled out of a room. When Roger learned that the man had died from complications of pneumonia, a "click" went off in his head. Roger knew that he himself had an advanced case of pneumonia and that it had been difficult to diagnose the disease because of his weight. Roger suddenly realized—and believed—that one way or another his overeating was going to kill him. This was Roger's spiritual message; and now he realized that he had an opportunity to learn from the crisis.

I see many overweight people who end up as cardiac deaths. Clinical studies show that obese people move less than thinner people, which contributes to heart problems; also, many heart attacks occur within a short time after a high-fat meal. Movement and light, healthy-fat meals are two ways of contributing to a healthy heart. If it hadn't been the pneumonia that scared Roger into the realization that his weight was dangerous, it might have been a heart attack, and he might not have been as lucky. As it was, Roger left the hospital cured of his pneumonia and determined to lose weight. The energy he had used in building his businesses and hiding the pain of his fat would now be channeled into losing weight. Just as he had previously given his entire attention to work and food, Roger now made losing weight his new obsession. Roger got the message. And listened.

As a cardiologist, I have seen many cases of heart attacks, near-death experiences, and, unfortunately, death itself. Some of those who survived got the transformational message. Some patients believed that their heart attacks were really spiritual gifts that would make them change their lives. They reframed their illnesses and found opportunities in these crises. Frequently, when one gets severely ill or experiences a near-death crisis, spiritual and/or emotional growth occurs. I have seen many patients dig deeper into themselves as a result of developing catastrophic illnesses. I believe this was the case with Roger.

While in the hospital, Roger had time to analyze his eating habits. He had been dieting for at least twenty years and nothing had worked, so he concluded that gimmicky diets don't work. The only diet he could count on was the age-old way of eating less and eating lighter. He didn't just worry about counting calories. Instead, he focused on lowering his fat intake. If he reduced the amount of red meats and oily foods he was consuming, he would need to increase fiber-rich foods in order to eat less and yet feel full. It just made sense.

So Roger set a reasonable goal. But he didn't deny himself everything. He would eat less bread and without butter except for the last bite, on which he would allow himself to smear just enough butter to get the full taste. After a short time, he was surprised to find that he no longer liked the taste of butter. It was too heavy, too oily, too strong.

Roger lost weight. The people who had known him his whole life didn't recognize him, and others he didn't know well would say, "I heard you lost weight, but I couldn't imagine losing this much! How did you do it?" Word spread, and everywhere Roger went, people asked him for weight loss advice. He explained to them the concept of eating healthy-fat and high-fiber foods, but many of them didn't understand about nutrition and fiber. He was thrilled about his own success in losing weight and wanted to help others. Just as he shed his fat and his fat lifestyle, Roger sold his grocery markets and opened a weight loss center where he could teach people about fat, fiber, and vitamins.

Like Roger, I believe in eating with awareness. The rest of this book will teach you how awareness, in itself, is the most important step in achieving optimum health.

CHAPTER Two

Fat in America

A recent article in the *Journal of the American Medical Association* declared a "fattening of America." Obesity is a major problem in our society; an alarming 30 percent of our population is obese.

Most researchers would agree that extreme degrees of obesity increase the risk of cancer and heart disease in both men and women. The health consequences of weight gain in women have recently been validated and are quite disturbing. In the February 8, 1995, edition of the *Journal of the American Medical Association,* study data clearly indicated that even a modest weight gain during adult life is associated with an increased risk of developing coronary artery disease. This recent information is especially germane to women who generally consider themselves to be "not too" overweight. Even being mildly overweight (ten to fifteen pounds) is a real problem.

The United States population is never at a loss for new ways to lose weight. We all know there is an abundance of diets available. Although some are more successful than others, any diet will work for a motivated individual. The odds of maintaining weight loss, however, are discouraging. Most diets result in the majority of individuals regaining their weight when they resume "normal" eating patterns. Studies show that only a small fraction of overweight people who succeed in losing weight are able to keep the weight off for more than a short period of time.

As we saw in the story of Roger, diets don't work. Dieting in general implies a temporary change in the way we eat, instead of a permanent shift in the way we view food and our relationship with it. Diet also implies deprivation. When one utilizes deprivation, food is not a friend, but rather an enemy. Typically people think that self-sacrifice is the only way to achieve success, and that the enjoyment of food is a sin that leads to an overpowering sense of frustration and failure. This emotional roller coaster can be quite disturbing. An ideal diet comes from one's own consciousness and unique personality. Such insight and awareness of what is unhealthy, and what you can live with and live without, is really the key to losing weight.

For example, people who starve themselves or force themselves to eat unusual or unpalatable foods are bound to fail in the long run. Clinical studies have demonstrated that people who participate in these diets fail to achieve long-term weight loss and may often end up weighing *more*. A more practical approach would be to gradually increase and improve the quality of one's diet by eating a variety of healthy-fat/high-fiber foods that taste good. Just as most people can change from whole milk to 2-percent milk and eventually lose their taste for whole milk, similar changes may take place with just a little experimentation. We all have food preferences. The secret is to make adjustments in order to balance our favorite foods with healthier choices.

For example, one serving of premium ice cream contains two to three times the calories of a serving of frozen yogurt. Therefore the choice is to eat more frozen yogurt or less ice cream. This awareness is a small but crucial step in nutritional healing. A long-term weight loss program really means choosing a lifestyle that is palatable and somewhat calorie-deficient but enjoyable. If the choice is to substitute frozen yogurt for ice cream, over time the brain makes the gradual shift into believing that frozen yogurt is the same as ice cream.

GET OFF THE COUCH AND MOVE ANYTHING!

Keeping this energetic point of view in mind, we need to ask how the body conserves and expends energy. The body utilizes energy at rest as well as during exercise. This principle is reflected in one's basal metabolism rate (BMR), which is the rate the body uses energy to sustain the basic functions of life (breathing, heart rate, and so on). The BMR may vary from one individual to another as well as from one activity to another.

For example, an active person is likely to have a higher metabolic rate than a sedentary person, thereby resulting in a higher utilization of energy. One way to alter one's metabolic rate is to become more active. Unfortunately, many obese people do not expend much energy. In fact, you may notice a slow-motion quality about them. Frequently the overweight individual detests exercise, but *any* movement is precisely what is necessary for long-term success in weight loss.

Metabolic rate also varies with age and gender. The highest BMR is found in infants, who burn energy at a very high rate to fuel their rapid growth. There is a gradual decline in BMR in childhood and a further decline in adult life. Metabolic rates for women are usually lower than those for men, so women may need to consume fewer calories, except during pregnancy and lactation, when energy demands increase. Although there are calorie charts available, there is considerable variation in energy requirements among people—even for individuals of the same size, age, and gender. For example, for a one-hundred-thirty pound, moderately active woman, the daily caloric requirement is approximately 2,000 calories. However, there may be as much as a 20 percent variation for women with the same activity level and body size.

Recent medical findings on mechanisms that encourage the development and maintenance of obesity have focused not just on the consequences of eating too much, but also on the effects of expending too little energy. Two recent medical studies on the development of obesity in infancy and adulthood suggest that differences in activity may be the key point in obesity. In one study, clinical investigators measured the total seven-day energy intake and expenditure of a group of infants three months of age and related their results to weight gain during the first year of life. The data indicate that, keeping food intake constant, infants who are overweight on their first birthday have a 20.7 percent lower expenditure of energy than infants who are of normal weight. These findings suggest that both activity level and food intake are critical in determining weight gain at an early age, but the former appears to be more significant than the latter. The lesson for adults is that physical activity is probably more important in weight reduction than caloric intake. So the first factor in losing weight is to think in terms of increasing activity. If these energy expenditure findings apply to infants, they can also be applied to adults.

SOLVING THE WEIGHT-GAIN MYSTERY

It was once believed that the major cause of obesity was overeating. But if this were true, the easiest way to lose weight would be to eat less. As this is not so easy, it is clearly not the whole story. The causes of weight gain are numerous and complex. These include genetic, environmental, and psychosocial factors, as well as individual differences in eating patterns, resting metabolic rate, biochemical shifts, and the unusual phenomenon of "brown fat."

Brown fat is more metabolically active than stored fat and actually has the ability to burn energy, turning excess calories into heat. Some researchers believe that thin people who eat excessively and yet are not overly active may have a larger quantity of brown fat in proportion to stored fat, resulting in greater expenditure of energy. We all know individuals who seemingly eat all they want and yet remain thin despite the fact that they are not overly active. Brown fat may be the secret to this mystery. (Many people, however, do not have much brown fat and, instead, have undesirably high amounts of stored fat.)

Consider the fact that it takes approximately one hundred calories of energy to walk one mile. If we walk one mile a day, we will have an energy output of seven hundred calories per week. Multiply this by fifty-two weeks, and our calorie expenditure per year will equal 36,400 calories. Since a pound of fat contains approximately 3,500 calories, this daily one-mile walk is equivalent to the loss of approximately ten pounds of fat in one year if all other factors remain equal. Thus, by simple arithmetic, it becomes clear that the concept of energy balance is important to weight change.

Caloric intake is another major consideration in weight loss. When caloric intake is below the daily energy requirement, the initial loss in body weight results primarily from a depletion in the body's carbohydrate stores. For weight loss to continue, stored fat must be metabolized to fulfill the body's energy needs. In other words, by restricting food intake and/or by increasing physical activity, the body burns up fat.

Fad diets, however, don't work according to this principle. These types of diets tend to fool the body's biochemistry by manipulating proteins, carbohydrates, or fat, and are nutritionally unbalanced, usually advocating very high protein consumption, with and without high fat intake, and low carbohydrate consumption.

The Atkins Diet, for example, employs a high-protein, high-fat, low-carbohydrate regimen to achieve rapid weight loss. This results in a high blood level of free fatty acids that are insufficiently burned, thus producing ketones. Ketones make the blood more acidic, resulting in loss of appetite. The Scarsdale Diet is based on consuming a diet high in protein and low in fat. In this case the body metabolizes not only its stored fat but also the fat from other tissues as well. In addition, if you consume excess protein, especially if you are inactive, this protein can be converted to fat, and may actually work against your weight loss goals.

The most effective nutritional programs are those that are balanced and contain proper amounts of healthy fats, carbohydrates, and proteins. But there is a lot of information about nutrition out there, and it can sometimes be contradictory. Consider, for example, the confusion over the Great Fat Debate.

THE GREAT FAT DEBATE

Over the last fifteen to twenty years, medical experts have been telling us that we should significantly restrict our intake of fat. Fat, they claim, is the enemy, especially when coupled with lack of exercise. As a cardiologist who has seen the damage to blood vessels wrought by fatty streaks and occlusions, I too got caught up in the antifat movement. Cholesterol largely comes from saturated fats, and cholesterol is one of the biggest enemies of a healthy heart. The very-low-fat, or even no-fat, diets propagated by Pritikin, Ornish, and others have now come under attack and medical scrutiny. After researching, writing about, and witnessing first-hand the frequently unfavorable—even counterproductive—results of low-fat regimens, I have reassessed my position. While it is true that most fats are not beneficial, some are vitally important, such as the essential fatty acids found in fish, some plants, and flax. Without them, your body manufactures hazardous fatty acids that are broken down into harmful cholesterol, which damages your vascular system. There is no getting around it. A diet too low in certain fats can literally undermine all your efforts to create a healthy lifestyle for yourself. And if you put a low-fat plan together with a high-carbohydrate diet, then you have a recipe for insulin resistance, which really is the focal point of the Great Fat Debate.

INSULIN RESISTANCE

Insulin is a hormone secreted by the pancreas. It helps your body utilize sugar and carbohydrates. But when you have had too much insulin circulating in your bloodstream for too long, as is often the case when people stick to a high-carbohydrate, low-fat diet, the chronically high levels of insulin that build up store sugars and excess carbohydrates as fat. This so-called insulin resistance leads to a host of unfavorable events, including higher cholesterol and blood pressure, carbohydrate cravings, weight gain, and even premature heart disease. The insulin-resistance chain reaction goes something like this:

carbohydrate craving→ carbohydrate overload→ high blood sugar→ high insulin→ fat storage→ more carbohydrate craving

As you can see, an overabundance of insulin can cause the entire process to go awry. The well-known doctors Julian Whitaker and Robert Atkins are on opposite sides of the fence on this issue. Dr. Atkins is a proponent of the high-protein, high-fat, low-carbohydrate diet, while Dr. Whitaker endorses the low-fat, high-fiber diet.

If Robert Atkins is correct, insulin resistance affects some fifty million people in the United States. Many studies that show that overweight people (as well as type II diabetics) who consume large quantities of carbohydrates subsequently produce greater quantities of insulin. However, specialized receptor cells in their bodies lose their ability to respond to insulin, and thus the insulin is used inefficiently. Carbohydrates are utilized ineffectively and stored as fat. Atkins argues that a high-fat, high-protein diet loaded with "taboo" foods like bacon, steaks, and other red meats will lower your insulin levels, thereby causing you to derive energy from both stored fat and food. Because the body relies on the breakdown of fat to supply its energy needs rather than using carbohydrates for this, excess insulin release is curtailed.

Excess insulin is definitely a major contributing factor in hardening of the arteries. Remember, when insulin levels fluctuate, blood sugar levels also fluctuate, thereby creating a vicious cycle of carbohydrate cravings. Carbohydrate cravings, increased body fat, a decrease in blood levels of HDL (a beneficial lipoprotein), and high triglyceride levels are the hallmarks of insulin resistance.

Although Atkins is correct in his conclusions concerning insulin resistance and modifying insulin resistance with a low-carbohydrate, high-protein diet, he is out on a limb when he proposes a diet high in saturated fat, mostly derived from meat and dairy products. This type of diet tends to contain high levels of insecticides, pesticides, and radioactive elements, which in the long run may increase your risk of cancer of the bowel, prostate, and breast, as well as coronary artery disease. The typical Atkins diet also produces arachidonic acid, a long-chain fatty acid and metabolic by-product found in organ meats, saturated fatty meats, and dairy products; it enhances blood clotting and inflammation and constriction of the blood vessels. (The opposite is true with the omega-3 fatty acids, which encourage vasodilation and blood thinning. I'll be discussing this in other sections of this book.)

Another demon lurking in the background of the Atkins diet is a low amount of fiber. Meat just does not have enough dietary fiber. Although the Atkins diet may improve your cholesterol profile initially as a result of weight loss, and you may feel better and not hungry, the price your body pays for this over the long run is considerable.

But what about Julian Whitaker's point of view that the best diet is one that is high in carbohydrates and low in fat? Whitaker's reasoning is also correct and has been the medical profession's dietary gospel for years. Whitaker points out that many world cultures populated by vegetarians consuming low-fat, high-fiber diets demonstrate an absence or a low incidence of heart disease. In its pure form, this diet would be a healthy one. However, for most Americans, "modern" methods of food processing often translate into diets of refined carbohydrates with hydrogenated oils. The result is dangerous trans-fatty acids in the body—harmful fats— that can lead to heart disease. So while both approaches have their advantages and may work for a certain segment of the population, I have to come to the conclusion that it is time to update our approach to diet.

Before I give you my opinion on the Atkins and Whitaker points of view, I would like to comment on these dietary plans not only in terms of their carbohydrate and fat content but also in terms of other components such as fiber, phytonutrients, essential fatty acids, antioxidants, and trans-fatty acids. We need to review the effects of both diet plans on insulin resistance and consider the impact that excessive saturated fat has on the incidence of cancer. In order to distinguish which is the most healthy approach to weight management and good nutrition, we need to be able to look beyond the trees and at the forest. Remember, any food you put into your mouth contains not only carbohydrates, protein, and fats, but also many other elements, some good, some bad. Foods are like drugs; they can be therapeutic, but they can also have potential side effects.

Due to an increase in obesity throughout the population, an epidemic of insulin resistance in the United States, and an increase in heart disease, I have modified my approach to eating well by developing a more scientifically based diet that protects you not only from high surges of insulin but also nurtures your body at the same time. I believe it is time for the "medical experts" to rethink their approach to a balanced diet. I know that I have, and I predict that Drs. Atkins, Whitaker, Ornish, and others will soon modify their recommendations as well. Simply put, we need to eat a diet higher in protein, with healthy fats, lots of fiber, and we need to eat fewer processed foods, especially those containing sugars.

How do you know a good diet when you see one? After I discuss basic nutrition, you will see that the optimal diet is one that includes phytonutrients and fiber and balances healthy fats, carbohydrates, and protein; it is the modified Mediterranean diet, which I will discuss in chapter six.

OBESITY AND FUTURISTIC MEDICINE

In addition to viewing obesity in terms of caloric intake, levels of activity, and insulin resistance, it is also useful to explore the insights that genetic research can give us. Is obesity related to the genes? Recently researchers from Rockefeller University reported that they had identified and actually cloned an "obesity gene" found in mice. It is thought that the gene directs fat cells in the body to produce a hormone that tells the brain to suppress the appetite. Thus, if the gene is defective, this hormone will be absent or deficient, and no regulation of the appetite occurs. Although more research is needed to see how this applies to humans, it is conceivable that some individuals do have a defective "fat gene." Additional gene research has determined that there is tremendous variability in how people's insulin levels respond to a high carbohydrate load. For now, there is nothing we can do but wait for more investigations to be done. In the meantime, it is important to follow the rules of a healthy lifestyle and, for the overweight, to consider my diet recommendations, begin an exercise program, and find emotional support.

CHAPTER Three

Basic Nutrition: Back to School

In order to eat well, it's important that you understand some basics about how food affects your body. Although this may be more information than you care to know about right now, I hope you'll find yourself referring back to this chapter again and again.

Remember that the loss of excess fat results from expending more energy than you take in, and that energy is derived from calories. Food calories can be divided into three major components: proteins, carbohydrates, and fats, with alcohol as a fourth, less important contributor. When counting calories, we need to consider the percentages that come from proteins, carbohydrates, or fats in any given serving.

Each of these nutrients provides different amounts of energy (calories per gram or per ounce), measured through sophisticated clinical studies. The following provides useful values for comparison:

- Carbohydrates contain 4 calories per gram, or 112 calories per ounce
- Fat contains 9 calories per gram, or 252 calories per ounce
- Protein contains 4 calories per gram, or 112 calories per ounce

From this brief analysis, one can easily see that an individual can eat over twice as much carbohydrates or protein as fat and still have the same caloric intake. (Hard liquor has 7 calories per gram or 196 calories per ounce, which is usually only one cocktail; wine has approximately 20 to 25 calories per ounce.)

Foods are classified according to their caloric density. For example, three ounces of fish contains approximately 150 calories; three ounces of beef chuck contains approximately 300 calories. Such caloric densities are usually related to the amount of fat in the food. Fish contains relatively less fat than beef. Therefore, more fish can be eaten than beef for the same amount of calories. But more fish may not be needed to satisfy hunger, so one can reduce total intake and therefore lose weight.

We can see that it is important to know the fat content in food. Being nutritionally aware means choosing foods that provide the most nutrition with the least fats and calories. For example, approximately 50 percent of the calories in whole milk come from fat, while only approximately 18 percent of the calories in 1-percent milk come from fat. If most of us can make the gradual transition from whole milk (3-percent) to 1-percent milk, the amount of calories is reduced by nearly half. One-percent milk is less caloric-dense and therefore better for you. And remember the cardinal rule: *No deprivation and no loss of pleasure.*

A good weight loss program should not only be calorie-light but also contain healthy amounts of carbohydrates, fats, and protein. In considering a healthy diet or a healthy lifestyle, we again have to remember that deprivation is the oppositional force. When putting our meals together we strive for a reasonable balance of carbohydrates, fats, and protein, but do we know how to do this properly?

The answer to this question is simple. All of us have had different protein requirements depending upon our lean body mass, percentage of fat, and level of physical activity. Ordinarily, most scientists would agree that in order to prevent muscle wasting and repair damaged tissue, we need to ingest at least one gram of protein per kilogram (2.2 pounds) of our body weight daily. For example, an average 150-pound male will require a minimum of 65 to 70 grams of protein each day. It is important for each of us to know our own protein requirement in order to structure our fat and carbohydrate ingestion in a healthy manner. There have been many books written on this topic. One particular text that approaches diet scientifically is *The Zone* by Barry Sears, PhD. I think Sears has done a respectable job in suggesting a diet with higher protein and fats and modest amounts of carbohydrates. However, I do believe that Sears is recommending too much protein. He suggests that the typical American receive 30 percent of daily calories from fat, 30 percent from protein, and the remaining 40 percent from carbohydrates. This plan does endorse excessive quantities of protein. An individual who requires 2,000 calories a day would be consuming 150 grams of protein according to this formula. However, I endorse his recommendations to divide the protein evenly over three meals and two snacks as a sound strategy. If your protein intake is monitored and split up evenly during the day, less carbohydrate may be ingested at each meal, reducing the peak insulin levels that occur with higher carbohydrate meals. But I want to warn you not to be overly enthusiastic about excessive protein consumption.

If we consume too many calories, excess proteins will be converted to fat and stored in the body to be burned later for energy. Amino acids that can be transferred into sugars are called glucogenic, and amino acids that are broken down to fat are called ketogenic amino acids. Since most Americans consume more than two times as much protein as they need, excessive protein ingestion is an easily overlooked source of weight gain. The important thing you need to do is balance your portions of protein, fats, and carbohydrates at each meal. This includes breakfast, lunch, and dinner. Most people, in general, do not get enough protein with breakfast. I believe that throughout the day we should try to get 20 to 25 percent of our calories from protein, 30 percent from fat, and the remainder, or 45 to 50 percent, of the rest of the calories from carbohydrates. Like Sears, I agree that we should take in fewer carbohydrates and more fats, but I do not agree with his 30 percent protein requirement. Ornish, Pritikin, and the other low-fat or no-fat gurus are requiring too many carbohydrates and not enough healthy fats, thus enhancing insulin release. When you eat carbohydrates, try to use fewer carbohydrates with a high glycemic index. The glycemic index is the entry of sugar into the bloodstream. Digested cereals such as puffed rice or cornflakes as well as white table sugar, breads (either white or wheat), potatoes, carrots, corn, and bananas move into the bloodstream quickly and thereby "turn on" insulin production. If you must have these carbohydrates, try to combine them with others that have a low glycemic index to moderate the release of sugar. Soybeans, barley, lentils, peaches, plums, high protein pastas, beans, and skim milk are all foods with a low glycemic index that maintain a sustained release of sugar into the blood. Remember that insulin is predominately secreted by the pancreas in response to a carbohydrate load. Combining fats and protein at each meal with low glycemic carbohydrates will not provoke a high insulin response—the greatest risk factor in the development of the arteriosclerotic plaque that leads to coronary artery disease.

What is it about insulin that is harmful to the heart? First, you need to know four basic facts about insulin resistance:

1. High insulin surges (hyperinsulinism) cause the accumulation of smooth muscle cells in the lining of blood vessels, setting the stage for plaque buildup in the arteries.
2. High insulin levels cause arachidonic acid release, which turns on thromboxane, a potent vasoconstrictive, inflammatory, and prothrombotic prostaglandin that enhances inflammation, clotting, and high blood pressure.
3. Hyperglycemia is a risk factor for coronary artery disease.
4. Insulin resistance causes a decrease in HDL and an increase in triglycerides, thereby accelerating the process of coronary artery disease.

In fact, a triglyceride/HDL ratio of four or more is considered a serious risk factor for the development of coronary artery disease.

A balanced approach to diet is the most sensible plan for all of us. Mindfully balancing fats, carbohydrates, and protein at every meal is the best way to keep our insulin levels within what Sears calls the "tight zone."

NUTRITIONAL AWARENESS KEEPS POUNDS OFF, FAT OUT

Medical research indicates that weight gain is related not only to the total number of calories, but also to the total number of grams of fat in the diet. Reducing our intake of unhealthy fat is a cardinal ingredient in weight loss and good health. Generally, people have considerable resistance to reducing the fat intake in their diets. However, it is crucial to point out that fat intake should be kept to a maximum of about 30 percent to optimize weight loss and ensure a healthy lifestyle. In considering a nutritional awareness program, and particularly in losing weight, it is important to focus our attention on the number of grams of fat we consume daily. This can be done by reading labels and avoiding various cooking techniques that result in excess fat content.

Mushrooms, for example, are quite low in calories and derive less than 10 percent of their calories from fat, but if they are deep fried in oil or broiled in butter, the fat and calorie content is considerably higher. Onions get about 3 to 5 percent of their calories from fat, but fried as onion rings, this figure approaches 90 percent, making them calorie-dense and a poor choice when seeking a healthy, nutritional balance.

In calculating the percentage of calories from fat in a particular product, you must know the calories per serving and the number of grams of fat per serving. The calculation process goes something like this: Multiply the number of grams of fat by 9 (remember there are 9 calories per gram of fat) to determine the total number of fat calories in a food product. Next, divide the number of fat calories by the number of total calories in the serving. Now convert this to a percentage by multiplying by 100. The goal in losing weight and staying healthy is to primarily choose foods that derive less than 30 percent of their calories from fat.

Let's now focus attention on the calculations involving carbohydrates and protein. One has to keep in mind that each gram of protein or carbohydrate has 4 calories. The calculation for percentage of calories from protein and carbohydrates is similar to that for fat, but we need to multiply the number of grams of carbohydrates or protein by 4 instead of 9. Then divide the number of protein or carbohydrate calories by the number of calories per serving and again convert this to a percentage (multiply by 100). With simple arithmetic one can determine the percentage of calories from protein, carbohydrates, and fats in a particular food. For example, potato chips get approximately 60 percent of their calories from fat. The usual serving of ten potato chips has approximately 115 calories, 1 gram of protein, 10 grams of carbohydrates, and 8 grams of fat per serving. Multiply 8 grams of fat by 9 calories per gram, and this equals 72 calories. Next, divide the number of fat calories by the number of total calories, which is 72 over 115. Now convert this to a percentage by multiplying it by 100. The figure comes out to 62.6 percent of calories from fat. Since potato chips contain such a considerable quantity of fat, in this case even a small portion is detrimental to diet and health. At 115 calories and 8 grams of fat for ten chips, just imagine how many calories you can consume while watching television with a bowl of chips next to you and not even feel satisfied. It is important to understand that substituting foods that give us the same satisfaction but less fat will alleviate the feelings of hunger. Again, an important tool in losing weight is knowledge and awareness of the fat content in our diets. When determining what foods to eat, remember that the number of calories you get from fat should be slightly higher than the number of calories you get from protein. You must not be overzealous in your approach to protein, as too much protein over time could negatively impact on your body.

YOU AND YOUR *BUN*

The process of breaking down protein (amino acids) is called deamination. This can cause considerable metabolic stress to the body as an expenditure of energy when protein is used as a fuel source. During this process the nitrogen that is released from the amino acids is quickly converted into ammonia. Since ammonia is toxic to the body, it is changed into the breakdown product called urea. Blood urea nitrogen, or BUN, is a measure of kidney function and really is a product of the breakdown of nitrogen waste products in the body. In a balanced diet in which protein accounts for up to 25 percent of the total caloric intake, our bodies can dispose of the urea through the normal functioning of the kidneys. However, taking excess quantities of protein, amounting to 40 to 50 percent of total calories, will cause a buildup of urea, which requires a large amount of water in order for the body to process it efficiently. If we do not drink enough water, our body takes it from our tissues to dilute the urea, placing an enormous burden on the kidneys.

Such a scenario occurs in individuals on very high protein diets. Wrestlers trying to "make weight" frequently use this destructive technique. I did this during my college career, when as a wrestler I needed to maintain a weight approximately ten to twelve pounds lighter than my natural and healthy weight. Our coaches recommended a high-protein diet—and we wondered why we were continuously "dying of thirst"! Yes, I was able to make weight on every occasion, but at the expense of my kidney function. After nine years of wrestling in high school and college, my kidney function was slightly abnormal when I entered medical school. The toxicities induced by high protein metabolism coupled with a poor intake of fluid probably affected the status of my kidneys. Unknowingly I caused renal dysfunction in myself, which could have been extremely hazardous. Luckily for me, I stopped the high-protein diet before it had time to do lasting damage.

This warning aside, though, protein has many important functions in the body. It makes up muscles, ligaments, tendons, organs, glands, nails, hair, and some body fluids. Protein is also essential for growth. Amino acids are the building blocks of protein. Protein is composed of different amino acids, each with a specific function. There are two types of amino acids, the essential and the nonessential. The nonessential amino acids can be produced by the liver, and include approximately 80 percent of the amino acids we need. The remaining 20 percent must be obtained from outside sources. There are nine essential amino acids. If we do not consume foods with enough of the essential amino acids, the body may be unable to produce the protein it requires for healthy functioning. We all have read signs, particularly in elementary school cafeterias, with statements such as "Eating meat builds strong muscles." This is because meat is considered to be one of the best sources of protein. Unfortunately, meat also contains considerable quantities of hidden fat. Other complete protein sources include dairy products, eggs, fish, and poultry.

Although the need for protein in the United States is grossly exaggerated, the proper balance of amino acids is indeed crucial. For example, some individuals on weight loss programs, particularly fasting programs, do not consume enough protein. This can be injurious to their health. If the body does not take in sufficient protein and a correct balance of amino acids each day, then it will take what it needs from its own muscles. Yes, the body will find a way to produce protein—but it does not distinguish skeletal muscle from heart muscle. Therefore, overzealous fasting and dieting may lead to deterioration of the heart muscle, making a person susceptible to arrhythmias and perhaps even sudden death. In our hospital weight loss program, for example, we were particularly careful to maintain the minimum daily protein requirement for each individual. We frequently performed electrocardiograms on these participants to ensure that their hearts were functioning properly.

We all need a basic minimum of protein. Therefore it is important to select foods that are good sources of protein. Proteins may come from animal sources such as meat, fish, eggs, and milk, but they also can come from grains, vegetables, and fruits. Most of us now know that animal proteins in fish, turkey, and white meat chicken offer complete proteins and are lower in fat than red meats. Eggs contain protein and some fat, but do have high quantities of cholesterol. Vegetable sources of protein, though highly desirable, are often deficient in one or more of the essential amino acids. Thus vegetarians may need to supplement their diets with dairy products or consume certain combinations of foods to make complete proteins. Excellent vegetable sources of protein as well as carbohydrates include legumes (such as beans, peas, and lentils) and grains.

Carbohydrates make up the largest source of calories in our diet and should be the major source of nutrients. They are the primary energy storage molecules found in most living organisms. Carbohydrates come from the plant kingdom, and are found in the form of starch, one of the components of plant cell walls. Starch is a polysaccharide—a molecule made up of many sugar molecules linked together. Substances such as sucrose (table sugar), maltose (malt sugar), and lactose (milk sugar) are disaccharides, which contain two linked sugar molecules. Monosaccharides are the simple sugars, such as glucose and fructose; these contain only one sugar molecule.

Complex carbohydrates are the predominant feature of most diets. It is important to remember that complex carbohydrates should make up about 45 to 50 percent of our caloric intake. Complex carbohydrates are not absorbed quickly into the bloodstream; they must be broken down slowly by the digestive process. Once they are digested, these polysaccharides are converted into glucose, a form of sugar the body can easily use for energy. Fructose, a monosaccharide, is found naturally in fruit and honey and is easily converted to glucose. Sucrose, which also eventually breaks down into glucose, makes up approximately 25 percent of the total carbohydrates we eat and occurs naturally in most carbohydrates, especially in beet or cane sugar and maple syrup.

The primary function of carbohydrates is to provide energy for the body. If we consume more carbohydrates than we need, the extra glucose may be stored as glycogen in the liver. While the liver can break down glycogen in situations in which glucose is needed, it is best to consume carbohydrates on a daily basis to provide a continual energy source.

HOW MUCH SUGAR DO YOU EAT?

Simple carbohydrates are most often found in sweet foods such as pastries, cakes, and cookies, which are usually made with refined sugar, particularly cane sugar. The problem with eating large quantities of sucrose is that it contains calories but no vitamins, minerals, or fiber. Simply stated, although such sugar provides energy, it really has no positive effects except to satisfy our craving for sweets. Such simple carbohydrates should be kept to a minimum, as they add nothing to the body but calories.

One goal of nutritional awareness is to increase your own consumption of nutrient-dense foods and decrease your consumption of calorie-dense foods. Most Americans are unaware that three fourths of all the sugar we eat comes in processed foods. Although some of us still continue to use a little white sugar in our coffee or tea or on our cereal, the amount of "hidden" sugar in breads, soft drinks, candies, cakes, and doughnuts is extremely high. The average American, for example, consumes approximately a hundred pounds of sugar per year.

Consuming simple carbohydrates also causes metabolic stress to the body. Simple sugars require less direction and so enter the bloodstream more quickly than other nutrients. Remember that this rate of entry into the bloodstream is called the glycemic index. This quick entry causes stress on the pancreas, resulting in increased insulin secretion. Such high amounts of insulin are required to metabolize the sugar. This may result in metabolic swings in our body, alternating between periods of high blood sugar and then low blood sugar. These periods are often experienced as mood swings. During a coffee break, for example, we may consume coffee with sugar and perhaps a doughnut. The simple sugars in these foods result in an increase in insulin. After the initial surge of insulin, the blood sugar usually drops. For this reason, we may be hungry again not long after our coffee break. We may also experience fatigue and light-headedness. This sets up a vicious cycle; we may find ourselves snacking on yet another doughnut, followed by a very high-calorie lunch. Caffeine, which I will discuss later, is yet another ugly player in this game.

The advantage of eating more complex carbohydrates is not only that they have additional vitamins, minerals, and fiber, but also that they take longer to be metabolized. The more unrefined the carbohydrate, the slower the release of glucose into the bloodstream. In contrast, the more refined the sugar, the more quickly glucose is released into the bloodstream, resulting in higher surges of insulin and possibly later symptoms of low blood sugar, or hypoglycemia. This is the beginning of insulin resistance and the beginning of weight gain, as more calories are stored as fat. Thus simple carbohydrates as well as other high-glycemic carbohydrates should be kept to a minimum at all times, whereas complex carbohydrates should make up not only the majority of our total carbohydrate intake but also at least 45 percent of our diet. Diets high in complex carbohydrates include lots of fruits, vegetables, and grains, providing large amounts of fiber as well as nutrients. This is a key factor in any plan for good nutrition and health.

CHAPTER Four

Fiber Can Be Fun

This chapter could save your life.

Most doctors would agree that a diet high in fiber results in a reduced risk of developing many chronic diseases. The importance of fiber in human health has been demonstrated by large population studies. African people on high-fiber diets, for instance, have a very low incidence of coronary artery disease, colorectal cancer, diverticulosis, gallbladder disease, and constipation. Some of the "less developed" populations of Africa have an average cholesterol level of 90 to 100, and coronary artery disease is practically nonexistent.

Such "nonindustrialized" cultures tend to rely on roots, yams, corn, rice, and other grains. These complex carbohydrates, as previously discussed, are better for the body than the refined carbohydrates and simple sugars that are found in the processed foods many of us eat in the West. Raising animals for slaughter is also a relatively recent historical phenomenon. Was man ever meant to eat meat in great quantities? If we compare the teeth of a human to the teeth of a dog or cat, we can easily distinguish the absence in humans of large canines and sharp incisors meant for tearing. Carnivorous animals, those whose diets consist mainly of flesh, generally do not succumb to coronary artery disease. They have genetic protection, as they evolved to eat meat.

Most humans living in industrialized societies, on the other hand, have a diet composed largely of meats and fats and yet have a vascular system that is not accustomed to such abuse. Such a drastic change in the Western diet has been associated with a multitude of diseases, including dental caries, diverticulosis, large-bowel cancer, hiatal hernia, coronary artery disease, diabetes, gallstones, and obesity. Over the last two centuries there has been a profound change in the diet of peoples living in industrialized societies. Although hunter-gatherers did consume animal protein, they were dependent upon the migratory habits of herds, and therefore their meat intake was limited. The most drastic changes in Westerners' diets have included an increase in salt, fat, and sugar, and a decrease in protein, complex carbohydrates, and dietary fiber (table 1).

TABLE 1

Percentage of Calories from Fat, Complex Carbohydrates, Fiber, and Salt in Three Population Groups

	Hunter-Gatherers	Peasant Agriculturalists	Western Peoples
	Fat 15–20	Fat 10–15	Fat 40+
		Sugar 5	
	Starch 50–70	Starch 60–75	Sugar 20
			Starch 25–30
	Protein 15–20	Protein 10–15	Protein 12
Salt (g/d)	1	5–15	15
Fiber (g/d)	40	16–20	20

From *Medical Applications of Clinical Nutrition*. Copyright ©1983 by Keats Publishing, Inc. Published by Keats Publishing, Inc., New Canaan, CT. Used with permission.

Dietary fiber is the part of plant foods that our systems cannot digest. When it is ingested, it passes through the small intestine unchanged. How many of us, for example, have changed a baby's diaper only to find the outer shells of corn kernels still intact even though their nutrients had been absorbed? The absorbable portion of corn is starch. Insoluble (undigestible) fiber increases the speed of transit through the intestines. Insoluble fiber includes cellulose, heavy cellulose, and lignin—the supportive skeleton of plants, and the fiber found in most fruits and vegetables. Soluble fiber, on the other hand, includes pectins, gums, and mucilages. These entities make up the intercellular cement of plants and have several positive effects on the body that promote health and help prevent various disease states. Soluble fiber forms a gel-like material that inhibits cholesterol and LDL absorption and is effective in reducing blood glucose levels. The familiar phrase "An apple a day keeps the doctor away" makes a great deal of sense. Apples are a good source of pectin, as is the white lining under the peel and the pulp of grapefruit. Later I will discuss my natural cholesterol-lowering approach, which incorporates soluble and insoluble fiber.

Most complex carbohydrates contain both types of fiber. The predominant type of fiber depends upon the plant species. Wheat bran, for example, contains more insoluble fiber than soluble fiber. Oat bran, rich in gums, is considered a better source of soluble fiber. Insoluble fiber is also found in cabbage, broccoli, turnips, Brussels sprouts, kidney beans, green beans, chickpeas, nuts, whole-grain cereals, and breads made from whole-grain wheat, rye, oats, barley, and corn. Fruits, especially the skins, are also an excellent source of insoluble fiber. Soluble fiber is found in specific fruits such as strawberries, peaches, apples, and citrus fruits. Berries and seeds are especially rich in soluble fiber.

FIBER HELPS PREVENT COLON CANCER

The physiological effects of dietary fiber begin with the first mouthful of food. High-fiber foods are "chewy." Chewing stimulates the flow of saliva and the secretion of gastric juices. Such prolonged chewing also gives the brain a message of satiety. For example, if we chew brown rice, or a high-fiber cookie for that matter, the increased time it takes creates a "conversation" between the brain and the stomach. Since it may take several seconds, perhaps even several minutes, to ingest such high-fiber foods, the stomach has more time to register the feeling of fullness. High-fiber meals fill the stomach and provide a feeling of fullness, particularly when ingested with generous quantities of water. The combination of water and fiber swells the stomach, satisfying hunger quickly. Soluble fiber also delays gastric emptying.

In the small intestine, insoluble fiber slows the rate of digestion. In the large intestine, dietary fiber, particularly the insoluble form, increases the bulk of stools. Fiber has a water-holding capacity that prevents water from being absorbed through the mucous membranes in the large intestine. This helps prevent dry, hard stools, thereby alleviating constipation. In general, cereal grains containing cellulose and fruits and vegetables containing pectin serve as excellent bulk-forming natural laxatives. Fiber, as we previously stated, increases the fecal transit rate, and this may protect us against colon cancer—the more quickly waste is eliminated, the less time carcinogens have to form as the result of bacterial and chemical activity in the bowel.

Statistics from population studies all over the world suggest that a high-fiber diet is protective while a high-fat diet may enhance the risk of colon cancer. Consider the United States and Finland, two countries that have a high incidence of colon cancer. Both of these populations consume high-fat diets, but colon cancer mortality is significantly lower among Finns, who consume a much greater amount of cereal fiber than Americans. The problem with the "normal" American diet is that it contains too much fat and not enough fiber. The average American consumes between 11 and 17 grams of fiber daily. Because diet is an important contributing factor in colon cancer (it has been estimated that 35 percent of all cancers in the country are caused by improper diet), the National Cancer Institute recommends a daily consumption of at least 20 to 30 grams of fiber (table 2). I recommend 30, with 40 being the maximum. This is essentially twice the daily intake of a typical American. Since colon cancer, in general, is more prevalent in obese persons, a high-fiber diet is especially essential for this group.

As fiber gives bulk to food without providing additional energy, fiber-rich foods offer excellent advantages to the obese population. It is also an important consideration in the diabetic population as well. A diet rich in complex carbohydrates and fiber may improve blood sugar levels by offering a continuous supply of energy rather than short bursts, thus perhaps reducing the amount of medication required. The American Diabetes Association suggests that patients who have diabetes mellitus should double their fiber intake. It is important to consider that diets rich in fiber also contain less fat and cholesterol and fewer calories. This too is as beneficial as weight reduction is in treating diabetes.

TABLE 2

Recommended Daily Fiber Intake Compared with Current Intake

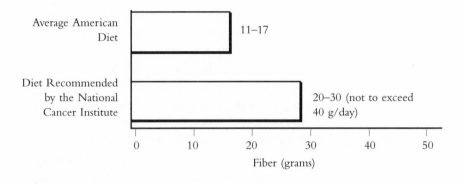

FIBER HELPS THE HEART

The benefits of fiber are also exceedingly important when one considers the causes of coronary artery disease. In experimental studies, soluble fiber sources (pectin, guar gum, and barley and oat bran) have been shown to reduce blood cholesterol levels when taken in generous amounts. We have all heard of the cholesterol-lowering effects of oats and oat bran. As little as 2 ounces of oat bran per day can reduce your cholesterol 7 to 10 percent. Actually, any oat product—oat bran, oatmeal, or even Cheerios, for that matter—is effective as a cholesterol-lowering agent.

Recently the media has questioned the validity of these claims for oat bran, citing some opinions that larger amounts may be needed to lower one's cholesterol. While this may be true, supplementing oat bran with other fiber-rich foods creates an additive or synergistic effect on the body. As little as one to one and one-half cups of beans daily, with some oat bran, can lower cholesterol by sixty points. I personally favor oat bran and oat products, particularly since they are excellent sources of soluble fiber and in clinical studies demonstrated definite reduction in LDL levels in many people.

Wheat bran, on the other hand, has a less significant effect on cholesterol because it is an insoluble fiber. However, wheat bran is considered by some to be the best bran to eat in order to reduce the risk of colon cancer. As previously mentioned, it helps to sweep away possible cancer-producing substances from the intestines by enhancing fecal bulk and increasing transit rate. Insoluble fiber acts in several ways to reduce blood cholesterol as well. This type of fiber may prevent the absorption of many chemicals into the intestines, particularly bile acids, which are necessary to form cholesterol in the body. By the same token, cholesterol may also be trapped by fiber and lost through the stools rather than absorbed. Pharmaceutical companies in this country have created substances that act in a similar way, but doesn't it make sense to just increase our intake of dietary fiber? Why take a synthetic drug if we don't have to? In addition, fiber-rich complex carbohydrates serve as a good alternative to foods high in fat; as recently noted in the *New England Journal of Medicine,* people who eat more food high in fiber eat less food high in fat. Therefore, it makes sense to increase the fiber in our diet. Western diets are too high in fat, sugar, and salt, and too low in fiber and starch. To put it simply, Americans need to eat more like the inhabitants of some of the less developed countries of the world.

The benefits of fiber are even greater than once thought. A recent article in the *Journal of the American Medical Association* in the spring of 1996 revealed that an increased dietary fiber intake, independent of fat intake, was extremely important in preventing coronary artery disease. The study showed a stunning 29 percent reduction in coronary artery disease for every 10-gram increase in cereal fiber. These remarkable results show benefits of fiber greater than previously known. It is very likely that a fiber intake may be working on other mechanisms in addition to cholesterol lowering. There is the possibility that some unknown factors associated with a high-fiber intake could be responsible for the reduction in coronary artery disease. Any foods, for example, with a high-fiber content are a tremendous source of phytonutrients including flavonoids, phytoestrogens, lignins, and carotenoids. Since these phytonutrients impact other cholesterol interactions, it can be assumed that these factors are also associated with a cholesterol-lowering effect. Thus, it is important to consider that food high in dietary fiber, rather than just fiber supplements alone, is the way to go.

Increasing intake of starch and fiber, reducing consumption of sugar and salt, and avoiding as much unhealthy fat as possible should not present any major difficulties. We do not deprive ourselves if we consume fiber. The risk/benefit ratio is exceedingly high. Although there are some potential adverse effects such as bloating, cramps, or flatulence, these symptoms are only fleeting and will disappear when our intestinal flora adjust to the change in the nutritional environment. One drawback of fiber-rich foods may be that they inhibit the absorption of minerals, including calcium and iron. For example, foods high in oxalates, such as chard, beets, and rhubarb, act to bind calcium. Soybeans also contain phytic acid, which acts to bind zinc. But vitamin and mineral supplementation, or the increased consumption of yellow and green vegetables (with the exception of spinach) and fruits, will help to replenish such minerals. Other rare potential hazards of fiber include the remote possibility of obstruction of the gastrointestinal tract, particularly in individuals who have undergone surgical procedures for peptic ulcer, stomach cancer, or ulcerative colitis. These individuals should consult their physicians before embarking on a high-fiber diet.

Remember, however, that many diseases can be reduced in severity or prevented by fiber, including not only diabetes, diverticulitis, and colon cancer, as mentioned, but also coronary artery disease. The risk/benefit ratio of fiber is overwhelmingly on the side of the benefit. By increasing the amount of fiber in our diet, we can gradually enhance the quality of our lives, feel better, and help to prevent many of the illnesses of modern man (table 3).

TABLE 3

Reported Benefits of Dietary Fiber

- Improvement in bowel function
- Reduction of serum cholesterol levels
- Displacement of fat, saturated fat, and cholesterol from the diet
- Improvement of blood sugar levels among patients with type II diabetes mellitus
- Treatment and prevention of diverticulosis
- Reduction of colon cancer risk

In table 4 you will find some quick and easy fiber foods that I recommend.

TABLE 4

Quick and Easy Fiber Combinations

Food Combinations	Dietary Fiber (grams)	Total Combined Fiber (grams)
1 raw carrot with	2.4	
1/2 cup raisins	4.9	7.3
1 pear with	5.0	
2 graham crackers	2.1	7.1
3 cups popcorn with	3.0	
1 cup dried figs	3.7	6.7
1/2 cantaloupe with	2.7	
3 dried prunes	3.9	6.6
1/2 cup blueberries with	2.5	
2/3 cup Shredded Wheat	3.3	5.8
1 baked potato with	3.7	
1/2 cup applesauce	2.0	5.7
3/4 cup oatmeal with	2.8	
1 mango	2.9	5.7
2/3 cup raisin bran with	3.6	
1/2 cup applesauce	2.0	5.6
1/2 cup brown rice with	2.4	
1 apple	2.9	5.3
1/2 cup corn (cooked) with	3.9	
1 slice whole-wheat bread	1.4	5.3

CHAPTER Five

Cholesterol: Myth, Fact, and Fiction

C holesterol is a topic of much conversation these days. The public is so frequently inundated by media reports and advertising regarding the health hazards of high cholesterol that this topic is of interest to both the healthy and the unhealthy alike. Almost every patient I have in my practice wants to know his or her cholesterol level—the young and the old, those with and without heart disease. But what is cholesterol? And why is there so much conversation regarding it?

Cholesterol is a fatty, waxlike substance that is both manufactured by the body and taken in through foods. It is needed in the production of hormones, cells, and bile salts. (For example, cholesterol is a necessary element in the production of the adrenal steroid hormone cortisone as well as the sex hormones.) Since our liver manufactures cholesterol, it would reserve enough to support the daily functioning of the body, even if we did not eat any cholesterol at all. Without cholesterol, our cells could not function. In small amounts, therefore, cholesterol is vital to our health and survival. But whenever a person eats beyond his energy requirements, a surplus of cholesterol accumulates in the blood. In addition, the liver uses the saturated fat we eat to produce even more cholesterol.

It is this gradual buildup of stored fat and cholesterol that increases the risk of atherosclerosis (hardening of the arteries), which consequently increases the risk of coronary artery disease and stroke, as well as peripheral vascular disease. When too much cholesterol gets into the blood, it may cause plaque to form in major blood vessels, resulting in a gradual hardening and narrowing of the arteries and heightening the risk of cardiac illness. There are many large population studies indicating that as one's cholesterol rises, one's risk of coronary artery disease also rises.

LOWER YOUR CHOLESTEROL AND LIVE

Consider the Japanese, whose diet consists mainly of rice, fish, and sea vegetables. This culture has the lowest incidence of coronary artery disease in the world. The American diet, on the other hand, includes considerable quantities of saturated fat (found in meats, oils, and dairy products). Americans have one of the highest rates of coronary artery disease in the world. The well-known Framingham study, for example, clearly demonstrates that there is a direct relationship between coronary artery disease and a typical American diet. This study began in 1948 and involved more than 5,000 subjects from Framingham, Massachusetts. The subjects were analyzed with respect to health habits such as diet, smoking, and high blood pressure. The results indicate that the higher the cholesterol intake, the greater the probability of developing heart disease. Currently, approximately one in four Americans has high cholesterol. The good news, however, is that if your blood cholesterol is high, you can reduce your risk of heart disease simply by lowering it.

A landmark study by the National Heart, Lung, and Blood Institute showed that the benefit from lowering cholesterol is considerable. In this trial, each 1-percent reduction in blood cholesterol was associated with a 2-percent reduction in coronary artery disease risk. Thus, participants who reduced their cholesterol by 25 percent reduced their risk of heart attack by almost one half. Other studies have also demonstrated that lowering cholesterol levels actually can reverse the buildup of blockages in coronary vessels. Since the medical literature so overwhelmingly shows a direct relationship between cholesterol and coronary artery disease, all reputable physicians should counsel their patients about the potential hazards of cholesterol. In fact, physicians do frequently recommend that patients know their cholesterol levels and take a more active role in healing themselves, particularly through dietary choices.

I have found that patients nowadays have become so aware and so knowledgeable about cholesterol that they not only want to know their total numbers, but also ask questions regarding HDL and LDL, lipoproteins that carry cholesterol in the blood. Blood is mostly water, and cholesterol is a fat. Since water and fat do not mix, cholesterol is carried in the blood in combination with proteins referred to as high-density lipoproteins (HDL) and low-density lipoproteins (LDL). HDL, commonly called "good cholesterol," is considered to be a type of cholesterol scavenger in the body. HDL picks up cholesterol from blood vessels and transports them back to the liver. LDL, on the other hand, infiltrates the blood vessel walls, thus increasing the risk of plaque buildup in the vessels. If the plaque buildup occurs in the coronary vessels, this could render an individual susceptible to heart disease. LDL is a noxious substance by itself. When it is combined with the toxic effects of cigarette smoking or the membrane-tearing effects of high blood pressure, a gradual inflammatory process results that causes a thickening of the vessel walls, which leads to gradual closure. Thus, the higher the LDL level, the more one is at risk for heart disease. Conversely, the higher the HDL level, the more protection one has from heart disease.

Cardiologists frequently look not only at total cholesterol, but also at the cholesterol fractions of LDL and HDL. Individuals who are at the most serious risk for developing coronary artery disease include those people with low HDL and high LDL. So doesn't it make sense to increase your HDL and lower your LDL? One way to increase HDL is by losing weight. Vigorous exercise is another effective way to raise HDL. Effective ways of lowering LDL also include weight loss as well as reduction of unhealthy fats in the diet, utilization of more dietary fiber, and cessation of cigarette smoking. Cigarette smoking is indeed a major cardiovascular risk factor, not only because of the toxic effects of tar and nicotine, but also because cigarette smoking enhances the harmful effect LDL has on the vascular wall. In a recent European study, smoking was found to increase the total cholesterol and cause a reduction in HDL, particularly in women.

EMOTIONS AFFECT CHOLESTEROL

In addition to smoking and diet, there are many other factors known to affect cholesterol. For example, emotions are a major consideration. Calming touch has been shown to actually lower blood cholesterol while stress increases it. Yes, it is true that excessive stress and tension can affect the regulation of cholesterol in your body, regardless of your intake through diet. Scientific studies have shown that accountants who are under severe pressure during tax season have considerable elevations in their blood cholesterol during the months of January through April. Following the tax season deadline of April 15, their cholesterol levels fall.

Perhaps one of the most interesting findings comes from a study of race car drivers done in England. Race car drivers take many chances and probably have an unconscious fear of death, which is one of the most intense emotions one can have. In this particular study, drivers who raced on the circuit had alarming increases in both cholesterol and triglycerides. Thus, their fear seems to be reflected in the high levels of blood cholesterol.

LOVE

But what about positive feelings such as love? Can they influence cholesterol? In one study, rabbits who received preferential care from their trainers had lower cholesterol levels and less plaque in their arteries than rabbits who were not cuddled. Touching and cuddling proved to enhance optimum health in these animals, and humans are no exception to this rule, either. As simple as it sounds, love indeed heals. In our Healing the Heart workshops, we clearly demonstrated profound decreases in cholesterol that were linked to contact, connectedness, and positive feelings. In these four- to seven-day workshops, cholesterol lowering was reported in every one of our participants, with some participants losing as much as 100 mg/dl of cholesterol in a mere four to five days of group support. Although these participants were on low-fat, high-fiber diets, their sudden, drastic reduction in cholesterol supports the notion of how emotional discharge can positively impact our health.

When we hold in our emotions and feelings, we create undesirable biochemical situations in our bodies that can render us more susceptible to cholesterol elevation. Unfortunately, most of us are unaware of these factors. In our Healing the Heart seminars, people are nurtured by a supportive environment; they feel connected to others and are comfortable letting their feelings out, and as a result, cholesterol levels fall.

Although digging into our hidden emotions can have a tremendous positive impact on our emotional and physical health, the commitment and vulnerability required to do this can be difficult for many of us. But I invite every one of you to consider looking into your emotional self. Growth may be painful but is well worth it in the long run.

CHECKING YOUR CHOLESTEROL

Levels of blood cholesterol can vary considerably among different individuals. How do you know if your cholesterol is too high? Recently a National Heart, Lung, and Blood Institute panel of experts came up with standard guidelines for doctors and their patients (table 5).

TABLE 5
National Cholesterol Education Program Guidelines

Blood Cholesterol Level	Category	Recommended Action
Greater than 240 mg/dl	High	See physician
Between 200 and 239 mg/dl	Borderline high	See physician
Less than 200 mg/dl	Desirable	Repeat cholesterol test in five years

Individuals with total cholesterol below 200 mg/dl appear to have a more favorable profile than individuals with cholesterol greater than 240. Patients at serious risk for coronary artery disease also include those with HDL levels less than 35 and LDL fractions greater than 160 (table 6). LDL levels below 130 mg/dl are considered desirable. HDL levels greater than 60 mg/dl are also considered protective.

Although HDL can be modified by exercise and weight reduction, most doctors would agree that the reduction of saturated fat is the most important way to lower levels of LDL. Saturated fats increase plasma cholesterol levels. Approximately 15 percent of total calories in the typical American diet come from saturated fatty acids, which is one reason Americans have such high serum cholesterol levels. Saturated fatty acids that have the greatest impact on raising cholesterol include lauric acid, myristic acid, and palmitic acid. Other nutrients, particularly alpha-

47

linolenic acid (an omega-3) and oleic acid (a monounsaturated fatty acid), may reduce LDL and its harmful effects.

TABLE 6

Classification of HDL, LDL, and Triglyceride Levels

HDL

More than 60 mg/dl	Protective
Less than 35 mg/dl	High risk

LDL

Less than 130 mg/dl	Desirable
Greater than 160 mg/dl	High risk

Triglycerides (Fat storage)

Less than 200 mg/dl	Desirable
200–399 mg/dl	Borderline high
400–1,000 mg/dl	High
More than 1,000 mg/dl	Very high (dangerous)

While there is some controversy about the mechanism of LDL reduction, it is undisputed that using omega-3 oils and monounsaturated fats, such as olive and almond oils, instead of saturated fats, such as butter, will reduce LDL levels. When the body takes in saturated fatty acids, the liver transforms them into blood cholesterol. Butter, for example, has little cholesterol, but it is approximately 70 percent saturated fat, so when it is ingested, the liver converts a portion of it to cholesterol.

CHOLESTEROL CULPRITS

Another way in which our diet choices can increase our cholesterol levels is simply through an excessive intake of calories. Obesity can also have the negative effect of lowering HDL levels. Weight loss, on the other hand, will help to reduce LDL levels while increasing HDL at the same time.

A major recommendation for lowering cholesterol is to reduce the total intake of calories. Again, this means reducing our total fat intake. Reducing the level of saturated fatty acids and replacing these acids with monounsaturated fatty acids and small quantities of polyunsaturated fatty acids is also recommended. Recently it was suggested that one should utilize more polyunsaturated fatty acids in the diet, but investigations have indicated that taking in a lot of polyunsaturated fatty acids may actually result in lowering HDL. This is an undesirable effect and one we wish to avoid. A better alternative is to use more monounsaturated fats such as olive oil. A more detailed description of polyunsaturated and monounsaturated fats will be given in a later chapter. For now, I ask you to focus your attention on the cholesterol-raising effects of saturated fat.

Saturated fat is found predominately in foods of animal origin, such as meat, butter, cream, cheese, and most other dairy products. Very high amounts of saturated fat are also found in chicken fat, beef fat, and particularly in organ meats such as heart, kidneys, and sweetbreads. Other saturated fats include coconut oil and palm oil, frequently used by manufacturers in processed foods and packaged baked goods. Coconut oil is approximately 99 percent saturated fat, actually containing higher percentages of saturated fat than butter or meat. It is important to recognize that these oils are used in nondairy creamers as well as commercially prepared whipped creams and vegetable shortenings in order to prolong shelf life and prevent rancidity. A good rule of thumb is to limit intake of commercially prepared baked goods, meats, saturated fats, and oils.

We should also reduce the intake of dairy products. Did you know that one of the most cholesterol-producing items in the American diet comes from milk? Milk fat, found in dairy products, including milk, butter, cheese, cream, and ice cream, contains high amounts of not only cholesterol, but also saturated fat. It is essential to reduce the amount of these items in the diet. For example, approximately 50 percent of whole milk's total calories are from fat. Thus it is best to gradually shift to 2-percent milk, which is preferable to whole milk but still gets about 36 percent of its calories from fat, down to 1-percent milk, which gets about 18 percent of its calories from fat. Skim milk is the most preferred. Skim milk and 1-percent milk really do not contain excessive amounts of fat, and they are also rich in protein and calcium, so it is not necessary to totally eliminate dairy products from the diet. It is strongly recommended, however, that individuals with high serum cholesterol and those who want to lose weight use either very low fat or skim milk whenever possible. Butter, cream, cheese, and ice cream should be eaten infrequently and only in small quantities, as they contain high levels of saturated fat and cholesterol. Low-fat substitutes are also available for all of these items.

Eggs are another culprit. Each egg yolk contains approximately 225 mg of cholesterol. Since the recommended intake of cholesterol is less than 300 mg per day, it is suggested that whole eggs be cut to a minimum. Egg whites, on the other hand, contain no cholesterol and are also an excellent source of protein. Egg substitutes contain no cholesterol, but some researchers say that they contain saturated fat. Since eggs contain considerable quantities of protein and particularly important minerals such as magnesium and sulfur (an extremely important mineral and anti-oxidizing element), I am not recommending that we remove eggs completely from our diet, even though the yolks contain much cholesterol. If you like to eat eggs, my recommendation would be to try boiled eggs or poached eggs, since they are not prepared with the excessive quantities of oil and fat that are commonly used to prepare fried or scrambled eggs. You could also use a nonstick skillet to prepare fried or scrambled eggs without fat.

Eggs can have a place in a healthy diet as long as we are aware of other sources of cholesterol in the foods we eat. The all-American breakfast of two eggs, bacon or sausage, buttered toast, and sweetened coffee has approximately 800 mg of cholesterol. Since two eggs contain approximately 450 mg of cholesterol, it is no wonder that the egg industry and the American Heart Association are at variance with each other. But don't forget that the rest of this breakfast contributes 350 mg of cholesterol. If you do eat eggs, choose foods low in cholesterol to eat during the remainder of the day.

SOME HEALTHY SUGGESTIONS

Organ meats have the highest cholesterol levels of all meats. Three ounces of sweetbreads, for example, contain approximately 2,600 mg of cholesterol! This is one item that should be absolutely forbidden to any health-conscious individual. Other items that I recommend be forbidden to people who want to stay healthy include processed meats such as bacon, salami, sausage, hot dogs, and bologna. These items should be avoided because of their high content of saturated fatty acids and calories, not to mention harmful nitrites and high sodium levels. Fast-food hamburgers are not a good choice, either; most hamburgers derive 50 percent of their calories from fat. All of the meats mentioned above are also high in cholesterol. Preferable meat choices would include chicken or turkey (without skin), although dark-meat chicken contains amounts of cholesterol comparable to those in beef. White-meat turkey, on the other hand, has lower amounts of cholesterol and saturated fatty acids than chicken and is recommended as a preferred meat substitute. Wild goose is another good alternative, as there is hardly any fat in the meat.

Although trimming the fat from meats and removing chicken skin does reduce the amount of fat and cholesterol, frequently the ingested cholesterol goes unnoticed, as in marbled meats. Such marbling in the meat contains high quantities of fat that are later converted to cholesterol and therefore should be avoided. If you insist on red meat, however, the best cuts are London broil or top round steak. You can ask the butcher to trim all the excess fat and grind the meat for hamburgers; these burgers will have approximately 4 to 5 grams of fat per serving, as opposed to the 25 grams found in chuck burgers. For my cardiac patients who like red meat, I frequently recommend a recipe (included in this book) for eye of round. Again, smart choices such as these are what nutritional awareness is all about.

Another alternative to meat is fish. Cardiologists usually recommend two to three helpings of fish per week to their patients. Fish is rich in beneficial omega-3 fatty acids, which are not found in significant quantities in most other foods (though there are small amounts in soybeans, walnut oil, and flax- and linseed oils). Most researchers agree that omega-3 fatty acids have the favorable effect of making the blood less sticky. This may help you live longer. A recent two-year study of male survivors of heart attacks showed that a moderate intake of fatty fish and fish oil decreased total mortality by 29 percent. While this effect occurred without any reduction in serum cholesterol levels (in this study), omega-3 fatty acids can cause a slight reduction of lipid levels and small decreases in LDL without affecting HDL cholesterol.

Population studies, particularly from the Netherlands and Greenland, seem to indicate that diets rich in fish products lower the incidence of coronary disease. The Japanese, who also ingest large quantities of fish, are protected from the epidemic of heart disease that plagues Western societies. Perhaps the cod liver oil your mother used to give you as a young child really *was* good for you!

Shellfish is considered by many nutritionists to be taboo because of its high cholesterol content. In reality, however, most shellfish do have acceptable levels of cholesterol, with the exception of squid. Squid contains approximately 250 mg of cholesterol per 100 grams. Crab, lobster, shrimp, oysters, and clams have lower levels. It is true that shellfish do contain more cholesterol by weight than poultry and even some red meats, but they are lower in saturated fats and have omega-3s as well. As a clinical cardiologist, keeping his data in mind, I would not restrict the amount of shellfish in the diet. It would be prudent, however, to use less squid and more fresh fish.

A word of caution, however, about fish, shellfish, and fish oils: Fish caught in coastal waters may be contaminated with pesticides, heavy metals, and PCBs. The recommendation here is to cut out as much of the dark meat from the fish as possible, as this is the fatty part. It usually occurs in the center of the fish and toward the tail. With careful trimming, many of these pollutants can be eliminated. It is important also to note the data on increased mercury levels found in deep-water fish such as tuna and swordfish. Although fish is an excellent source of protein as well as omega-3 fatty acids, one should use caution due to the possibility of heavy metal toxicity. Although I do not restrict omega-3 fatty acids from fish, these healthy fats can also be found in grain and vegetable sources as well as in walnuts and flax seed. Pumpkin seeds and soybeans supply small amounts of omega-3 fatty acids as well. Avocados are particularly high in total fat but contain omega-3 fatty acids. Grains, fruits, and most vegetables have no cholesterol, but some vegetable oils, such as coconut and palm oils, and many processed foods are high in saturated fat and should be avoided. So, as previously stated, be sure to read labels!

Fat, Good Fat, and Bad Fat

Austrian-born singer Ernestine Schumann-Heink struggled through the orchestra pit in a cramped Detroit concert hall, knocking over music racks with every step. "Sideways, madam," the conductor urged in alarm. "Sideways!"

"Mein Gott!" cried the singer in reply. "I haff no sideways!"

On another occasion, Enrico Caruso saw her seated in a restaurant with a very large steak on her plate. "Stina," he said, "surely you are not going to eat that alone?"

"Of course not alone," she laughed. "Mit potatoes!"

In the typical Western diet, fat is responsible for nearly half of the total calories consumed each day. While some dietary fat is necessary, both to supply us with energy and for the proper functioning of the body, it is important not only to understand why fat intake should be limited to around 30 percent of total calories, but also to understand which fats are the healthiest.

Until now I've been talking about fat as a food, but let's consider for a moment fat as . . . well, *fat*. The kind you have on your body. Body fat has its uses—among other things, it serves as an insulator, and it also helps protect more delicate tissues from injury—but in general, most Americans have too much body fat.

SINK OR SWIM

In a passive exercise study of women at the New England Heart Center, we determined the amount of fat in several areas of the body. In our study, we concluded that exercise in combination with a high-fiber/healthy-fat diet actually reduced body fat. Significant reductions in body fat were noted, particularly in the suprailiac (waist) and triceps (back of upper arms) areas. While there is some disagreement among the experts, it is safe to say that 20 to 25 percent of body fat for men and 20 to 30 percent of body fat for women is considered the maximum range for a healthy person. One can be slightly out of this range and still be healthy, but it is my belief that less body fat is more acceptable. We should strive to keep our body fat within an acceptable range (table 7).

Most of us are unaware of how many calories we should eat, much less how many grams of fat we should consume. The following table gives you a helpful index regarding your daily caloric needs as well as the total fat allowance. For the purposes of this chart, your caloric needs are determined by your activity. For example, if you are very active, multiply your weight in pounds by the number 16. If you are moderately active, multiply by 15. If you are inactive, multiply by 14, and if you are sedentary, multiply by 12. Someone like myself, weighing approximately 150 pounds and being moderately active, would need 2,250 calories, with a maximum fat intake not to exceed 75 grams.

TABLE 7

Maximum Allowable Fat Intake for Moderately Active
Men and Women

Ideal Body Weight (lbs)	Calories	Fat (g) per day
120	1,800	60
130	1,950	65
140	2,100	70
150	2,250	75
160	2,400	80
170	2,550	85
180	2,700	90

190	2,850	95
200	3,000	100
210	3,150	105
220	3,300	110
230	3,450	115
240	3,600	120
250	3,750	125

We also need to know that as we get older our body fat increases. This is why the older we get the easier it is to float in water. I remember that when I was a collegiate wrestler I had less than 10 percent body fat. I was also taking scuba diving lessons at the time. During the scuba diving certification process, it was apparent to everyone in the class that I did not need lead weights to get me to the bottom. I indeed had negative buoyancy—I sank like a rock! Neither could I float as other people could. I really thought there was something wrong with me; perhaps I had heavy bones or lead in my pants. What I really had was less body fat than everyone else, and since fat is lighter than muscle, the others floated. Thus the ability to float is directly related to the amount of body fat we possess. As we get older, at least one thing gets easier—floating!

One of the many things that gets more difficult as we age is keeping body fat off, since our metabolism slows down considerably. As a cardiologist, I know that keeping body fat within an acceptable range is an important secondary measure to help win the war against heart disease. And the amount of body fat you have depends to a large extent on how many calories you ingest in the form of fats in food.

An important reason to avoid excessive amounts of fat—especially saturated fat—in our diet is that it plays a major role in the development of heart disease. As I've pointed out, fat intake is related to levels of total cholesterol as well as HDL and LDL. Reducing the amount of fat you eat will improve your blood levels of total cholesterol, HDL, and LDL, and will reduce your risk of heart disease.

Another major reason to cut down on fat, especially animal fat, is that it contains significant amounts of pesticides, hormones, and other toxins. These toxins are found in small quantities in vegetable products, but as you go up the food chain, these small quantities accumulate in animals and become concentrated in their fatty tissue. While significant quantities of these toxins are found in dairy products, the highest amounts of pollutants are found in animal flesh. Thus, if we limit our consumption of animal fats, we also limit our exposure to these dangerous chemicals (table 8).

TABLE 8

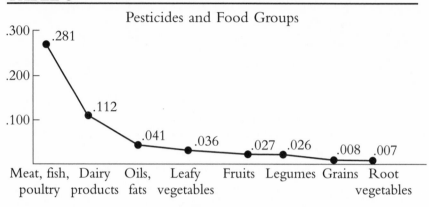

Pesticides and Food Groups

Source: *Runner's World.*

Reducing the risk of cancer is yet another reason for us to decrease the amount of fat in our diet. There are several studies that show a causal relationship between high fat intake and an increased incidence of cancer. Population studies as well as animal studies have presented convincing evidence that a high fat intake increases one's chances of developing cancer, particularly of the prostate, breast, and colon. For example, researchers from the Harvard School of Public Health found that men with lower fat intakes had lower rates of precancerous polyps in the colon, as compared with men with higher fat intakes.

In addition to the health hazards I've just mentioned, high-fat diets are also associated with obesity, diabetes, and gout. It's clear that you stand to benefit from being nutritionally aware and from controlling not just your total fat intake, but also the kinds of fat you ingest.

KINDS OF FAT

Fat is a chemical combination of carbon, hydrogen, and oxygen atoms (table 9). *Saturated fats,* which are found in all animal products as well as in tropical oils such as coconut oil and palm oil, contain a high proportion of hydrogen atoms. They tend to be solid at room temperature. Saturated fats are the worst threats to the cardiovascular system, since they are converted to cholesterol in the body and will raise cholesterol levels significantly if consumed in excess. *Monounsaturated fats* have relatively fewer hydrogen atoms; these fats come from plant sources and tend to be liquid at room temperature. A good example of a monounsaturated fat is olive oil. A large body of research indicates that monounsaturated fats pose the least problem for the heart. *Polyunsaturated fats,* such as sunflower oil, corn oil, cottonseed oil, and canola oil, also come from plant sources and also are liquid at room temperature. They have the fewest number of hydrogen atoms.

TABLE 9

Representation of Chemical Bonds in Saturated, Monounsaturated, and Polyunsaturated Fats

Saturated	Monounsaturated	Polyunsaturated
H H H H H H	H H H H H H	H H H H H
-C-C-C-C-C-C-	-C-C-C=C-C-	-C=C-C=C-C
H H H H H H	H H H H	H

Hydrogenated fats, which are often found in processed foods and commercial baked goods, are vegetable oils that have had extra hydrogen molecules added to them to make them solid at room temperature and also to extend shelf life. These extra hydrogen atoms make them less heart-healthy. There has also been some evidence that trans-fatty acids, compounds produced during the hydrogenation process, may raise LDL levels, reduce HDL levels, and increase the amount of LP(a) in the blood, all of which may increase the risk of coronary artery disease. LP(a) is an ugly lipoprotein that has been shown to be a risk factor for developing heart disease.

It's important to remember that both mono- and polyunsaturated fats do contain small quantities of saturated fat. Don't forget also that all fats are extremely calorie-dense; one tablespoon of any oil contains 14 grams of fat. So, I recommend that you keep the consumption of oils to a minimum, but if you need to use oil, I recommend olive oil as the most healthy choice. Extra-virgin olive oil is best, as it is cold-pressed and of the highest quality.

POLYUNSATURATED FATS: THE PARADOX

Many people like the light taste of polyunsaturated fats, such as canola oil. These fats have also been promoted as being better for you than other types of fats, but I believe they are not as good for you as monounsaturated fats. It is paradoxical that while polyunsaturated fats will indeed lower LDL levels when substituted for saturated fats, large intakes of polyunsaturated fats are associated with a lowering of HDL levels as well, which is not beneficial to the cardiovascular system. In addition, polyunsaturated fats are essential for the proper functioning of cell membranes throughout the body; however, they are easily oxidized, making the cells more vulnerable to harmful changes that may lead to degenerative diseases, such as heart disease, cataracts, and Alzheimer's—perhaps even cancer. This susceptibility to oxidation, with all the negative effects it entails, is the reason why I don't recommend oils such as canola oil.

MONOUNSATURATED FATS: THE GOOD FATS

Like polyunsaturated fats, monounsaturated fats such as olive oil and almond oil lower LDL levels when compared with saturated fats. They do not, however, appear to lower HDL, the beneficial lipoprotein, as polyunsaturated fats tend to do.

The populations of the Mediterranean consume large amounts of olive oil in their diet. They also have lower mortality rates from heart disease than people in other regions of Europe. Inhabitants of the island of Crete, for example, have an insignificant rate of heart disease as compared with several Western European countries. The data in one study indicated that not one person on the entire island of Crete died of a myocardial infarction over one particular ten-year period. Yet the average cholesterol level of the islanders was over 200. While there may be many factors contributing to the low incidence of heart-disease-related mortality in Crete—as well as in the entire Mediterranean region—one factor seems to stand out. Given the documented evidence on the positive effects of monounsaturated fats on LDL and HDL levels, it seems likely that the Mediterranean diet, rich in olive oil, plays a significant role.

ESSENTIAL FATTY ACIDS

Essential fatty acids (EFAs) are chemicals that the body needs to make hormones and other compounds that are necessary for life itself. However, the body cannot produce all the EFAs it needs by itself; some kinds must be consumed in food. Because EFAs have both negative and positive effects, they provide an excellent example of how we can help ourselves be healthier by being nutritionally aware.

Many EFAs play a major role in causing or exacerbating disease. For example, there is a group of compounds derived from activated EFAs called eicosanoids. Some of these can wreak havoc in the body, causing allergic and immunological problems, stimulating inflammation, and causing blood vessels to constrict and blood to clot abnormally. But not all eicosanoids are bad. Some increase the oxygen content of blood; others prevent platelets from becoming too sticky. Arachidonic acid, which I've mentioned earlier as something to avoid, is indeed very bad for you when it reaches excessive levels in your body, but in appropriate quantities it is absolutely essential for the proper development of the central nervous system in babies and young children.

The crucial roles that EFAs play are one reason why fat intake should not be restricted to extremely low levels, especially in children. When not enough fat is consumed, deficiencies in certain EFAs can occur. For example, if we do not get enough of two EFAs called linoleic acid and linolenic acid, our bodies may produce an abnormal fatty acid called mead fatty acid, which can cause additional cholesterol production and ultimately lead to hardening of the arteries.

While most cardiologists recommend a low-fat diet for the prevention or reduction of coronary artery disease, they may overlook the substantial evidence we now have concerning the link between low linolenic/linoleic fatty acid intake and coronary artery disease.

We must not be too overzealous in our approach to fats. Soybean products, seeds, nuts, tofu, flaxseed oil, oatmeal, and fish provide an excellent source of omega-3 oils needed to maintain homeostasis in the body, especially in the cardiovascular system. Earlier I discussed the health advantages of the omega oils. We can group these essential fatty acids into various classes. Omega-3 fatty acids are long-chain N-3 fatty acids (eicosapentaenoic [EPAs] and docosahexaenoic acids [DHAs]). DHA is found in breast milk. Severe deficiencies of DHA, like deficiencies in arachidonic acid, can cause visual and cerebrovascular dysfunction in children up to two years of age. The omega-3s are absolutely vital to life, but what about the other omega oils?

I have already told you about olive oil, which is, in essence, an omega-9 oleic fatty acid. Omega-9s are neutral fatty acids or monoun-saturated fats that do not significantly affect insulin release or participate in eicosanoid production.

Omega-6s are necessary for the production of both good and bad eicosanoids, but an excess of omega-6s has its downside. The problem with omega-6 essential fatty acids is that an enormous amount of omega-6 may be absorbed into the body from the diet. Not only are omega-6s found in many of the vegetable oils we commonly use, but they are contained in the trans-fatty acids found in margarine and in partially hydrogenated oils, which are found in almost all processed foods. Re-member that an excess of omega-6 intake can stimulate an overproduc-tion of arachidonic acid. Since many vegetable oils contain considerable quantities of linoleic acid (an omega-6 oil), deficiencies of linoleic acid are uncommon. However, you must remember that the polyunsaturated acids containing linoleic acid, such as safflower oil, corn oil, peanut oil, and even canola oil, are all prone to excessive lipid peroxidation (lipid peroxidation occurs when fat is metabolized in the presence of oxygen). So while they are a good source of linoleic acid, these polyunsaturated fats are easily oxidized and are therefore a tremendous source of free radical stress in the body. It is overwhelming free radical stress that accel-erates premature aging.

Flax- and grapeseed oils contain much alpha-linolenic acid (ALA). Alpha-linolenic acid may cause a repression of the enzyme Delta-6 desaturase, inhibiting the transformation of linoleic acid to the activated gamma-linolenic acid (GLA). However, ALA can be quite supportive to the body's physiology. Some studies have shown, for example, that the ALA found in flaxseed can lower total cholesterol, including LDL. In *The Zone,* Dr. Sears is critical of linolenic acid, but I disagree. There is just too much positive research supporting the health benefits of ALA.

Consider that a typical Greek male between the ages of fifty-five and fifty-nine has one eighth the incidence of coronary artery disease as his American male counterpart. Although Greeks consume a typically Medi-terranean diet, the tradition of eating purslane (wild plants containing alpha-linolenic acid) may be responsible for the low incidence of coro-nary artery disease in Greece. Since ALA can reduce the production of GLA, it can be the gatekeeper for limiting the synthesis of all the eicosanoids, including the bad ones. Since the bad eicosanoids, such as thromboxane, are largely responsible for cardiovascular disease, the use of ALA may not be a bad idea. One of the best ways to manipulate your eicosanoids is to take the good ones in and keep the bad ones out. Probably the best way to do this is to consider taking flaxseed oil, evening primrose oil, borage oil, or black currant oil, all of which will enhance GLA. Consuming fish, especially cold-water fish like salmon, will supply the body with rich sources of EPA. Remember that fish oils are direct antagonists to arachidonic acid and that DHA and EPA are the omega-3 oils that reduce LP(a). Keep in mind also that LP(a) is a toxic lipoprotein that causes blood clotting and inflammatory responses in the blood. Over the last one hundred years, there has been an overabundance of omega-6s and an insufficiency of omega-3s in the American diet. To promote our own good health, we must reverse this trend. If we do, the chance of developing coronary artery disease will decrease.

Another means of reducing arachidonic acid is either to avoid it in the diet through a reduction in meat and dairy products or to reduce the amount of activated insulin ingested. If Dr. Sears is correct in assuming that too much insulin is responsible for turning activated GLA into arachidonic acid, then the best way to reduce such bad eicosanoids in the body is to suppress insulin. The optimum strategy to achieve this goal is to maintain a moderate-carbohydrate/higher-protein diet with healthy fats.

If you consume healthy fats along with generous portions of protein and modest portions of carbohydrates, your body will naturally increase good eicosanoids while simultaneously reducing bad eicosanoids. By achieving a healthy balance of carbohydrates, healthy fats, and protein in your diet, your body will produce favorable prostaglandins and thereby enhance your cardiovascular health.

BE NUTRITIONALLY AWARE

We can help our bodies stay in balance by consuming fats wisely. As I previously mentioned, I recommend using olive oil whenever possible. The oils naturally found in fish are also healthy fats; if you like fish, eat two to three servings per week, and if you don't, you can consider supplementing your diet with flaxseed oil capsules. Flaxseed oil is an excellent way to help your body regulate its production of hormones while reducing LDL cholesterol at the same time.

Avoid saturated fats, and minimize your use of polyunsaturated oils. The trans-fatty acids that are found in hydrogenated vegetable oil products (such as margarine and many commercial baked goods) should be avoided as well.

Reading labels when you shop is a necessary part of being nutritionally aware. The new food labels give us lots of information, but sometimes they don't tell us the whole truth. For example, a label may say that a certain product contains no cholesterol, but that does not necessarily mean that it doesn't contain saturated fat—which, as you recall, is converted in the body to cholesterol. As another example, the word *hydrogenated* on a label should tell you that the fats in that particular product are not the healthiest choice. Be sure you know the proportions of saturated fat, monounsaturated fat, and polyunsaturates in the oils you buy (table 10).

TABLE 10

Fat Content of Commonly Used Fats and Oils (approximately 1 tablespoon)

Type of Fat or Oil	Saturated Fat (g)	Monounsaturated Fat (g)	Polyunsaturated Fat (g)
Almond oil	1.3	9.1	3.6
Beef fat	7.1	6.0	0.5
Butter	9.0	4.1	0.6
Canola oil	0.8	8.4	4.4
Chicken fat	4.2	6.4	3.0
Coconut oil	11.7	0.8	0.2
Corn oil	1.7	3.4	7.9
Cottonseed oil	3.6	2.6	6.9
Flaxseed oil	1.3	2.2	10.5
Grapeseed oil	1.6	2.4	9.9
Lard	5.6	6.4	1.6
Margarine	2.0	5.0	4.0
Mayonnaise	2.0	3.0	7.0
Olive oil	1.9	9.8	1.2
Peanut oil	2.6	6.2	4.1
Pumpkinseed oil	1.2	4.8	8.0

Type of Fat or Oil	Saturated Fat (g)	Monounsaturated Fat (g)	Polyunsaturated Fat (g)
Safflower oil	1.3	1.7	10.0
Sesame oil	1.8	6.4	5.7
Soy oil	2.0	3.1	7.8
Sunflower oil	1.4	2.8	8.7
Walnut oil	2.2	3.9	7.8

Avoid (Bad Fats)	Substitute (Good Fats)
Beef fat	Fish oil
Butter	Almond oil
Coconut oil	Olive oil
Lard	*Flaxseed oil
Palm oil	*Grapeseed oil
Margarine	Evening primrose oil
All hydrogenated oils	Black currant oil

*Contains significant quantities of ALA.

In addition to organizing your menu around fats, it is also important to keep tabs on the fiber content. Remember that by increasing the fiber content and reducing the fat content, weight loss may be considerable (table 11). When considering weight loss, you need to know your daily intake of fat. Remember we are not counting total calories but only the grams of fat. I try to take in less than 75 grams of fat per day. This is the equivalent of two quarter-pound cheeseburgers found in many of the fast-food restaurants. Keeping the intake of grams of fat to a respectable level will not only reduce total body fat, but will also reduce caloric intake.

In our previous discussions we mentioned that excess calories are predominately stored in the body as fat; you're familiar with the type of fat that is around the waistline, thighs, and backs of our arms. Cardiologists refer to it as the triglycerides in the body, but in simple terms this is our body fat. Body fat can be determined by anthropometric measurements using calipers. Accumulation of body fat is a simple mechanism. We either eat too much or we exercise too little.

Remember also that fats are only one part of a healthy diet. Consuming generous portions of protein and modest portions of carbohydrates will also help your body to function as optimally as possible, as will getting enough fiber. As you will see, the modified Mediterranean diet will give you all of this and more!

TABLE 11

High-Fiber Healthy-Fat Food

Food	Serving Size	Fiber (g)	Fat (g)	Calories
Health Valley Chili	5 oz.	12.2	3	160
All-Bran cereal	1/3 cup	8.6	1	70
Multi-grain Pancake Mix (Arrowhead Mills)	3 pancakes	8.0	2	290
Prunes	5 large	7.9	Trace	115
Oatmeal	1/3 cup	7.0	2	110
Chickpeas	1/2 cup	6.2	Trace	115
40% Bran Cereal	1/4 cup	6.0	1	95
Kidney beans	1/2 cup	5.8	Trace	110
Pinto beans	1/2 cup	5.3	Trace	115
Split peas	1/2 cup	5.1	Trace	115
Pears	1 pear	5.0	1	110
Raisins	1/2 cup	4.0	Trace	220
Broccoli	1 spear	4.5	Trace	55
Lima beans	1/2 cup	4.4	Trace	105
Green peas	1/2 cup	4.1	Trace	65

THE MODIFIED MEDITERRANEAN DIET

The Mediterranean diet, with certain modifications, is the optimum diet in the fight against heart disease and cancer. The Mediterranean diet not only contains more healthy fats, but also lots of fiber, good sources of protein, and many of the nutrients, antioxidants, and phytonutrients we need for optimum health.

Studies show that northern European populations such as those of Scotland and Scandinavia have a far greater incidence of coronary artery disease than do the Mediterranean populations of Greece and Italy. Why is this so? I believe it is because there is something heart protective in the Mediterranean diet. Research studies have shown the value of the relatively high-fat (30 percent of calories from fat) Mediterranean diet. In one popular study the survival rate of heart attack patients was remarkably higher in those consuming a typically Mediterranean diet supplemented with alpha-linolenic acid (which acts like an omega-3 fatty acid); the control group (eating a lower-fat diet) actually had more heart attacks. Let's take a closer look at what you can do to achieve the maximum benefits from your diet.

The Mediterranean diet is rich in antioxidants and favorable fats, such as the essential fatty acids found in plants and seafood. It also includes considerable amounts of fish and shellfish products containing the omega-3 oils. Remember that omega-3 fatty acids are essential to life and cannot be manufactured by your body. They must be consumed in the diet. Alpha-linolenic and omega-3 fatty acids are the most important essential fatty acids for the protection of cardiovascular health.

Fish, flaxseed, and Mediterranean plants rich in omega-3 fatty acids not only help prevent the formation of sticky clumps of platelets in blood vessels, but also lower blood-clotting fragments called fibrinogen, thus keeping the blood "slippery" and the arteries open, thereby preventing clots. In addition, they help to lower blood levels of cholesterol, triglycerides, and blood pressure, further reducing your risk of heart disease. Remember that DHA, which is found in fish and shellfish, lowers blood levels of a lipoprotein called LP(a). Remember that high levels of LP(a) are associated with an increased risk of coronary artery disease in both men and women.

There have been many studies documenting a link between the consumption of omega-3 fatty acids and a lower incidence of coronary artery disease. For example, the Inuit people of Greenland consume large amounts of fatty marine animals such as whales, seals, and fish, yet they have a very low incidence of coronary artery disease. A twenty-year analysis of the eating habits of Dutch men has also found that the risk of heart disease dropped as the consumption of fish increased. In more recent studies, omega-3s from plant sources (flax) were associated with a lower risk of stroke. Since the Mediterranean diet contains abundant quantities of fish and shellfish and significant amounts of omega-3 fatty acids from vegetables, nuts, and seeds, it is reasonable to assume that there is a connection between an abundance of these essential fatty acids and a low incidence of coronary artery disease.

The Mediterranean diet also relies on olive oil, which appears to be the major source of fat in the Mediterranean countries of Greece, Italy, and Spain. Again, olive oil is a monounsaturated fat that does not cause excessive insulin release; it preserves HDL levels and may also lower levels of LDL. Olive oil also has blood-thinning (and therefore anti-clotting) properties; it also has an antioxidant effect. The combination of olive oil, a monounsaturated fat, with omega-3 fatty acids may provide considerable cardiovascular protection.

The Mediterranean diet also contains large amounts of fresh fruits, vegetables, and legumes, which provide not only many antioxidants, but also many phytonutrients. Phytonutrients are natural disease fighters that plants have developed over the years to protect them against disease and insects. Research has shown that phytonutrients yield similar benefits to people. There are many types of phytonutrients: flavonoids, carotenoids, polyphenols, terpenoids, carbinols, indoles, and sulphoraphanes, to mention a few. Research on phytonutrients has shown that people who eat more fresh fruits and vegetables have a lower incidence of heart disease and cancer.

In addition to containing many fruits and vegetables, the Mediterranean diet also includes legumes such as lentils and chickpeas, which will also decrease insulin levels. Legumes are an example of a food high in complex carbohydrates with a low-glycemic index.

Every carbohydrate, from peaches to pasta, has a different glycemic index that governs the rate of glucose entering the bloodstream. That is, some carbohydrates are absorbed quickly, while others are absorbed slowly. The pancreas responds by secreting high levels of insulin to counteract the glucose load caused by high-glycemic carbohydrates. Legumes also contain fiber. Fiber, as you know, slows the absorption of carbohydrates even further, thereby decreasing insulin secretion even more.

But what about pasta? For years I was a strong proponent of pasta. However, with all the information concerning insulin resistance that has recently appeared in the medical literature, I am now consuming fewer pastas made with highly processed wheat, including semolina. These pastas have too many grams of carbohydrate and not enough protein. Thus, they are considered a moderate-glycemic carbohydrate and will stimulate insulin release.

But what can you do if you really like pasta? Is there a way to keep it in your life? Yes, but the answer involves balancing the moderate-glycemic pasta with equivalent portions of protein and fats. Metabolically, the worst thing you can do is to have a huge portion of pasta, a salad, and lots of bread. That's what I did for years, setting off the vicious cycle of blood sugar, insulin spikes, and carbohydrate cravings. But remember that you can escape this damaging chain of events by eating approximately 45 to 50 percent carbohydrates, 20 to 25 percent protein, and 30 percent healthy fat at every meal.

Because I love pasta and am unwilling to give it up, I called one of my nutritional consultants, Dr. Steven H. Novil, at the Academy of Antiaging Medicine in Chicago. He told me about low-glycemic pastas such as Jerusalem artichoke and spelt (rye pasta). Both contain complex carbohydrates with a lower glycemic index, more fiber, and slightly more protein than traditional varieties. But if you are a traditionalist and cannot change the type of pasta you consume, you can simply scale down your portions of pasta and add some clam sauce or chicken, obtaining a desirable balance of higher protein, moderate carbohydrates, and healthy fats.

Another modification to the Mediterranean diet that I recommend is to eat eggs. Eggs will give you not only more protein—in fact, they are the most perfect source of protein—but also essential antioxidants such as magnesium and sulfur. Unfortunately, as mentioned in an earlier chapter, egg yolk contains lots of cholesterol as well as arachidonic acid; however, the antioxidant capability of sulfur helps to neutralize this problem. I enjoy eggs and eat from two to four of them a week.

You must also be aware of overprocessed grains such as white flour. When grains are highly processed, their consumption can increase insulin secretion. You need to consider instead whole grains such as barley and buckwheat, legumes, lentils, chickpeas, and vegetables such as asparagus. Lentils and asparagus both contain high quantities of folic acid and high levels of alpha-linolenic acid. Plant proteins have a cholesterol-lowering effect. Thus a high fruit and vegetable intake is strongly recommended. However, you must use some caution. For example, white potatoes, sweet potatoes, white rice, and other high-glycemic foods should be kept to a minimum. Try to limit your consumption of breads, pastries, bagels, and other products made with white flour. All breads, indeed all grains, are susceptible to mold. Breads also contain yeast, which is a fungus. An overconsumption of fungi in susceptible individuals can weaken the immune system.

In summary, how do you choose a diet that's right for you? Consider the Mediterranean diet with the modifications I have suggested (table 13).

Remember, if you include pasta in your diet, consider the alternatives that I have mentioned, and use the philosophy "less is more." If you don't like fish, consider taking flaxseed oil capsules or eating vegetables high in alpha-linolenic acid such as asparagus. And add soy to your diet. You can do this by consuming foods such as tofu, miso, or soy milk. Since whole milk from cows contains tremendous quantities of arachidonic acid, I prefer using soy milk in my decaffeinated coffee. Not only does it taste great, but I also have the comfort of knowing that I am protecting my heart at the same time. Other suitable but less ideal choices would include skim milk or even 1-percent milk.

This modified Mediterranean diet will improve insulin resistance, give you more energy, and help you lose weight. However, you can also lower your insulin levels by exercising regularly and by keeping stress to a minimum. Thus, like your choice of diet, your choice of lifestyle will also have a positive impact not only on your insulin levels, but also on your general health and well-being (table 12).

TABLE 12

Benefits of a Mediterranean Diet

1. Low in saturated fat, high in fiber, creating less insulin resistance
2. Antioxidant rich in vitamin C, beta carotene, vitamin E, magnesium, and L-glutathione
3. Carotenoids, flavonoids, and polyphenols
4. Low in dairy and meat products, resulting in less arachidonic acid
5. Higher alpha-linolenic acid content
6. More beneficial essential fatty acids
7. Legumes such as lentils and chickpeas, resulting in insulin level decrease
8. Olive oil, preferred fat over margarine (trans-fatty acids)
9. Red wine—the French Paradox, quercetin effect
10. Fish and shellfish containing EPA and DHA

TABLE 13

The Sinatra Mediterranean Diet

Decrease your intake of high-glycemic carbohydrates in such foods as white rice, as well as in processed foods containing flours, such as breads, cereals (like cornflakes, frosted flakes, puffed wheat, and sweetened granola), pastries, bagels, and flour-based pastas.

Increase your consumption of oatmeal and higher fiber pastas such as spelt and Jerusalem artichoke instead of using traditional pastas made with semolina flour.

Decrease your intake of vegetables with a high-glycemic index, such as potatoes, corn, peas, and carrots. Avoid highly processed canned vegetables.

Increase your consumption of fresh vegetables with a low-glycemic index. Top veggies include asparagus, broccoli, kale, spinach, cabbage, Brussels sprouts, and legumes (like lentils and chickpeas). They provide alpha-linolenic acid and phytonutrients, the natural disease fighters of the world.

Decrease your intake of fruits with a high-glycemic index, like bananas, raisins, mango, and papaya. Drink less fruit juice, especially orange and apple juice, and dilute what you do drink with water.

Increase your consumption of a variety of low-glycemic fruits like grapefruit, cherries, peaches, plums, kiwi, and rhubarb. Pears, apples, cantaloupes, and grapes are also suitable; however, they contain more sugar.

Decrease your intake of large amounts of red meat and especially organ meats as much as possible because of their high levels of arachidonic acid. Flavor sauces or soups with small amounts of meats such as lamb, chicken, turkey, or beef. Also consider seasoning your

Increase your consumption of protein in the form of fish (including shellfish), a food high in omega-3 oils, and soy products (including tofu, soybeans, and tempeh). Don't avoid eggs completely, since they are a perfect source of protein and provide essential anti-food with nutrient-rich herbs like garlic, chives, sage, oregano, and parsley.

oxidants such as magnesium and sulfur.

Decrease your intake of dairy products (especially those containing whole milk), since they are high in saturated fat and arachidonic acid.

Increase your consumption of soy milk. Low-fat cottage cheese, low-fat yogurt, feta cheese, and small amounts of grated Parmesan are also permissible.

CHAPTER Seven

The Good, the Bad, and the Ugly: Water, Salt, Alcohol, and Caffeine

A re you a drinker? I hope so.

The human body is mostly made up of water. Water is involved in almost every bodily function, including digestion, absorption of nutrients, and excretion. Water also helps maintain proper body temperature. Since water is continuously lost through urination, elimination, eating, and breathing, it is important to replenish the body's supply each day. Most researchers agree that drinking at least eight glasses of water a day is necessary for good health. And water is also crucial to weight loss. Studies have shown that a decrease in water consumption will cause an increase in fat deposits, while an increase in water can actually reduce the amount of fat in the body.

The mechanism is simple. If the kidneys cannot function properly due to dehydration, some of the burden must be taken up by the liver. Since the liver metabolizes stored fat for energy, it cannot work at full capacity if the kidneys are compromised. Therefore, the liver metabolizes less fat, so more fat remains in the body, which in turn results in weight gain.

Water is an extremely important catalyst in weight loss. For example, in our hospital-based weight loss program, each participant must drink large quantities of water continuously. If adequate water is not consumed, dehydration would occur and weakness and lethargy would result. Since water is a major factor in fat metabolism, it makes sense for an overweight person to drink as much water as possible. In addition to helping rid the body of toxins, water can help relieve constipation as well. When the body gets too little water or too much salt, or if the patient is given too much diuretic, the body will take water from its internal sources. The colon is one such source, and the result is constipation.

Drinking enough water not only is essential to weight loss, but also is essential to good health. In medical school, I trained with one of the top kidney experts in the United States. He was one of the original pioneers in the field of kidney dialysis. When we used to make rounds in the hospital wards, my professor would never pass a water fountain without drinking. By watching him I learned a lot. He continuously drank water to give his kidneys the nurturing they needed. If that was good enough for a professor of nephrology, it was certainly good enough for me. I tried to remind myself as much as possible about the medical consequences of deficient water intake. In summary, we need to drink at least eight eight-ounce glasses of water every day. This is about two quarts of fluid. During a weight loss program, we should drink at least one glass of water with each meal and a glass at least one hour prior to the meal.

SHAKE THE SALT HABIT

Excess sodium in the diet creates unnecessary fluid retention in the tissues, even edema (swelling), and depletes stores of water in other parts of the body such as the colon and upper gastrointestinal tract. In high concentrations it disturbs the mineral balance in the body. Too much salt in our diet can cause fluid buildup, thereby causing blood pressure to rise, and high blood pressure can lead to heart disease. The National Cholesterol Education Program recommends a sodium intake of less than three grams per day. Excessive salt intake has been linked to disease not only in urbanized societies, but also in less developed societies as well. Caribbean peoples who cook their foods in seawater, for example, had much higher levels of blood pressure than those who cooked in freshwater. In order to get rid of excess salt in the body, we need to drink more water. Since water is forced through the kidneys, it eliminates the excess sodium.

Unfortunately, salt does not come only from the salt shaker. Processed foods are the source of much of the sodium in the average American diet; much of that salt is "hidden." Again, we need to read labels. For example, some commercially prepared soups contain almost a gram of sodium per can, and a fast-food hamburger may also contain at least one gram of sodium. A large kosher dill pickle contains more than one gram of sodium. Hidden salt also lurks in items such as ketchup and even breakfast cereal. Overconsumption of processed foods and a lack of nutritional awareness leaves us vulnerable to an overabundance of sodium in our diet. We need to be aware, for example, that additional sodium is often added to food items such as bread products, smoked meats and fish, and olives not just to enhance flavor, but also as a preservative.

Since sodium occurs naturally in most foods, there is virtually no danger of our body not getting enough. You really don't need any additional sodium chloride (table salt). Salt is not a food; it has no nutritional value. The only time I would suggest the use of salt is in the case of individuals who lose a lot of sodium chloride through excessive perspiration. Elderly patients who suffer from low blood pressure and who do not have heart disease may also be permitted to use salt. Yet the best way for these individuals to increase salt intake would be to consume fruits and vegetables. Celery and sea vegetables, for example, contain sodium chloride in its natural form.

LAST CALL FOR ALCOHOL

Alcohol is a source of empty calories, that is, it provides no vitamins, minerals, or other essential nutrients. This is certainly one type of beverage that should not be used by anyone trying to lose weight. Alcohol is not a food, but rather a drug. In fact it may be considered a poison. It causes metabolic damage to the body and depresses the immune system. As a clinical cardiologist, I can attest to the amount of heart disease that alcohol causes. I have seen hundreds of patients with no previous known history of heart disease come into my office with heart muscle disease. The most common cause of such disease—in the absence of factors such as coronary artery disease, viral illnesses, or valvular problems—is alcohol.

There are countless studies on the relationship of alcohol to cardiovascular disease; but one study in particular showed that at least two ounces of hard liquor per day can cause deterioration of the heart muscle over a short period of time. In this study a group of volunteers drank two ounces of vodka per day; the control group drank water. At the end of the experiment microscopic analysis showed that those who had consumed alcohol sustained heart muscle deterioration.

Alcohol can damage almost any organ in the body. The heart, the brain, and the liver are perhaps the most vulnerable. Much of my medical internship and residency included treating alcoholics. The number of diseases common among alcoholics is incredible: pneumonia, liver disease, arthritis, eating disorders, delirium, dementia, and nerve and muscular disorders are just a few of them. And the emotional destruction that alcohol causes is as profound as the physical destruction.

Another important fact to consider in relation to alcohol is the effect it has on sleep. Alcohol is probably the leading cause of insomnia. While alcohol may serve as a depressant, causing the body to appear as though it is in a deep sleep, the sleep pattern is not a good one. After ingesting alcohol, particularly in combination with sugar, many people have difficulty falling asleep because of the vasodilative effects of alcohol and the rapid heart rate that follows.

One of the most common things I see in my office is alcohol-induced cardiac arrhythmia. Patients come in with many different scenarios: skipped, irregular, or rapid heartbeats. Other causes may be emotional distress, which is frequently compounded by the use of alcohol as a remedy. Overall, I would recommend avoiding hard alcohol altogether.

THE FRENCH PARADOX

While hard liquor should be avoided, wine, on the other hand, has been used in moderation as a healing remedy for centuries. Records dating back four thousand years refer to the dietary and medicinal uses of wine. Wine contains polyphenols—agents that kill viruses and bacteria. Polyphenols, like some vitamins, also have antioxidant capabilities, namely, the ability to tie up free radicals that harm cells. One particular polyphenol found in red wine is quercetin, a bioflavonoid known for its antioxidant and antihistamine properties and touted as the main ingredient in the "French Paradox."

The paradox in the French Paradox is that the French seem to have high serum cholesterol but a low incidence of coronary artery disease. In fact, in one major clinical study involving various cultures from all over the world, France was second only to Japan in having the lowest incidence of heart disease. If the typical French diet includes lots of cheese, cream sauces, pâtés, and other high-fat foods, why should the French have such a low incidence of coronary artery disease? The answer seems to lie in their consumption of red wine.

Many researchers believe it is the consumption of red wine that counteracts the large amounts of fat in the French diet. But what is it about red wine that makes it so medicinal? Current studies indicate that quercetin and other compounds called tannins protect the body from harmful cholesterol. Tannins, found in the skin and seeds of grapes, give wine a characteristic color. Red grapes contain considerably more tannin than white grapes.

After these observations about the French Paradox were published in the medical literature, other investigators tested the tannin–quercetin hypothesis. For example, some experimental groups consumed red wine before a meal, while others drank other types of alcohol, such as vodka or a placebo. It was clearly demonstrated that one to two glasses of wine— red wine only—before dinner can sustain antioxidant activity for up to two hours. Antioxidant activity protects cells and prevents the oxidation of cholesterol, which leads to plaque buildup.

A more recent Dutch follow-up study showed similar findings. It clearly demonstrated that older men, aged sixty-five to eighty-five, who consumed greater quantities of onions, green apples, and green tea (foods high in quercetin), had a reduced death rate. Not only do bioflavonoids protect one against heart disease, but they also have been shown to act as a defense against cancer.

Some investigators have also suggested the use of an evaporated wine residue to be used as a salve in treating cold sores and herpes simplex infections. The low alcohol content in wine may offer yet another healing advantage. Recent investigations have supported the hypothesis that light alcohol consumption may actually reduce the risk of coronary artery disease, perhaps by favorably influencing HDL and blood-clotting mechanisms. Wine, however, is alcohol, and like caffeine needs to be used in moderation. Keep in mind that although the French have a low incidence of coronary artery disease, they have the highest incidence of cirrhosis of the liver.

COFFEE TALK

Caffeinated beverages such as coffee and tea were once widely utilized as drug therapy by physicians in Western Europe. In 1859, for example, caffeine was commonly used as a treatment for respiratory disorders and written up in the medical journals as the prescription of choice for bronchial asthma. The pharmacological properties of caffeine are similar to the xanthines, a group of compounds that stimulate the central nervous system and the heart, relax muscles (especially the bronchial tubes), and stimulate the brain. Caffeine also acts like a diuretic, resulting in increased blood flow to the kidneys, and allowing more water to be excreted; you can see how drinking a cup of coffee and then getting stuck in a traffic jam could have some undesirable consequences.

The average American consumes approximately two to five cups of coffee a day, totaling 200 to 300 mg of caffeine. Decaffeinated coffee does contain caffeine but in very low quantities. Caffeine is also found in chocolate, cocoa, and many soft drinks, although a cup of tea usually contains less than half the caffeine in a cup of coffee (table 14).

TABLE 14

Average Caffeine Content of Selected Items

BEVERAGES

Soft Drinks	Serving Size	Caffeine (mg)
Cherry cola (diet or regular)	12 oz.	48.0
Coca-Cola or Diet Coke	12 oz.	46.0
Cola (decaffeinated)	12 oz.	0.2
Dr Pepper	12 oz.	37.0
Diet Pepsi	12 oz.	36.0
Mountain Dew	12 oz.	54.0
Pepsi	12 oz.	38.0
Coffee	Serving Size	Caffeine (mg)
Brewed, regular	6 oz.	103.0
Brewed, decaffeinated	6 oz.	3.0
Instant, regular	1 rounded teaspoon	57.0

Coffee	Serving Size	Caffeine (mg)
Instant, decaffeinated	1 rounded teaspoon	2.0

Tea	Serving Size	Caffeine (mg)
Brewed, commercial	5 oz.	20–50
Brewed, imported	5 oz.	25–80
Instant	5 oz.	10–20
Iced tea	12 oz.	70
Crystal Light iced tea	8 oz.	11

Chocolate Beverages	Serving Size	Caffeine (mg)
Chocolate-flavor mix	2–3 teaspoons	8
Chocolate syrup	2 tablespoons	6
Cocoa/hot chocolate	4 teaspoons	6

Candy	Serving Size	Caffeine (mg)
German sweet (Bakers)	1 oz.	8
Semi-sweet (Bakers)	1 oz.	13
Milk chocolate (Cadbury)	1 oz.	15

Over-the-Counter Drugs (per tablet)	Caffeine (mg)
Anacin	32
Excedrin	65
No-Doz	100

Young children who drink colas can suffer from the symptoms of excessive caffeine intake, including irritability, hyperactivity, and insomnia. In my own clinical practice, I have seen scores of patients with problems related to caffeine intake. For example, I remember a case involving a twenty-five-year-old male with a history of a psychiatric disorder who was taking tranquilizers for mood control. He was referred to me for cardiologic evaluation because of an exceedingly high heart rate, frequently greater than 120 beats per minute, and a blood pressure as high as 220/120.

An in-depth medical history revealed that he was drinking ten cups of coffee per day. He was also drinking considerable quantities of colas. This individual suffered not from a drug-induced heartbeat problem, but from caffeinism—a condition in which the heart rate and the blood pressure increase, and the patient feels very irritable and hyperactive.

Patients suffering from caffeinism frequently complain of erratic heartbeat, with skipping or fluttering. Often they will have insomnia. Many other patients with cardiac-induced arrhythmias find that caffeine will aggravate their symptoms. The treatment is simple: Reduce or eliminate caffeine intake.

Because caffeine is a diuretic, too much of it can wash out the body's vitamins and minerals. In addition, excessive caffeine intake has been found to result in a reduction of the body's supply of calcium, magnesium, and potassium.

Caffeinated beverages, especially coffee, have also been known to enhance gastric acid secretion and aggravate ulcers. Every physician knows that if a patient is suffering from excess acid production or abdominal discomfort, it is important to instruct them to avoid caffeine, alcohol, nicotine, and aspirin, since these are the four most common compounds that harm the gastrointestinal tract. Caffeine, like nicotine and alcohol, is considered a drug. Therefore we must weigh the potential benefits versus the hazards. Some physicians believe coffee is harmful and should be avoided altogether. For the asymptomatic individual, limited quantities of caffeine may be acceptable. The benefit for some people may be improved mood, alertness, and concentration. The trade-off, however, could be lethargy and fatigue as a result of the low blood sugar that may occur in the hour after coffee consumption. I know that during my days as an athlete and particularly during my days as a medical student, I relied on caffeine to keep me mentally alert and physically sharp over the short term. Coffee is definitely considered a pick-me-up.

On the other hand, we can risk poisoning our bodies with too much caffeine. Please understand: Caffeine is indeed a drug with considerable side effects. I would recommend consuming no more than one to two cups of coffee per day and none after 3:00 P.M. Decaffeinated coffee and tea should also be consumed in moderation.

In summary, caffeine, like alcohol, needs to be used with caution. As mentioned previously, water is the best beverage, and it is definitely a major player in the search for optimum health; but as you know, many water supplies are contaminated with heavy metals, chlorine, and other environmental pollutants. If you don't use water filters or high-quality bottled water, it's a good idea to have your water analyzed.

CHAPTER
Eight

The Truth about Free Radicals, Vitamins, and Antioxidants

I'd like to share a letter to the editor I wrote to my local newspaper in Connecticut, responding to an article about whether or not to take vitamins.

As a physician, father, cook, and author who has researched the medical literature, I can tell you that although there is no substitute for a balanced diet, the fact remains that vitamin and mineral deficiencies do exist in our population. Many of our soils have become worn out; water has become polluted, industrial and automobile emissions pollute the environment, heavy metal toxicities and nuclear waste are poisoning much of the earth. These many toxins create metabolic stress. One way of protecting our bodies is by binding free radicals with antioxidants.

For example, if excessive fat is consumed during a meal at our favorite fast-food restaurant, if excessive radiation is taken in at the beach, if toxic fumes from traffic are inhaled, or if heavy metals are absorbed (in drinking water, for example), the body becomes involved in a biochemical war for self-protection. Our immune systems attack the invading toxins, leaving behind the by-product of these biochemical reactions to accumulate in our bodies. These wastes may trigger hormonal changes that may lead to symptoms of allergy, palpitations, nausea, and shortness of breath, to mention a few. Such occurrences may lead to biological changes, disease, and aging. This is where vitamins and minerals become crucial.

Although eating fresh fruits and vegetables on a daily basis would help, it is accepted that transport and storage can diminish vitamin content in some produce. In the article printed in this paper, it was stated that it is preferable to eat a fresh orange rather than take supplements. How fresh is fresh? Has that orange been laced with chemical agents or pesticides? Many vitamins and minerals are not prevalent in the diet, specifically coenzyme Q_{10}, vital to people suffering from cardiovascular problems. Though coenzyme Q_{10} is abundant in beef heart, pork, mackerel, and sardines, not many of us thrive on that particular diet. Additional complications exist for those on antibiotics, oral contraceptives, corticosteriods, or overusing alcohol or caffeine. These are only some of the evils which deplete our bodies' vitamin and mineral levels.

Consider also those who have undergone major bypass surgery and been placed on a heart-lung machine. The process of circulating blood through this device destroys vitamins, minerals, and coenzyme factors. Many more circumstances and rationales exist for needing supplementary vitamins and minerals in our modern world, none of which are disputed by the Japanese. Since coenzyme Q_{10} went on sale in April, 1974, approximately six million people in that country take the supplement annually. As a clinical cardiologist and also a modified vegetarian who consumes large amounts of grains, produce, and herbs, I will continue to take vitamins and minerals and recommend them to my family and patients.

As a layperson and particularly as a young doctor, I never held vitamins or minerals in high esteem. After all, I always felt I ate well, so why should I use supplements, when I consumed grains, fresh fruits, and vegetables? Being a doctor, I thought I knew what was beneficial. But once again, my patients were my best teachers. Frequently I needed to prescribe drugs for various conditions, but sometimes those drugs didn't work. While occasionally I had to ask myself if my patients were taking the medications, more often I knew that they had accepted my advice and followed instructions. It was only after careful scrutiny and much investigation that I discovered that many of my patients were not adequately absorbing their medications. I knew that due to diminished hydrochloric acid in their stomachs, some people could not absorb medicine. Could the same thing happen with foods? If so, how would we know? Through becoming ill? It became increasingly clear to me that not all the agents we put into our bodies will be absorbed. Even if we were to absorb all the nutrients we eat, is this enough to sustain our bodies in today's environment? Over the last several years, as I continued to read and practice preventive medicine, I gradually began to believe more and more in the healing powers of vitamins, minerals, and naturally healthy foods. Deficiencies in essential nutrients can cause bodily changes that may be overlooked by patients and physicians alike. In my own case, I had psoriasis on my elbows and knees for years. After taking vitamin and mineral preparations I had personally developed, within one year many of my symptoms disappeared. Although I still suffer occasional flare-ups, my skin in general is much healthier in these localized areas. It was only by trial and error that I learned I was not fully benefiting from all the nutrients I thought I was getting, even though I was eating well. Although there are no clinical studies to prove such effects, in my case this was highly significant. It seems as though even if we are not sick, we may unknowingly be in a state of less than perfect health.

ASK FOR HIGH-GRADE FUEL

I like to think of the body as a Porsche with a finely tuned engine requiring a high-performance fuel to operate; when the fuel is of inferior grade, the engine may stall and sputter. When the engine has no fuel, it stops. The human body reacts in a similar fashion. We need food and nourishment to keep our engine going. However, without proper nutrition—if we consume insufficient nutrients, or even poor-grade nutrients—our bodies will not function efficiently.

This reasoning can also be applied to many vitamin and mineral formulas that are presently on the market. Some formulas have high-grade nutrients, while others contain inferior-grade nutrients as well as inferior delivery systems.

The problem with most of us is that we believe we are getting all the vital nutrients we need from our diet. But is this true? Overcooking foods or microwaving them may alter the foods' vitamin and enzyme content. This is particularly true for the elderly, who frequently cannot get out to purchase fresh fruits and vegetables and who may use microwaving as their preferred way of cooking. Microwaving can seriously reduce B vitamins in food. Recently it has been discovered that many suffer from large deficiencies of B vitamins, especially in the elderly population. I am very skeptical of microwaves and don't have one in my house.

Habits such as microwaving are in a sense similar to using a low-grade fuel. Freshness can also be fleeting. Frequently, fresh produce will lose much of its vitamin value because of storage, shipping, and handling. Asparagus, for example, loses up to two thirds of its vitamin C after just two days at room temperature.

Although the vitamins and minerals found in natural whole foods will give some of us protection against illness, I believe that supplementation enhances our health. It is a little-known fact that certain vitamin and mineral supplements can significantly protect individuals against the increasing dangers of radiation and chemical pollutants. As a clinical cardiologist, I have seen numerous articles on the beneficial effects of beta carotene, vitamins C and E, and selenium. These nutrients are frequently referred to as antioxidants, which protect our bodies from the formation of free radicals sometimes associated with the diseases of modern man.

FREE RADICALS AND DISEASE

While we cannot readily see what is happening inside the body, we can see common effects of oxidation, such as the browning of a freshly cut apple or the rusting of metal. In the human body, oxidation can be the result of normal metabolism or the work of external factors such as radiation, air pollution, and alcohol or heavy-metal intoxication, to name a few.

Free radicals are highly reactive molecules produced during such oxidation. They interfere with enzymatic reactions, attack cells, membranes, even DNA itself. The body, trying to protect itself, becomes involved in a biochemical war between the invading free radicals and the immune system. During such biochemical battles, toxic wastes of combat accumulate in the body, producing enormous metabolic stress.

Our industrialized and overpolluted environment also creates a continuous attack on our bodies, adversely affecting us in numerous ways. For example, metals such as iron, lead, and cadmium are increasingly present in our drinking water. In Manchester, Connecticut, where I live, our water has been tested and found to have too much lead. In addition to harmful metals, increasing radiation—not just from industrial technology, but also from our old friend, the sun, via a receding ozone layer—places enormous stress on the body.

Other man-made risk factors such as emissions, cigarette smoke, and other pollutants in the air we breathe, insidiously poison our bodies. Electromagnetic contamination is another factor. Flying in an airplane at thirty thousand feet, or worse yet sitting near a jet engine on a plane, creates a firestorm of free radicals in our bodies. Free radicals are also generated by walking past our refrigerators, watching TV up close, sitting down at a computer, and probably cooking with microwaves. These electromagnetic waves are invisible but they continually zap us.

Another factor is the radiation that is emitted from the ground. There is considerable investigation into the impact of radon on the formation of free radicals and its role in the development of lung cancer. Radon is found deep in the earth in rocks, over time working its way to the surface and into our homes, infiltrating our bodies. For example, I have a patient with lung cancer who never smoked, but his home was contaminated with radioactive radon. He is currently part of a statewide study to determine the degree of the relationship between radon and lung cancer. Environmental toxins that can produce free radicals are all around us.

The increasing amount of fats in our diets also causes relentless biochemical reactions that are toxic to the body. Free radicals can be produced by the body itself during the oxidation of food, especially fats. During the burning of fats (oxidation) and especially if the fat is rancid, an alarming number of free radicals are produced. Consider all the free radicals you have in your refrigerator, like the leftovers sitting in a sea of fat. Consider the margarine that has turned a strange color, or the butter that's soft, warm, and rancid. And remember the mayonnaise jar that is half full? The air in the jar may be turning the mayonnaise rancid. These little things, totally overlooked by most of us, provide the raw materials to create dire reactions in the body.

While the effects of free radicals on health and disease are not completely understood, free radicals are believed to cause biological changes over time resulting in aging or the acceleration of a variety of chronic diseases, such as heart disease, cancer, and cataracts. For example, in cancer, free radicals may disrupt DNA, leading to tumor growth, and in heart disease the oxidation of LDL is now believed to be a prime factor in atherosclerosis. Although more research is needed to establish causality between free radicals and disease, multiple studies have shown the benefits of an antioxidant defense system.

ANTIOXIDANTS

Antioxidants act like friendly guardians or bodyguards neutralizing free radicals. Sacrificing themselves in chemical reactions, they engulf free radicals before they can do their damage to the body. Antioxidants protect DNA, cellular membranes, and even various enzyme systems involved in the metabolism of fats and carbohydrates. Thus, the integrity of every cell in the body depends on the balance of free radicals and antioxidants.

Biological antioxidants can be single nutrients such as beta carotene, vitamin E, vitamin C, or selenium, among others. Or they can be elaborate antioxidant enzyme systems (such as glutathione peroxidase or superoxide dismutase). Although antioxidant enzyme systems are thought to be genetically predetermined, the concentration of antioxidant vitamins and minerals is directly related to diet and supplement intake.

This free radical/antioxidant theory appeals to me as a doctor. Many of us not only eat high-fat diets that can form free radicals, but also are exposed to harmful metals, chemicals, drugs, pesticides, and the various forms of electromagnetic contamination and radiation I have discussed.

A personal example may be useful here. As a clinical cardiologist, I frequently encounter radiation. Performing cardiac catheterizations and inserting pacemakers requires working with X-ray devices, which produce radiation. The patient gets a small dose, but so does the doctor. One of my particularly long cases took over four hours, with seventy-five minutes of fluoroscopy. Even with the use of a lead apron and collar (to protect the thyroid gland), I received considerable radiation contamination through this one procedure alone. Since radiation accumulates over time, many small doses add up and can certainly be disruptive to the body. In my particular case, I stopped performing cardiac catheterizations after finding hemorrhages in my corneas I believe were related to radiation.

Since eye diseases run in my family, I took a personal interest in nurturing my eyes. I researched literature about the healing properties of vitamins, minerals, and antioxidants for the eyes. I found one study indicating a diet rich in vitamin A supported healing in the eyes. In a group of over fifty thousand female nurses, those who took the highest quantity of vitamin A and others who used vitamin C supplements over a long period of time had a 30 percent reduction in cataracts. Why are these vitamins effective? Antioxidants help to prevent the oxidation of protein in the lens, which leads to the formation of cataracts. Since cataracts are a common part of the aging process, this study was eye-opening for me, to say the least.

Another eye condition in which antioxidants may be of use is age-related macular degeneration, or AMD. This is the leading cause of blindness in people over the age of sixty-five. The macula is the most sensitive part of the retina and previous observational studies and animal experiments have demonstrated that antioxidants benefit the retina. The outer retina is rich in polyunsaturated fatty acids and is highly susceptible to free radical attack and oxidation. Antioxidants and other nutrients help maintain the cellular membranes of the blood vessels that supply the vulnerable macular region of the retina.

Lutein and zeaxanthin are pigments found in the retina that filter out harmful blue light, which accelerates the oxidation process. Lutein is found in spinach, collard greens, apricots, corn, red peppers, and peaches. As levels of the carotenoids in lutein and zeaxanthin are significantly decreased in advanced AMD, it makes sense to incorporate these nutrients in an effort to protect our precious eyesight. I personally try to eat apricots, spinach, or other sources of these excellent carotenoids almost every day. In addition, I take a daily multivitamin and mineral supplement containing mixed carotenoids, vitamin C, vitamin E, and zinc, all of which have been shown to be protective for the eyes.

How much vitamin and mineral supplementation is enough? We need to be aware that the recommended daily allowance (RDA) was instituted approximately fifty years ago by the U.S. Food and Nutrition Board as a guideline for the daily amount of vitamins and nutrients necessary to prevent illnesses directly due to vitamin deficiency, such as scurvy, beriberi, and so on. The RDAs, however, are considered only to be minimum doses that ward off such conditions, and these diseases are rare today. It has become apparent that larger doses of vitamins (but not megadoses) may provide more protection for the body. The RDA may not be enough, given today's electromagnetically contaminated and chemically polluted environment. We need to consider a larger dose than the RDA in order to provide ourselves with an optimal daily allowance that is health enhancing.

WHAT DOES *RDA* MEAN?

In the following chart, the RDAs listed represent the bare minimum of essential nutrients that the average person needs.

Vitamins	Children Under 4 Years		Adults and Children 4 Years and Older	
Vitamin A	2,500	IU	5,000	IU
Vitamin D	400	IU	400	IU
Vitamin E	10	IU	30	IU
Vitamin C	40	mg	60	mg
Folic Acid	0.2 mg		0.4 mg	
Vitamin B-1	0.7 mg		1.5 mg	
Vitamin B-2	0.8 mg		1.7 mg	
Vitamin B-12	3	mcg	6	mcg
Niacin (B-3)	9	mg	20	mg
Pantothenic Acid (B-5)	5	mg	10	mg
Minerals				
Calcium	800	mg	1,000	mg
Phosphorus	800	mg	1,000	mg
Iodine	70	mcg	150	mcg
Iron	10	mcg	18	mcg
Magnesium	200	mg	400	mg
Copper	1	mg	2	mg
Zinc	6	mg	15	mg

When considering nutritional supplementation, remember that taking vitamins and minerals in their proper balance is important. For example, high doses of single B vitamins may cause depletion of other B vitamins, and too much of the mineral zinc may interfere with the absorption of iron, causing anemia. It was observed in the *Journal of the American Medical Association* that large numbers of elderly patients may be ingesting too much zinc. Consequently, a careful history of zinc ingestion is necessary when evaluating elderly patients for anemia. We also need to be aware that some vitamin supplements, particularly vitamins A and D, can cause serious illness if taken in excessive dosages. Once again, the key is moderation. The following list points out some potential dangers from excessive supplementation.

Hazards of Megadoses of Vitamins and Minerals

1. *Vitamin A:* A fat-soluble vitamin stored in the body. Taking vitamin A in doses higher than 50,000 IU per day may cause weight loss, skin difficulties, bone pain, bleeding, and other symptoms.
2. *Vitamin D:* Another fat-soluble vitamin. When taken in doses greater than 3,000 IU per day, it may cause kidney impairment, weight loss, and thirst.
3. *Vitamin E:* Rarely, bleeding may occur. Use caution if you are taking more than 200 IU of vitamin E a day and also taking Coumadin (a blood thinner); check with your physician before taking a higher dose of vitamin E.
4. *Vitamin C:* Caution needs to be used with this vitamin in patients on hemodialysis or with chronic renal failure. Vitamin C will enhance the absorption of iron. Approximately 2 percent of the population may have an iron overload state in which the body contains too much iron. If you are taking more than 1,000 mg of vitamin C per day, I recommend having your iron level evaluated by your physician.
5. *Iron and Copper:* Potent oxidants. Do not take them unless recommended by your physician.
6. *Calcium:* Avoid if you have renal failure.
7. *Zinc:* More than 100 mg per day may cause immunosuppression, which may make people more susceptible to infections.
8. *Selenium:* More than 300 to 400 mg per day may cause anemia, poor appetite, and liver cirrhosis.
9. *Beta carotene:* Use with caution in the presence of alcoholic liver disease, cigarette smoking, or exposure to asbestos.
10. *Vitamin B-6:* More than 300 mg daily may cause liver and neurologic toxicity.

Later in this chapter and the next, I will give you specific recommendations concerning vitamin and mineral supplementation. Since beta carotene is water soluble and a precursor of vitamin A, I prefer using beta carotene over vitamin A. Unless your physician is treating you for osteoporosis, I would not use more than 400 IU per day of vitamin D. Although I recommend coenzyme Q_{10} to most everyone in my practice, caution should be utilized in nursing mothers. I would also not administer coenzyme Q_{10} to small children, as they have healthy livers and their bodies should contain sufficient quantities of it.

ADVANTAGES OF SUPPLEMENTATION

Now that I have told you about the downside of excessive dosing of vitamins and minerals, I want to discuss with you the many advantages of antioxidants, vitamins, minerals, and targeted nutritional supplementation. Unfortunately, the medical profession in general has not been very supportive of targeted nutritional supplementation. There has been much negativity and personal bias on this subject. I know this is true, because I was biased against vitamins in the late 1970s.

Why has this been true for so many health professionals? Historically, few doctors have been trained in the field of nutrition, and until recently only a few professionals believed that supplemental vitamins would be beneficial. There were very few scientific studies demonstrating the health benefits of supplements in humans. It was believed that a balanced diet would supply all the vitamins and nutrients needed to prevent various vitamin deficiency diseases such as scurvy, beriberi, and rickets which we rarely see today.

Such was the thinking of earlier decades. However, the 1990s began to show us that antioxidants, minerals, and nutrients in significant doses can help prevent certain other diseases. In the past couple of years, there has been an explosion in the medical literature about vitamin and mineral supplementation. You cannot pick up a medical journal today without seeing a reference to vitamins, minerals, or antioxidants. Numerous well-controlled scientific studies have shown impressive prevention benefits, especially for the antioxidants (beta carotene, vitamin C, vitamin E, coenzyme Q_{10}, selenium, and others). Consider the following facts about prevention of heart disease, cancer, and cataracts:

1. There has been an increasing accumulation of research supporting the use of coenzyme Q_{10} in the treatment of cardiovascular disease and cancer. Multiple case studies have shown marked improvement in congestive heart failure, and case reports indicate that 300 to 400 mg daily of coenzyme Q_{10} has been associated with the remission of breast cancer.
2. In a California study, a vitamin C intake of greater than 300 to 500 mg

per day seems to increase life expectancy due to a decrease in heart attacks and various forms of cancer.

3. High-vitamin diets reduce cataract risk. In a study of over fifty thousand female nurses, those with the highest intake of vitamins C and A had a 39 percent lower risk of cataract formation.

4. Vitamin E has been shown to play a major role in the prevention of atherosclerosis in men and especially women. As presented recently in the *New England Journal of Medicine,* a 26 to 41 percent reduction in heart attacks occurred after a two-year period in which participants took 100 to 400 IU of vitamin E per day.

5. In a Chinese study of twenty-nine thousand participants, the ingestion of beta carotene, vitamin E, and selenium resulted in a 13 percent reduction in esophageal and gastric cancer, and a 9 percent reduction in deaths as compared to the population not taking supplements.

6. Vitamin E supplements promoted regression of coronary artery disease in men following coronary bypass surgery.

7. Beta carotene studies have shown that this antioxidant results in a decrease in tumor size in patients with oral leukoplakia (precancerous mouth lesions).

8. There is strong evidence that high dietary intake of vitamin C offers protection against non–hormone-dependent cancers of the esophagus, larynx, oral cavity, pancreas, stomach, rectum, breast, cervix, and lungs.

9. Positive health benefits have also been demonstrated for numerous other vitamins and minerals. Hundreds of articles have appeared in medical journals over the past few years on these topics, and there are many large population studies and clinical trials presently under way that will yield further information concerning vitamins, minerals, and antioxidants. Although vitamin and mineral supplements are no substitute for a proper diet, they are a beneficial, nontoxic, and easy way to promote optimum health. Unfortunately, even the rare individual who eats a balanced diet (about 9 percent of Americans) that includes five to nine servings of fresh fruits and vegetables a day does not get the larger amount of these nutrients demonstrated in scientific studies to be effective.

While supplemental vitamins and minerals are the easiest way to make up the deficit, the problem is that most supplements are unregulated as to potency and absorption. The Center for Science in the Public

Interest in Washington, D.C., found tremendous variability in potency when fifty vitamin preparations were analyzed. Furthermore, many vitamin preparations are hard to absorb, and so much of the product goes into and out of the body without many of the nutrients being absorbed into the bloodstream. Choosing the right vitamin and mineral formula is a complex yet crucial task.

A FLAWED BUT FAMOUS STUDY

Choosing the right vitamin and mineral formula is difficult not only for the general population, but also for investigators performing major clinical studies. For example, you may have heard of a famous Finnish study in which beta carotene supplements seemed to cause lung cancer. The disclosure of these results hit the media like an explosion. This study got more press than any other study in the history of medicine. The question is, why? One reason may be that the results of this study appeared just before the passage of the famous Hatch-Richardson Bill regarding the purchase of vitamin and mineral supplements.

The study population in the Finnish trial included approximately twenty-nine thousand male smokers in Finland. Most of these individuals had been smoking for thirty years. Since the average fat content of the Finnish diet was at about 38 percent of total calories, most participants had high cholesterol levels. In addition, many of the participants drank considerable quantities of alcohol. Although this study had other serious flaws and limitations from the beginning, one might ask why researchers would choose a population with such serious risk factors for heart disease and cancer and try to resurrect them at the eleventh hour with antioxidant supplements (the supplements were also of low quality and low dosage).

The trial showed the following results: The men taking vitamin E had fewer lung cancers, but the results were not significant statistically. The men taking beta carotene had 18 percent more lung cancers, which was statistically significant. The men taking vitamin E had 34 percent fewer prostate cancers and 15 percent fewer colorectal cancers. The men taking beta carotene had slightly more cases of cancer (other than lung cancer), but that was not statistically significant.

The researchers could not find a reason why smokers taking beta carotene were observed to have more cancers. My own personal interpretation of this study includes a major concern about the choice of the vitamins and minerals. I previously mentioned that a Chinese study in which participants took beta carotene, vitamin E, and selenium showed that these subjects had reduction in cancer. The supplements used in the Chinese study were manufactured in the United States. Consistent with good manufacturing practices, these vitamin supplements did not contain quinoline yellow (yellow dye #10) which is not certified for use in this country as a food additive. However, all formulas in the Finnish study were colored with quinoline yellow, and were not manufactured in the United States under stringent regulations.

Since the Finnish study is at variance with all other clinical studies and had such unexpected results, the question about the impact of quinoline yellow remains. Laced with quinoline yellow, could vitamin E and beta carotene become ineffective, lose potency, or even become harmful? And no one has looked at the biochemical interaction of quinoline yellow and beta carotene in animal studies. We need to look at the impact quinoline yellow has on these food nutrients.

Nevertheless, the Finnish study has had a tremendous negative impact on people in this country. People seem to forget that it is at variance with over two hundred published population studies showing a lower risk in cancer and cardiovascular disease in people consuming antioxidants, vitamins C and E, and beta carotene. People forget also that even the authors of the Finnish study were skeptical of the results, stating "An adverse effect of beta carotene seems unlikely, in spite of all the statistical significance, therefore the finding may be due to chance."

My reason for discussing this flawed study with you is to raise your awareness about the usefulness and possible limitations of not only supplements but also the studies that evaluate them. As the Finnish study was doomed to fail from the beginning because of poor-quality ingredients and poor design, we must certainly question its results.

VITAMINS

Vitamins are a group of organic compounds that regulate the metabolism of carbohydrates, protein, and fat. Vitamins are considered micronutrients and act as a catalyst for chemical reactions in the body. Frequently a vitamin will be described as a coenzyme because it works with enzymes in assisting biochemical functions. Since vitamins cannot be produced by the body we must get them through the diet and/or in vitamin and mineral supplements.

Some vitamins such as A, D, E, and K may be fat soluble and do not need to be replenished on a daily basis, as the body can store them in the adipose tissue. The water-soluble vitamins such as B vitamins and vitamin C must be ingested on a daily basis as they cannot be stored in the body.

Vitamin A and Beta Carotene

Vitamin A is essential to prevent night blindness and the formation of cataracts. It is also important in the development of healthy bones, skin, hair, and mucous membranes. It enhances immunity and is important in the maintenance and repair of epithelial tissue (skin and mucous membranes). As an antioxidant, vitamin A helps protect against the adverse effects of radiation and chemical pollutants. Although high doses of vitamin A can be utilized to treat infections and conditions of physical or emotional stress, supplements of vitamin A should not be taken in high dosages for a long period of time. There have been cases on record where megadose therapy resulted in liver damage, skin rash, and brain dysfunction.

Provitamin A, or beta carotene, is a precursor of vitamin A and is converted into vitamin A by the body. Beta carotene is a yellowish compound contained in carrot juice, cantaloupe, watercress, and other fruits and vegetables, especially those with yellow, orange, or dark green hues. Unlike megadoses of vitamin A, beta carotene has been shown to have few toxic side effects. In a recent study by Harvard medical experts, it has been shown that taking beta carotene in a dose of 50 mg (approximately 80,000 IU) every other day over a twelve-year period did not produce any harm. The tendency to turn the skin a slight yellow-orange color when taken in very high doses may occur. Beta carotene is safe to use except in uncontrolled diabetics and hypothyroid individuals, as they have difficulty metabolizing beta carotene.

Beta carotene has become the focus of much research. In large population studies, people eating foods high in beta carotene had fewer heart attacks than those taking less beta carotene. Both vitamin A and beta carotene are extremely important to the immune mechanisms of the body and may help to fight the common cold and other flu-like illnesses. Beta carotene also has been reported to protect the lungs from ozone and smog in polluted city environments and is helpful in combating the toxic effects of automobile emissions.

The RDA for vitamin A or beta carotene is 3,000 IU for children and 3 mg or 5,000 IU for adults. We usually get plenty of vitamin A in our diet. Foods that contain considerable quantities of vitamin A include carrots, beets, capers, sweet potatoes, spinach, Swiss chard, broccoli, dandelions, garlic, kale, parsley, red peppers, yellow squash, turnip greens, and watercress. For an animal source of vitamin A, I recommend fish liver oils, particularly cod liver oil. I do not recommend eating calves' liver or other organ meats. Though I'm sure that vitamin supplements would be preferable, one tablespoon of cod liver oil contains 11,000 IU of preformed vitamin A. Similarly three and a half ounces of carrots offer approximately 11,500 units of vitamin A. As a supplement, I suggest 12,500 to 25,000 units of beta carotene per day. It is also important to note that antibiotics, cholesterol-lowering agents, some laxatives, various antacids, and excessive quantities of alcohol or caffeine may interfere with vitamin A absorption.

Vitamin B-1 (Thiamine)

My first exposure to a patient with vitamin B-1 deficiency occurred during my internship. A man in his mid-fifties came to the hospital with congestive heart failure. His arms and legs were very swollen. This man was an alcoholic. Although he responded to treatment for heart failure, he did not appear to improve significantly until he received vitamin B-1. Thiamine enhances circulation and is needed for normal functioning of the heart muscle and smooth muscle of the gastrointestinal tract. It is also an important constituent of the central nervous system. Vitamin B-1 is administered to many patients with alcoholism as it protects the brain. If not taken in the diet deficiencies may occur. Excellent sources of B-1 include brown rice, whole grains, peas, wheat germ, soybeans, dried beans, Brussels sprouts, oatmeal, prunes, raisins, and sunflower seeds, to mention a few.

Vitamin B-2 (Riboflavin)

Riboflavin is necessary for antibody production, cell respiration, and metabolism of fats, carbohydrates, and proteins. Signs of riboflavin deficiency include cracks and sores at the corners of the mouth. It has also been suggested by researchers that riboflavin may alleviate allergic conjunctivitis, a common problem for hay fever sufferers. Riboflavin is also beneficial for the skin, nails, and hair. It may be helpful in controlling dandruff. High doses of riboflavin (100 mg) when taken in combination with other B-vitamins and magnesium have been known to prevent and reduce the discomfort of migraine headaches. Sources of riboflavin include whole grains, spinach, poultry, fish, meat, asparagus, broccoli, Brussels sprouts, currants, and sea vegetables. It is also important to know that oral contraceptives and estrogen may increase the need for riboflavin, and that this is one particular vitamin that is easily destroyed by overcooking and the use of alcohol. Incidentally, riboflavin is responsible for the bright yellow urine you may have noticed after ingestion of multivitamins.

Vitamin B-3 (Niacin)

Niacin is an important vitamin for blood circulation, energy production, and functioning of the nervous system. In large doses, it is helpful in lowering cholesterol. I already told you something about my personal experience with niacin. I took niacin in powdered form, and immediately developed a "niacin flush"—tingling of the skin accompanied by a hot flash. Some people dislike this reaction, but others like it, and some even use niacin to enhance sexual pleasure; some of my patients discovered this by accident and now take dosages of up to 500 mg at bedtime. Deficiencies in niacin may cause abnormalities in the central nervous system. Excellent sources of niacin include meat, broccoli, grains, dried beans, potatoes, tomatoes, and nuts. Vitamin B-3 in its long-acting form should not be taken in large quantities, as it may damage the liver.

Vitamin B-5 (Pantothenic Acid)

Pantothenic acid, also referred to as vitamin B-5, is known as the "anti-stress vitamin" because of its crucial role in energy metabolism. In situations of severe emotional and physical stress, it is not uncommon for some individuals to need an additional 500 mg of pantothenic acid per day. Although the human requirement for pantothenic acid is not known, 10 mg is considered sufficient. However, more of the vitamin is required after injury, while under stress, or during antibiotic therapy. Although symptoms of pantothenic acid deficiency are rare, considerable amounts of the vitamin are lost in the processing, canning, and cooking of foods, especially in acidic or alkaline solutions.

The brain contains the highest concentration of pantothenic acid in the body; therefore, a deficiency of pantothenic acid, as with all the B vitamins, would include symptoms such as fatigue, depression, and insomnia. Alcoholics may be particularly prone to B-vitamin deficiency, especially if foods high in B-5 are not consumed. Excellent sources of pantothenic acid include whole grains, meat, cabbage, cauliflower, beans, eggs, ocean fish, and poultry.

Vitamin B-6 (Pyridoxine)

Vitamin B-6 is important for the regulation and formation of blood cells. It is required for the synthesis of nucleic acids. Some investigators have reported that vitamin B-6 helped some individuals recall dreams. It is also used to calm the effects of premenstrual syndrome and is helpful in the treatment of allergies and asthma. In weight loss, B-6 has been reported to be a useful nutrient as well. The use of 200 mg of B-6 on a daily basis has been helpful to some of my patients with carpal tunnel syndrome. Since vitamin B-6 has absolutely no toxicity at this dosage, it may be a suitable alternative to surgery, particularly since people may respond to dosages as low as 40 to 100 mg per day.

Oral contraceptives and estrogen may increase the need for vitamin B-6. A urologist may prescribe vitamin B-6, as it is useful in preventing calcium oxalate gravel in the urinary tract. In short, vitamin B-6 is an important coenzyme in the metabolism of amino acids that can affect our mental and physical health. Most foods contain small amounts of vitamin B-6. The best sources include brewers' yeast, carrots, fish, meat, peas, sunflower seeds, avocados, and green peppers. As a supplement, I recommend 20 to 40 mg per day.

Vitamin B-12 (Cyanocobalamin)

Vitamin B-12 is necessary for the formation of blood cells. It is also necessary in the maintenance of a healthy nervous system. A prolonged absence of vitamin B-12 may cause pernicious anemia. This is a type of anemia that may cause weakness, lethargy, and damage to the nervous system. One of my elderly angina patients had a vitamin B-12 absorption problem, and almost underwent coronary artery bypass surgery because of severe coronary disease. We discovered, however, that his angina could have been provoked by a low blood count as a result of B-12 deficiency. After he received B-12 injections, he felt considerably better and had fewer angina symptoms. He currently receives monthly B-12 injections which have completely corrected the problem. This treatment has continued for ten years, and at the age of eighty-four, he still has a good quality of life. Sources of vitamin B-12 include all animal proteins, cheese, eggs, milk, tofu, and sea vegetables. Since B-12 is not present in most vegetables, vegetarians need to be cautious and supplement B-12 in their diet. Oral contraceptives and estrogen may also increase the need for B-12. As a supplement, I recommend 20 to 40 mcg daily.

Folic Acid

Over the past couple of years, this B vitamin has received tremendous attention in the medical literature. The U.S. Public Health Service has recently recommended that every woman of childbearing age take in 400 mg of folic acid daily, since it has been shown to have a positive impact on reducing the frequency of birth defects in the spinal cord and central nervous system, such as spina bifida. Folic acid has also been shown to decrease the incidence of cervical cancer in women, so it is not unreasonable to recommend this vitamin to large segments of the female population. But what about males? Do they need folic acid too?

The most exciting research in cardiovascular literature in recent years has involved—you guessed it—folic acid. Why has folic acid become so fashionable? Coronary artery disease, peripheral vascular disease, and vascular disease in the brain may now be considered diseases of aging, and these are exacerbated if the body does not have sufficient folic acid. Deficiencies of folic acid can occur because of microwaving and over-processing foods, and poor dietary habits. Another problem is red meat, which contains the amino acid methionine. In order for methionine to be properly metabolized, the body needs sufficient quantities of folic acid and other B vitamins. If these vitamins are lacking, methionine cannot be broken down properly, and the dangerous amino acid homocysteine results. Homocysteine is extremely toxic to the walls of the blood vessels and capillaries, causing cell membrane inflammation. The blood vessels become vulnerable to LDL, and plaque is deposited on the blood vessel wall, thus causing atherosclerosis. This can also occur in young people. In recent studies, it has been demonstrated that high levels of homocysteine in the body cause premature vascular disease, including stroke and heart attack.

The antidote to all of this is folic acid (and, to a lesser degree, vitamins B-6 and B-12). Although it is wise to eat less red meat, it is perhaps wiser still to take a B-vitamin supplement containing all of this protection. Since these data are very new and have only been published in recent years, perhaps three quarters of the physicians in this country including cardiologists have not yet assimilated them. One problem in our society today is the poor eating habits of teens and young adults who fail to consume foods rich in folic acid. My recommendation is to give folic acid in doses of at least 400 mcg daily to everyone, including young children over the age of eight. Chewable natural vitamins can be found in most health food stores.

Other B Vitamins

Other B-complex vitamins include biotin, choline, inositol, and para-aminobenzoic acid (PABA). These vitamins are found in many of the foods mentioned as good sources of vitamin B-12, with the exception of PABA, which is found in molasses, liver, and kidneys as well as whole grains. PABA is an antioxidant that may protect against sunburn and various skin cancers.

Generally, there are no known toxicities if the B vitamins are taken in small amounts. In mega amounts, however, one has to utilize caution. It is also important to note that alcohol and caffeine as well as birth control pills and estrogen can increase the need for B vitamins.

Vitamin C

Vitamin C has been the subject of considerable controversy ever since Linus Pauling first publicized it as the "cure for the common cold." Numerous research studies have indicated that vitamin C improves the immune system. In animals, for example, vitamin C has been shown to offer some protection against high doses of radiation. Perhaps the most famous and noteworthy effect of vitamin C is preventing the disease of scurvy. Scurvy is an illness in which subcutaneous bleeding occurs along with loss of appetite, tender joints, and low-grade anemia, accompanied by slow wound healing. Centuries ago, sailing ships used to carry limes in order to prevent scurvy among the crew. Recently, there was a case of scurvy at a major university center in a young man who had been eating out of cans for six months. He came to the doctor complaining of bleeding and funny "corkscrew-type" hair. This modern case of scurvy was caused by eating only processed foods, with no fresh fruits or vegetables. Vitamin C was the antidote.

Vitamin C is a powerful antioxidant that is necessary for tissue growth and repair, particularly in the gums. Vitamin C also plays a critical role in the absorption of iron, which is necessary for the formation of red blood cells, thereby preventing anemia. Doctors frequently will administer vitamin C in combination with iron, for vitamin C creates an acidic pH in the stomach so that iron-bound compounds can be absorbed. Vitamin C is also an essential constituent in the metabolism of amino acids, particularly tyrosine and phenylalanine. When an individual is under psychological and emotional stress, vitamin C may become depleted from the adrenal glands. Foods rich in vitamin C or vitamin supplements may help to prevent the body from reacting negatively to prolonged stress. Some clinical studies have also demonstrated a reduction in serum cholesterol with vitamin C supplementation. Since the body cannot manufacture its own vitamin C, supplementation must be obtained through the diet, or in nutritional supplements. Since most vitamin C is water soluble and can be excreted through the urine, it must be taken on a daily basis.

Although evidence linking vitamin C to a reduced risk of cardiovascular disease is still coming in, it is already well known that many people who have lower vitamin C levels are at an increased risk for heart disease. If one scrutinizes the research, the groups most at risk for heart disease, such as men, the elderly, diabetics, and hypertensives, have lower vitamin C plasma levels. In addition to these groups, smokers are especially deficient in vitamin C and should seriously consider taking vitamin C as a supplement.

In other clinical studies, vitamin C has been shown to decrease platelet stickiness. Another interesting function of vitamin C is that it raises the body's level of glutathione. In a double-blind study performed at the University of Arizona, experimental subjects placed on 500 mg of vitamin C daily showed a 50 percent increase in glutathione levels. Glutathione is a powerful antioxidant in itself and is perhaps one of the body's most potent free radical scavengers. Thus, vitamin C may help glutathione levels and improve overall antioxidant status.

Common sources of vitamin C include bell peppers, broccoli, squash, cabbage, strawberries, lemons, kale, citrus fruits, currants, parsley, onions, radishes, rosehips, spinach, Swiss chard, tomatoes, turnip greens, and Brussels sprouts.

Once again, it is important for us to remember that oral contraceptives and corticosteroids may reduce the levels of vitamin C in the body. Alcohol is also an antagonist to vitamin C. Although vitamin C toxicity is rare, kidney stones could occur if vitamin C is taken in large doses and not accompanied by adequate hydration. In doses higher than 5,000 mg daily, some side effects may occur. Excess urination, diarrhea, or skin rashes may be experienced. I suggest 300 to 600 mg per day.

Vitamin D

Vitamin D is the bone vitamin. A deficiency of vitamin D may impair bone growth and development. This is commonly seen as rickets in children and osteomalacia in adults. Vitamin D also enhances the maintenance of healthy teeth. The principal source of vitamin D is exposure to the sun's ultraviolet rays. Regular sunshine, perhaps as little as half an hour per day, is all that is necessary to activate vitamin D production in the body. A deficiency of vitamin D could result from lack of exposure to the sun, especially if the vitamin is not taken in the diet. Nursing home inhabitants, for example, who do not go out into the sun, are susceptible to vitamin D deficiency. This is an important consideration, since vitamin D is not self-activated and requires conversion by the liver from either its natural or supplemented form.

It is also important to note that in the elderly, vitamin D can help in overall treatment of osteoporosis, an illness resulting from gradual loss of bone, predominantly in the spine and hips, that affects 50 to 60 percent of all women over the age of fifty. When treating osteoporosis, it is important to know the overall health of the patient. Many of these individuals may have kidney and liver disease and are frequently diabetic. Thus vitamin and mineral supplementation is critical in this population.

As vitamin D is a fat-soluble vitamin and is stored by the body, it may be toxic if taken in megadoses. This can be particularly serious in children or individuals with kidney disease. Certain drugs, such as steroid hormones, interfere with the action of vitamin D in the intestines; others, such as cholesterol-lowering drugs, may also interfere with the absorption of vitamin D. The dietary sources of vitamin D include fish oils and ocean fish, particularly fatty fish like halibut, salmon, mackerel, and bluefish. It is also found in abundance in eggs, liver, milk, sweet potatoes, and sunflower seeds. I suggest an intake of 400 IU daily.

Vitamin E

Vitamin E is gaining more and more popularity with cardiologists. It is a fat-soluble antioxidant present in the LDL particle. An article concerning vitamin E and its positive effect on angina was published in the prestigious medical journal *The Lancet*. Although the mechanism by which vitamin E has a protective effect on the heart is not well established, recent research indicates that vitamin E is an important antioxidant that may help protect unsaturated fatty acids from breaking down and causing the formation of free radicals. Vitamin E may help reduce the deleterious influence of LDL on cellular membranes, preventing the oxidation of LDL, the cardinal step in atherosclerosis. In addition, it has been reported to reduce the long-term effects of aging and may be used as an adjunct in cancer treatments.

Over the last two to three years, vitamin E has been the subject of careful scrutiny. There have been multiple studies regarding its role in cancer and cardiovascular disease. Perhaps the most noteworthy study involved 87,000 women and showed a 41 percent reduction in risk of heart disease among women who took vitamin E supplements for more than two years. There was also a significant improvement in risks with a dosage as low as 100 IU and even more improvement at the 200-IU level. In a follow-up study involving almost 40,000 men, similar findings were found. However, the vitamin E intake for men showed the lowest risk was at 400 IU. Thus men may need higher levels of supplementation than women.

In a study of patients who had undergone coronary artery angioplasty, researchers in Atlanta demonstrated that patients taking vitamin E had less risk of recurrent narrowing (restenosis) of the blood vessels. Since restenosis rates for angioplasty are high, I am working with some major medical centers to assess the efficacy of multimineral combinations in preventing reclosure of the vessels following balloon angioplasty.

Perhaps the most exciting news about vitamin E came out of a June 1995 paper in the *Journal of the American Medical Association*. In this study of 156 men aged 40 to 59 with a previous history of coronary artery bypass surgery, those subjects given supplementary vitamin E intake greater than 100 IU per day had less new coronary artery blockage than did subjects given a placebo or those given less than 100 IU per day. The data were also confirmed by cardiac catheterization, a procedure that takes pictures of the coronary vessels. This was indeed a landmark study, for the results indicate a positive association between supplemental vitamin E intake and reduction in coronary artery disease.

Previous studies also demonstrated that a higher level of vitamin E in the blood results in less frequent occurrence of heart disease symptoms such as angina and even reduces the death rate. Several population studies have also confirmed that people who take in higher amounts of vitamin E in their diet have a lower incidence of coronary artery disease. Although most cardiologists I know take vitamin E, I am sure this information will persuade even the most resistant cardiologists and other physicians to consider vitamin E supplements. The 1996 Cambridge Heart Antioxidant Study involved 2,000 patients with coronary artery disease. Those who used natural vitamin E showed a 77 percent decrease in the risk of a nonfatal heart attack. This effect became apparent two hundred days after the beginning of therapy.

The favorable effects of vitamin E on the immune system were also demonstrated in an animal study. Two groups of mice were exposed to what normally would be a lethal dose of radiation. One group was given vitamin E and the other was not. All the mice who were irradiated but not given vitamin E succumbed to the radiation. The experimental group given the vitamin, however, had an increase in survival rates, thus demonstrating the protective effects of vitamin E against radiation and on the overall immune response. Vitamin E has been shown to be effective against many common pollutants in the environment, such as nitrosamines (carcinogens found in many processed meats), chlorine, mercury, and carbon monoxide. When combined with beta carotene and vitamin C, vitamin E is extremely helpful in neutralizing the deleterious effects of industrial pollutants and toxic heavy metals. Another exciting discovery about vitamin E and diabetes was announced in October 1995. Of the 1,000 men in this study, the ones with the lowest vitamin E levels had approximately four times the risk of developing diabetes. Vitamin E protects the pancreas from free radical oxidative stress, thus protecting the glandular tissue.

Vitamin E has also been reported to be effective in thinning the blood, eliminating leg cramps, and aiding in the prevention of cataracts, as well as decreasing the breast tenderness and swelling experienced with premenstrual syndrome. The best sources of vitamin E include vegetable oils such as wheat germ oil and peanut oil. Green leafy vegetables, nuts, seeds, dry beans, brown rice, and whole wheat are other good sources of vitamin E. Vitamin E is found in fats, oils, and margarines. Therefore, if you consume a low-fat diet, you may not get the RDA of vitamin E.

As a supplement, approximately 200 to 400 IU of vitamin E per day is suggested to enhance the body's health and immunity. Although not all the mechanisms of vitamin E are clear, medical research has revealed yet another secret of vitamin E in health. It has recently been verified that vitamin E's role may be accentuated by the use of coenzyme Q_{10}.

Coenzyme Q_{10}

Coenzyme Q_{10} is a vitamin that has the ability to regenerate oxidized vitamin E and recycle it in the body. Before cataloguing its other functions, I'd like to share with you a letter I sent to the editor of the *Journal of the American Medical Association* about the use of coenzyme Q_{10} in congestive heart failure:

> Targeted nutritional supplementation with fat-soluble and water-soluble minerals is important adjuvant therapy in patients with congestive heart failure. As a clinical cardiologist who works on a day-to-day basis with many patients both from the physiological and psychological point of view, I fully support the inclusion of psychological and nutritional approaches in the overall care of the patient. In addition to what was mentioned in this article, I would recommend the addition of coenzyme Q_{10} to patients with diminished left ventricular function. I have had the opportunity to treat thousands of patients with coenzyme Q_{10} and for a large number there has been a significant improvement not only in left ventricular function, but also in quality of life. I have even had heart transplant patients refuse transplantation following the use of coenzyme Q_{10}. Although these are anecdotal cases, there have been at least fifty major articles published in the last ten years in reputable journals on the use of coenzyme Q_{10} in cardiac related diseases, especially congestive heart failure and idiopathic dilated cardiomyopathy.
>
> The contractive ability of the heart depends on the functional capacity of myocardial cells to expand and contract. Congestive heart failure often involves insufficient myocardial contractive forces. Literally heart failure is an energy-starved heart. The cardiologist cannot focus only on fluid retention but must also pay attention to the biochemistry of "pulsation." It is important to consider the molecular and cellular components of the heart.
>
> When it comes to the heart, cardiologists need to think bioenergetically. This is where coenzyme Q_{10} comes in. Although coenzyme Q_{10} has major therapeutic mechanisms in myocardial injury, it has also been demonstrated to scavenge free radicals produced by lipid peroxidation, stabilize cellular membranes, and prevent depletion of the metabolites necessary for the resynthesis of ATP in mitochondria. As the oxygen-based production of energy takes place in the mitochondria, it is not unusual that the coenzyme Q_{10} concentration of myocardial cells is approximately ten times greater than brain or colon cells. Cardiac muscle is one of the few tissues in the body to be continuously aerobic, thus requiring ATP support. Coen-

zyme Q_{10} enhances ATP/ADP production in mitochondria, thus helping to drive the "machinery" of the cell.

As side effects of coenzyme Q_{10} are rare, I suggest this as another nutritional additive to the treatment of congestive heart failure, cardiomyopathy, and in those patients with abnormal systolic and diastolic dysfunction. Certainly one set of researchers in Naples, Italy, has concluded that treatment of every 1,000 cases of congestive heart failure patients with coenzyme Q_{10} for one year could reduce hospitalizations by 20 percent. In this era of cost containment, this is indeed remarkable.

I first learned about coenzyme Q_{10} several years ago in an article appearing in the *Annals of Thoracic Surgery* in February 1982. In this particular study, a control group and an experimental group were designed to investigate the impact of coenzyme Q_{10} on cardiovascular function in patients on heart-lung machines during open heart surgery. Coenzyme Q_{10} increased cardiac output and overall heart efficiency.

Although this study was highly provocative, my openness to such vitamin and mineral therapy at that time was, to say the least, nonexistent. As a well-trained traditional cardiologist, I saw no need for such nutritional supplementation, particularly since drugs such as diuretics and myocardial stimulants were considered highly useful. It took four years of experience, growth, and humility to teach me that vitamins and other natural remedies can be a useful adjunct to traditional medical therapies. I began using coenzyme Q_{10} on my patients in 1986.

Congestive heart failure is a term that cardiologists use when the heart muscle is weakened. When the heart muscle becomes so weak that it cannot pump the blood effectively to the organs of the body, patients may develop swelling of the ankles, lack of appetite, fatigue, and shortness of breath on activity. Sometimes the pumping ability of the heart is so impaired that the blood, instead of being pumped out of the heart, backs up into the lungs. When this happens, patients will complain of shortness of breath not only during activity but also sometimes while at rest, especially when lying down. Congestive heart failure means that the tiny myocardial cells are so exhausted that they cannot contract effectively enough to create sufficient pumping action that will effectively circulate the blood around the body. Congestive heart failure is indeed the most frustrating and challenging dilemma of my profession.

Over the last twenty years, I have seen thousands of patients with congestive heart failure. For some, the diagnosis is obvious: A large heart attack destroyed a considerable quantity of heart muscle, and the contracting ability of the heart is so severely impaired that the remaining viable myocardial cells eventually become exhausted and can no longer sustain the pumping action of the heart.

A long-standing history of high blood pressure can also reduce myocardial function. Valvular disease, frequently induced by childhood rheumatic fever, as well as viral illness and toxins such as chronic alcohol abuse, can likewise impair the functioning of the heart muscle. Some of the cardiomyopathies have also been found to be the result of vitamin deficiencies such as beriberi. The rare cardiomyopathy of pregnancy may be related to nutritional deficiencies also.

As a clinical cardiologist, I can also attest to numerous cases of unexplained heart failure. These are individuals who have cardiomyopathy of an unknown nature; that is, in these individuals there was no known cause for the heart muscle to weaken. There was no history of diabetes, heart attack, high blood pressure, alcohol abuse, rheumatic fever, or severe viral illnesses. Some patients just develop weakening of the heart for no apparent reason.

Although some patients with cardiomyopathy improve, the majority of these individuals deteriorate. For the cardiologist, the treatment of heart failure is similar to the oncologist's treatment of life-threatening cancer. Although we can find drugs to help control the symptoms, there is really no known cure for cardiomyopathy. Like incurable cancer, heart failure frequently ends in death. In one of the most heartbreaking weeks of my practice, I lost five male patients to congestive heart failure. Many of these patients had also been my friends for several years. But one of my colleagues gave me a book, entitled *The Miracle Nutrient Coenzyme Q$_{10}$,* by Emile G. Bliznakof, MD, and Gerald L. Hunt. I also met a renowned cardiologist, Dr. William Frishman, who not only knew about coenzyme Q$_{10}$ but had also published a major article on Q$_{10}$ in a cardiovascular pharmacology journal. He proceeded to tell me that coenzyme Q$_{10}$, in his clinical studies, was considered therapeutic not only in congestive heart failure but also in cardiac arrhythmia and high blood pressure. My interest was now overwhelming, and I was determined to learn all I could about the nutrient.

Coenzyme Q$_{10}$ is a vitaminlike substance that is similar in structure to vitamin K. Like vitamin E, it is a powerful antioxidant. In humans, coenzyme Q_{10} is found in high concentrations in various organs, particularly the heart. In cells, the highest concentration of coenzyme Q_{10} is found primarily in the mitochondria, the powerhouses that supply energy to the cell.

The function of coenzyme Q_{10} is to stabilize cell membranes and act as an antioxidant and free radical scavenger. It prevents the depletion of products necessary for the production of cellular energy by stimulating the formation of ATP at the mitochondrial level. Coenzyme Q_{10} is critical for the production of energy and the healthy functioning of the cell.

Since coenzyme Q_{10} is necessary for the optimal functioning of the cell, can a deficiency of it impair energy production? The answer to that question is yes. Can cardiovascular malfunction such as congestive heart failure be caused by a deficiency of coenzyme Q_{10}? The answer to that question is also yes.

The father of coenzyme Q_{10} research, Dr. Karl Folkers, demonstrated that patients with cardiovascular disease are deficient in this nutrient. He found that levels of coenzyme Q_{10} in cardiac patients are lower than in age-matched controls. Moreover, through autopsy and biopsy studies on both diseased and healthy human hearts, Folkers has also determined that once internal levels of coenzyme Q_{10} drop to 25 percent below normal, disease may develop. If levels drop to 75 percent below normal, serious pathology and even death may occur. Although more research needs to be done, Folkers predicts that coenzyme Q_{10} therapy will one day be an accepted international treatment for congestive heart failure. I personally use the nutrient in every one of my patients with congestive heart failure if they are willing to take it. Recently I have been using much higher doses, even giving some very ill patients 300 to 400 mg per day.

Japanese and more recent American studies have shown the favorable impact of giving coenzyme Q_{10} to individuals with congestive heart failure. By increasing the level of intrinsic cellular energy, it has a direct and beneficial effect on the energy-depleted muscle cells of the failing heart. Since it protects critical cellular components from low oxygen states, the administration of coenzyme Q_{10} enhances energy production in cells that are literally starving for energy. Since it has been demonstrated that levels of coenzyme Q_{10} decline with advancing age, perhaps idiopathic cardiomyopathy may be related to a deficiency of cellular and mitochondrial coenzyme Q_{10}. For some unexplained reason the body's ability to extract this nutrient from natural food sources declines with the aging of the organs, the liver being the most significant. Thus, coenzyme Q_{10} supplements may be a significant healing remedy in selected populations, especially the elderly.

In experimental animal studies, coenzyme Q_{10} protected heart cells from the damaging effects of oxygen deficiency. Multiple clinical studies also show that coenzyme Q_{10} protects individuals from the chest pains or discomfort doctors frequently refer to as angina pectoris. For example, studies of patients with angina pectoris have shown a longer duration of pain-free exercise time in patients treated with coenzyme Q_{10}. In addition, the enzyme has been found to be an anti-arrhythmic agent. The cardiovascular literature has demonstrated that coenzyme Q_{10} effects a reduction in blood pressure as well.

Apparently some hypertensive patients may be deficient in coenzyme Q_{10}. In one placebo-controlled, double-blind study, patients given supplements demonstrated a reduction in both systolic and diastolic blood pressure over matched controls. More and more I have been using coenzyme Q_{10} as a natural approach to lowering blood pressure, with favorable results.

Coenzyme Q_{10} has also been used in the treatment of other disorders. For example, some forms of muscular dystrophy have been known to respond to coenzyme Q_{10} therapy. In addition, it has been used in the treatment of periodontal disease. The nutrient has also been used to treat immunodeficiency diseases; its use in AIDS patients is under investigation, with preliminary research showing a positive impact.

Weight reduction is another useful attribute of coenzyme Q_{10}. In my practice, I have seen patients who adhered to their diet, but could not lose weight, possibly the result of a lower metabolism. In one European study, obese patients were recognized as being deficient in coenzyme Q_{10}, raising the question whether the nutrient could be useful in selected individuals with a presumed low metabolism. An anecdotal case comes to mind. Mary was in her fifties, and came to our weight reduction program out of frustration. She had tried several weight loss programs, but she had been unable to lose weight. After two weeks on our program, Mary had still not lost weight. I sensed her tremendous despair; she was really trying.

After carefully going over her program, it was apparent that she was indeed staying on the diet. At this point, I suggested some dietary supplements. I placed her on a regime with coenzyme Q_{10}, vitamin B-6, zinc, chromium picolinate, and a multivitamin and mineral complex. She was told to take these supplements after every meal. She persisted in her regimen and, to her surprise, lost five pounds in the following week. Perhaps she may have had a low metabolism and in addition a subtle deficiency of nutrients.

Clinical research has also revealed the beneficial effects of coenzyme Q_{10} in brain disorders, aging, and allergies. Coenzyme Q_{10} has the ability to counteract histamines and may have considerable utility in the treatment of asthma. It has also been used to help shrink breast cancers and even reverse metastatic cancer in some patients.

The usual doses of coenzyme Q_{10} may range from 30 mg one to three times daily, to as high as 300 to 400 mg in the treatment of congestive heart failure, and 90 to 180 mg for angina and hypertension. The highest doses are used in treating congestive heart failure. In clinical studies where 150 mg has been used, no significant side effects have occurred. In a large study of over 5,000 patients taking a dose of 30 mg, abdominal discomfort was reported in twenty patients, and loss of appetite in twelve. Since coenzyme Q_{10} is neither a protein nor a foreign substance, only rare side effects are to be anticipated.

The best sources of coenzyme Q_{10} are beef and pork. Other good sources include mackerel, salmon, sardines, eggs, wheat germ, spinach, and broccoli. Since the highest concentrations are found in red meats, particularly organ meats, people who avoid these foods, especially cardiac patients, may have a deficiency. Therefore, supplements may be necessary, particularly for the elderly or those on vegetarian diets.

I personally take between 90 and 180 mg of coenzyme Q_{10} per day. I take the vitamin for several reasons: to bolster my immunity, prevent the oxidation of LDL, and to improve my allergies.

My experience with my patients has also been extremely rewarding. To this date, I have placed over 10,000 patients on coenzyme Q_{10} therapy. I also have recommended the nutrient for several patients with cardiac arrhythmias who were reluctant to take standard antiarrhythmic drugs because of persistent side effects. One patient who suffered from a panic disorder was continuously plagued by cardiac irregularities. It was not uncommon for him to go to the emergency room because of an irregular heartbeat. After adding coenzyme Q_{10}, vitamins, and herbs to his diet, the problem diminished. For hundreds of patients with congestive heart failure, the addition of this coenzyme had a considerable impact on their quality of life. Many other patients with high blood pressure have been able to lower their doses of medication with the addition of coenzyme Q_{10}. Some were even able to discontinue all their hypertension medications during treatment.

Thus, in the cardiovascular patient, coenzyme Q_{10} may serve as a valuable adjunct therapy, with minimal risk of any side effects. In addition to the treatment of heart disease, it may have beneficial effects in cancer and obesity, as well as immunodeficiency disorders. It is also interesting to note that coenzyme Q_{10} has been officially approved by the ministry of health in Japan and is on the formulary in all Japanese hospitals. It is also on the formulary at Manchester Memorial Hospital in Connecticut.

Coenzyme Q_{10} on the hospital formulary was extremely important for one elderly woman who survived a life-threatening transfer to our facility at her son's request. Her son, a Ph.D. scientist, was wise enough to believe Q_{10} to be his mother's only hope in the face of the failure of traditional medicine. Physicians where she had been on life support for ten days refused to administer Q_{10} because of their lack of knowledge, fear, and bias against nonconventional supplementation.

I treated this woman with 450 mg Q_{10} daily (in her feeding tube), IV magnesium, antioxidants, vitamins, and minerals. Within a few days she was weaned off the ventilator, eventually walking out of the hospital two weeks later. Although the nursing care was outstanding, I credit her recovery to coenzyme Q_{10}. Her son believes so as well.

Since there is overwhelming medical evidence supporting the use of coenzyme Q_{10}, and negligible, if any, risk, my recommendation is that this nutrient be utilized in treating many of the common degenerative, nutritional, and infectious diseases of our day.

So, where can you get coenzyme Q_{10}? And how much does it cost? I was able to find it in perhaps two thirds of the health food stores I visited. When pure coenzyme Q_{10} is purchased in capsules, make sure that it is yellow in color, its natural hue. It is also available in a softgel capsule; its bioavailability will be significantly improved with this type of delivery system.

The price of this supplement varies from one store to the next. The usual cost for fifty 30 mg capsules is approximately $15 to $20. When purchasing coenzyme Q_{10} make sure it has not passed its expiration date.

In summary, coenzyme Q_{10} is an exciting recent medical discovery. It is certainly right up there with antibiotics and insulin. It is a widely prescribed heart medication in Japan, Sweden, Italy, and Denmark.

However, in the United States, coenzyme Q_{10} is not taken seriously by the majority of the medical community.

At the Ninth International Symposium on Coenzyme Q_{10} in Ancona, Italy, in May 1996 (where I lectured on coenzyme Q_{10} and congestive heart failure), approximately two to three hundred physicians and scientists from all over the world presented medicinal as well as biochemical data on coenzyme Q_{10}. However, only a handful were from the United States, indicating the lack of awareness among physicians in this country. At the international level, coenzyme Q_{10} has been held in high esteem for its cardiac-healing capabilities, and it is my hope that eventually this nutrient will be a standard treatment for supporting the heart among American cardiologists.

Nine

Minerals, Botanicals, and Enzymes

G ood nutrition doesn't begin and end with vitamins. Minerals, like vitamins, perform many functions in the body, particularly at the cellular level. Herbs have been used medicinally for centuries, though they are little appreciated by Western medicine today. And enzymes and friendly bacteria help nutrients do their work by enhancing their absorption by the body. While a full discussion of all the different varieties of minerals, botanicals, enzymes, and friendly bacteria is beyond the scope of this book, I will describe some of the most useful ones in this chapter.

MINERALS

Minerals are important components of bone and blood, maintaining healthy nerve and organ function. Minerals are inorganic substances that have their origin in rock formations deep in the earth and eventually erode into soil. The minerals are absorbed from the soil by plants and eventually find their way into the rest of the food chain. Eating whole foods and consuming the skin of vegetables whenever possible instead of peeling them will allow you to receive the full mineral benefit of the foods you eat.

It is important to note that once minerals are absorbed into the human body, they may be in competition with one another. For example, excessive zinc can deplete the body of copper, while high calcium levels may affect magnesium and manganese absorption. We also need to consider that people on high-fiber diets may risk mineral deficiencies when their mineral intake is low or borderline low. Plant foods, especially cereal grains, contain phytate, a binding agent that forms insoluble compounds with certain minerals and thus hinders their absorption. Also, high-fiber diets may decrease the time it takes for food to pass through the intestines, resulting in a decrease in mineral absorption. Thus, high-fiber diets and/or vegetarian diets may require additional mineral supplementation. When taking mineral supplements, it is important to take a multimineral supplement rather than individual minerals, unless recommended by your physician.

Calcium

Calcium is necessary for good bone and tooth development. It also plays a major role in cardiac electrical conduction and in the transmission of impulses through the nerves. Calcium is also necessary for muscle contraction and blood clotting.

Calcium deficiencies may cause muscle cramps, cardiac arrhythmia, brittle nails, tooth decay, and numbness in the arms and legs. The most critical period for adequate calcium intake is in childhood, when the skeleton is developing. The recommended daily intake of calcium for children is 800 to 1,200 mg per day (table 15). It is also crucial for women to make sure to take the RDA of this mineral, since they are at risk for developing osteoporosis, particularly in the postmenopausal period; recently the RDA of calcium has been increased to 1,500 mg for postmenopausal women.

Calcium taken in the diet slows the loss of bone mass associated with aging. Recent evidence indicates that providing calcium supplements to postmenopausal women diminishes the rate of bone mass loss both with and without accompanying hormone replacement. Whatever their age, both women and men should aim to meet the recommended dietary allowance of calcium.

The absorption of calcium depends on several factors. Usually only 20 to 30 percent of the calcium taken in through our diet is absorbed into the blood. Caffeine may limit its absorption. Foods grown in calcium-deficient soil may also not have enough calcium present to be absorbed.

The best sources of calcium include dairy products, seafood, green leafy vegetables (except lettuce), asparagus, broccoli, cabbage, molasses, and sea vegetables (table 16). Sea vegetables are among the richest sources of calcium and magnesium in the world. One ounce of wakame (a type of seaweed), for example, has approximately the same amount of calcium as eight ounces of milk. Other wonderful sources of calcium include figs, dates, parsley, prunes, and sesame seeds. Utilizing sesame seeds as an accent in our foods is extremely healthful. Sesame seeds can be used in marinades for fish or chicken as well as in salads or on a bowl of rice. One cup of sesame seeds has as much calcium as three cups of milk.

Cheeses also provide tremendous amounts of calcium, but they are also a major source of fat. Cream cheese, for example, provides significant quantities of calcium (8 to 10 percent of the RDA) but also has approximately 10 to 11 grams of fat per one-ounce serving.

TABLE 15

Recommended Daily Dietary Allowances for Calcium

Population Group	Calcium RDA
Children, 1–10 years old	800 mg
Children and young adults, 11–24 years old	1,200 mg
Adults, 25–50 years old	800 mg
Adult men, 51 years old and older	800 mg
Pregnant and lactating women	1,200 mg
Postmenopausal women	1,500 mg

Food and Nutrition Board, National Academy of Science/National Research Council.

Similarly, ice cream provides abundant calcium but also has considerable fat. Some gourmet ice creams, for example, may contain as much as 34 grams of fat per serving with 150 mg of calcium. Low-fat frozen yogurt, on the other hand, contains very little fat and the same amount of calcium. Skim milk and very low-fat milk products are excellent sources of calcium that do not contain excessive fat. Here again, awareness is necessary. All milk, regardless of whether we are discussing whole milk, 1- or 2-percent milk, or skim milk, provides about 300 mg of calcium per cup.

When taking calcium supplements, it is important to remember to take them in divided doses and before bedtime. Too much calcium, however, can be harmful. Prolonged excessive intake of calcium and vitamin D (in amounts well above the RDA) has been shown to cause hypercalcemia, which can adversely affect one's blood pressure as well as kidney function. It is also important to note that excessive calcium may impair the absorption of magnesium, zinc, and manganese. Calcium supplements should be utilized with caution by anyone with kidney disease or advanced diabetes.

Zinc

Zinc, an essential trace mineral, has many functions. It is most important in supporting the prostate gland and in the growth of the reproductive organs. Patients with diets low in zinc have been found to have an increase in acne and prostatitis. Low levels of the mineral have also been found in individuals with prostate cancer.

Zinc is equally important to the immune response, particularly in the healing of wounds. It is necessary for the absorption and maintenance of vitamin E and the B-complex vitamins, and it plays a key role in helping the body eliminate toxic metals such as aluminum, lead, and excess copper.

Zinc is found in abundance in fish, meats, poultry, and whole grains. Alcohol consumption, diuretics, excess calcium, diarrhea, or eating disorders may lower zinc levels.

Research has shown that a deficiency in zinc may be related to excess fat storage and may contribute to weight gain. In a state of zinc deficiency, sugars may be only partially metabolized, thus leading to their increased availability for conversion to stored fat. In a study of overweight children having low levels of zinc, weight loss was retarded until zinc was supplemented in the diet. Therefore, zinc supplements may be indicated for individuals who remain resistant to weight loss after a thorough medical examination and modification of lifestyle and nutritional habits. I suggest 15 to 30 mg of zinc per day.

TABLE 16

Recommended Foods High in Calcium

Cereals	Nuts and Seeds
Oatmeal	Sesame seeds
Cheeses	*Vegetables*
Feta	Asparagus
★Ricotta, part skim	Broccoli
	Cabbage
Fruits	★Daikon
★Figs	Soybeans
Dates	Turtle beans
Prunes	Collards
Raisins	★Kale
	Kelp
Milk/Yogurt	Parsley
★Skim milk	Wakame
Yogurt, non-fat and low-fat	★Tofu
★1-percent milk	White beans
Other Foods	
Molasses	

★Foods highest in calcium are marked with an asterisk.

Magnesium

Magnesium, along with potassium (which we will discuss next), is extremely important in heart function. Magnesium is involved in over three hundred enzymatic reactions in the body. In the last few years, medical trials have demonstrated that a magnesium deficiency is strongly correlated with multiple medical problems. Low magnesium is one of the most underdiagnosed serum electrolyte abnormalities in clinical practice today. It is a factor in several medical conditions, including insulin-dependent diabetes, heart failure, Crohn's disease, and alcoholism.

Magnesium deficiency is frequently seen in individuals with other electrolyte abnormalities such as low potassium, sodium, and calcium. It is also found in individuals on diuretics as well as in those taking one of a number of commonly prescribed medications for gastrointestinal distress (table 18). In the athlete, magnesium stores may be severely depleted as a result of long-term physical training.

Over the last thirty years, researchers have demonstrated that a deficiency of magnesium can lead to atherosclerosis in animals. Other clinical studies demonstrated that people who consumed hard water—that is, water high in magnesium and calcium—had a lower risk of heart attack. It appears from these clinical studies that magnesium helps protect the heart. In the 1990s, magnesium has become an extremely popular adjunct in the management of patients who have suffered acute heart attacks.

Magnesium deficiency can result in a host of cardiological disorders, including life-threatening arrhythmias, heart muscle disease, and potentially fatal heart attacks (table 17). As a cardiologist, I cannot overemphasize the importance of magnesium. It is well known, for example, that magnesium deficiency will significantly exacerbate the arrhythmias caused by low serum potassium, especially in patients taking an excess of digitalis preparations (digoxin, Lanoxin). Depletion of both potassium and magnesium is commonly present in heart patients, and treatment involves administering both agents.

TABLE 17

Potential Cardiovascular Consequences of
Magnesium Deficiency

- Cardiac arrhythmias (abnormal rhythm)
- Atherosclerosis
- Cardiomyopathy (weakness of the heart muscle)
- Coronary vasospasm (chest pain)
- Heart attack
- Sudden death

In a study conducted in France, the link between magnesium deficiency, free-radical damage, and LDL was established and implies the involvement of magnesium deficiency in hardening of the arteries. As many Americans consume less than the RDA of magnesium, increasing intake of magnesium-rich foods and/or taking supplements may help reduce the risk of marginal deficiency, cardiovascular complications, and even high blood pressure.

Recently the medical literature has also cited low red-blood-cell magnesium levels as a potential cause of chronic fatigue syndrome. This syndrome is characterized by the presence of fatigue for more than six months, impairment of memory and concentration, and a variety of other symptoms such as muscle aches or tenderness, joint pain, headaches, and depression. Although the specific cause remains unknown, a generalized immune deficiency seems to be a major factor. Some viral illnesses have also been known to cause chronic fatigue syndrome. Usually the treatment of such a condition includes rest, alleviation of stress, and vitamin and nutritional therapy. In one study, a group of chronic fatigue syndrome patients was treated with magnesium while another group received placebos. The magnesium-treated patients had improved levels of magnesium in their red blood cells and reported heightened energy levels when compared with the others. Recent data also suggest that magnesium administered intravenously has "cured" migraine headache within minutes up to 50 percent of the time.

In another magnesium study, supplementation was proven to be an effective treatment for the symptoms of premenstrual syndrome. In this double-blind, placebo-controlled study, both pain and mood change were positively affected by oral magnesium preparations.

Magnesium serves as a coenzyme for approximately 80 percent of the enzymes in the body and is the fourth most abundant element in the human body. Researchers believe that magnesium levels may decrease as a result of stress, anxiety, or lack of physical activity. A major factor that contributes to magnesium deficiency, however, is a reduction in available dietary magnesium, due in large part to a low concentration of magnesium in our water and soil. The consumption of overprocessed foods also appears to reduce the amount of magnesium in the diet. In addition, there are numerous medical conditions that produce a net loss of magnesium from the body (table 18).

In the absence of renal disease, magnesium supplements may be taken without fear of adverse reactions. Magnesium chloride is a good choice because it is well absorbed. The best sources of magnesium in the diet are sea vegetables, sesame seeds, figs, green leafy vegetables, fish, meat, seafood, brown rice, soybean products, whole grains, bananas, apricots, nuts, and seeds (table 19). As a supplement, I recommend 140 to 250 mg per day, and for any cardiac patient with or without high blood pressure, at least 400 mg a day.

TABLE 18

Causes of Magnesium Deficiency

1. Excessive Urinary Loss
   Diuretics
   Alcohol abuse
   Diabetic ketoacidosis
   Postobstructive diuresis
   Hypercalcemia
   Syndrome of inappropriate antidiuretic hormone secretion
2. Decrease in Intestinal Absorption
   Prolonged gastrointestinal suction
   Surgical resection of the bowel
   Diarrheal states
   Various bowel diseases
   H-2 receptor antagonist therapy (Tagamet or Zantac)
3. Decreased Intake
   IV therapy inadequate in magnesium
   Protein-caloric malnutrition
   Starvation
   Bulimia

TABLE 19

Recommended Foods High in Magnesium

Cereal and grains	Nuts and Seeds
All-Bran cereal	*Pumpkin seeds
Brown rice	Sesame seeds
	Sunflower seeds
Fish	
All seafood	Vegetables
Fruits	Adzuki beans
	Black beans
*Figs, dried	*Kelp
Apricots	Spinach
Bananas	Wakame

*Foods highest in magnesium are marked with an asterisk.

Magnesium also has one other vital protective function in the body. It helps to counteract aluminum toxicity, which is gaining attention in both the medical and lay literature. A few years ago in England, industrial contamination of the water supply with aluminum caused a small outbreak of central nervous system problems similar to Alzheimer's disease; more recently there has been further evidence suggesting that there is a connection between excessive aluminum in the environment and the development of lesions in the brain associated with Alzheimer's disease. Like many of the other environmental toxins, aluminum may accumulate in the body over a long period, eventually taking its toll on health.

Aluminum is a toxic metal; unfortunately, it is still being used in drugs and cosmetics, baking powder, food additives, and packaging, as well as pots and pans. It is also found in our water. Aluminum has no known benefit to the human body. In addition to the possible connection with Alzheimer's disease, aluminum may cause other central nervous system disturbances as well as enhance the development of osteoporosis.

It makes sense to avoid aluminum as much as possible, particularly since the environment is so overwhelmed by it. My recommendation would be to exchange any aluminum cookware for stainless steel or glass. I recommend avoiding food and beverages that come in aluminum cans. Read labels to avoid compounds containing aluminum, like baking powder. Eat a diet high in fiber and foods that inhibit aluminum absorption, including almonds, spinach, and rhubarb. The B vitamins, particularly B-6, are also recommended. In addition to a high-fiber diet, magnesium, calcium, vitamin C, and zinc are helpful nutrients in counteracting aluminum toxicity.

Potassium

Potassium is a mineral that truly concerns physicians. The effects of either low potassium or high potassium can be life-threatening. Since potassium is necessary to the healthy functioning of nerves, cells, and membranes, it is an important electrolyte to monitor. Low potassium is a major cause of cardiac arrhythmia; diuretics for the treatment of high blood pressure or congestive heart failure may interfere with potassium absorption and excretion. Although potassium supplementation is usually not necessary, individuals on diuretics or laxatives or who have excessive diarrhea may require extra potassium. Caution should be taken, however, in those individuals with renal insufficiency, as additional potassium in these people's diets may not be excreted by the kidneys. You should be able to get all the potassium you need from your diet. The highest levels of potassium are found in sea vegetables, fruits, vegetables, fish, lean meat, poultry, garlic, raisins, bananas, apricots, and whole grains (table 20). Coffee and alcohol may deplete potassium in the body. If you consume these beverages, it is important to maintain a proper potassium intake.

Potassium, calcium, and magnesium deficiencies have all been incriminated in blood pressure elevation. In my natural approach to blood pressure control, adequate supplementation of these minerals is crucial.

TABLE 20

Recommended Foods High in Potassium

Cereals	Lobster
All–Bran	Mackerel
Bran Buds	Mussels
Raisin bran	Perch
	Salmon
Dried Fruits	Snapper
Dates	Sole
*Figs	Swordfish
*Prunes	Trout
*Raisins	Tuna
Fresh Fruits	*Meats and Poultry*
Apricots	Beef rib eye
Bananas	Beef eye round
Cantaloupe	Goose without skin
Nectarines	
	Milk and Yogurt
Fish and Shellfish	Yogurt, non–fat or low–fat
Anchovies	
Bass, freshwater	*Nuts and Seeds*
Bluefish	*Soybean nuts
Catfish	
Clams	*Vegetables*
Crabs, blue	*Avocado
Flounder	Bamboo shoots
Haddock	Beet greens
Halibut	Chickpeas
	Garlic

Potato with skin
Sea vegetables
Sweet potato
Swiss chard

Beans
★Adzuki beans
Black beans

Kidney beans
Lentils
★Lima beans
Pinto beans
Natto (soybean product)
Turtle beans
★White beans

★Foods highest in potassium are marked with an asterisk.

Selenium

As an antioxidant, selenium actively scavenges free radicals. It is important to the immune system and has been regarded as protective against cancer and heart disease. Asia has considerable quantities of selenium in its soil, making the Asian diet rich in the mineral; not surprisingly, cancer and heart disease occur considerably less often in Asian cultures than in the West. Studies have shown that people who consume selenium, whether in food or in supplement form, develop fewer cancers, particularly of the breast, colon, and prostate.

In the United States, there is an inverse relationship between rates of breast cancer and selenium content in the soil. For example, Ohio tends to have the highest incidence of breast cancer and the lowest amounts of selenium in the soil. Conversely, the Dakotas have the highest soil concentrations of selenium and a lower incidence of breast cancer.

A selenium-rich diet has been proven in animal studies to reduce skin tumors when these animals were exposed to massive doses of ultraviolet light. The results seem to indicate that increasing selenium intake may significantly reduce the risk of developing UV-induced skin cancer.

When combined with vitamin E or coenzyme Q_{10}, selenium's efficacy is much greater, making it a very powerful antioxidant. This type of synergy was suggested in a small-scale study of heart attack patients. Those patients receiving a combination of selenium and coenzyme Q_{10} had a better index of survival one year following their heart attack. The data were gathered from sixty-one patients during the year following their heart attacks. Six patients (20 percent) of the control group died of repeat heart attacks, while only one patient (3 percent) died from the group taking the selenium/coenzyme Q_{10} combination. Although this was only a limited sample, it does suggest the cardiovascular protective possibilities of coenzyme Q_{10} and selenium.

Selenium also protects against environmental pollutants such as lead and cadmium and can help mitigate the toxic effects of mercury, which is prevalent in dental fillings, cosmetics, pesticides, and saltwater fish, particularly tuna and swordfish. Prominent sources of selenium include fish, sea vegetables, whole grains, wheat germ, garlic, onions, chicken, brown rice, and broccoli. There are no known side effects at levels less than 300 mcg per day. The recommended daily dose of selenium is approximately 50 to 200 mcg per day.

Iron

Iron, in simple terms, is essential for the production of hemoglobin, which is found in red blood cells. Since iron is the mineral most prevalent in blood, a lack of it causes anemia. Deficiencies in iron result in symptoms such as fatigue, pallor, and dizziness. Other symptoms of a lack of iron include brittle hair, hair loss, and ridging of the nails.

Several factors influence the amount of iron absorbed in the diet. A degree of hydrochloric acid (natural stomach acid) must be present in the stomach in order for iron to be absorbed. Vitamin C can also increase iron absorption by as much as 30 percent. Iron absorption can be decreased by antacids, aspirin, caffeine, and some food preservatives.

The most common cause of iron deficiency results from bleeding, either through the gastrointestinal tract or through excessive menstrual bleeding. Iron deficiency is more likely to occur in rapidly growing teenagers as well as menstruating women. Iron supplementation is recommended in pregnancy as well as in cases of chronic blood loss. The RDA for iron is 10 mg per day for men and postmenopausal women and 18 mg per day for nonmenopausal women. Since we can obtain much of the iron we need from our diet, it is not recommended that healthy men and postmenopausal women take iron supplements. Young women, however, could benefit from taking iron on a daily basis, especially when pregnant.

Iron overload can go unnoticed and may be quite insidious in its onset. Since iron is stored in the body, excessive iron taken over a considerable period of time can cause problems, particularly in the liver, heart, and pancreas. Individuals who ingest considerable quantities of iron in their drinking water in addition to taking iron supplements may develop headaches, shortness of breath, and fatigue—symptoms of iron overload. Using iron cookware is yet another source by which one can ingest additional amounts of iron. Earlier I discussed with you the cautious use of excess vitamin C in situations of iron overload. If your serum iron and other iron indices are elevated, you need to be careful about ingesting iron and vitamin C. It is best to see your physician if you are in doubt about the iron stores in your body.

The best sources of iron include sea vegetables, green leafy vegetables, whole grains, lean meats, eggs, poultry, dates, prunes, beans, lentils, parsley, peaches, raisins, brown rice, molasses, and sesame seeds.

TABLE 21

Recommended Foods High in Iron

Cereals and Grains	*Fruits*
Oatmeal	*Figs, dried
Bran Buds cereal	Peaches
Bran flakes	Prunes
Product 19 cereal	Dates
Brown rice	Raisins

Fish	*Nuts and Seeds*
Clams	Sesame seeds
Oysters	Pumpkin seeds, dried

Vegetables	*Miscellaneous*
Artichokes	Eggs
Chickpeas	Lean meats (including steak
Great Northern beans	and poultry)
Kidney beans	*Prune juice (best for iron)
Lentils	Sea vegetables
Lima beans	
Spinach	
Tofu	
Turtle beans	
White beans	

*Foods highest in iron are marked with an asterisk.

Iodine

Iodine is especially important in the healthy functioning of the thyroid gland. It calms the body and relieves nervous tension. Although it is needed only in trace amounts, iodine deficiencies can occur, particularly if drinking water is chlorinated. If too little iodine is taken in the diet, it affects the nervous system. Some of the possible signs of deficiency are the inability to think clearly, irritability, and difficulty sleeping. Iodine deficiency may also result from soil that does not have sufficient iodine. The best sources of iodine include sea vegetables, saltwater fish, Swiss chard, watercress, turnip greens, mushrooms, bananas, cabbage, and onions.

Mineral Supplements and You

There are many important minerals that the body utilizes in normal functioning. Many of these are trace elements that are extremely useful for the everyday functioning of the body. Because of this, many manufacturers produce supplements that contain combinations of minerals. While I am quite impressed by the quality and complexity of the formulas and delivery systems of many of these supplements, quite a number contain questionably large amounts of metals such as iron and copper.

Although some manufacturers do not place iron in their formulas because of its oxidant properties, many multivitamin and mineral preparations do include, in my opinion, excessive quantities of iron. Naturally, if iron supplementation is required for iron deficiency anemia or in menstruating or pregnant women, then it could be taken without any undue side effects. However, since iron, as we previously mentioned, is stored in the body and accumulates over time, it is one mineral that should not be consumed unless prescribed by a physician. In my view, men who don't have any evidence of chronic blood loss should not take any iron unless it is clearly demonstrated that they are iron deficient.

Copper is another oxidant that should be limited to small quantities. The RDA for copper is 2 mg per day. Although copper is needed to make red blood cells, we tend to get all the copper we need from our drinking water, as it usually travels through copper pipes in our schools, homes, and workplaces. Frequently multivitamin and mineral preparations will include copper in their formulas. Although I am not recommending that you stay away from such formulas, keep in mind that, as with iron, an overconsumption of copper could occur. Therefore I recommend you choose vitamin and mineral formulas that are devoid of these metals or contain much less than the RDA requirements.

BOTANICALS

For centuries herbs have been used for medicinal purposes. The Chinese have long believed that certain plants support good health and prolong life. Present-day Europeans use many herbal remedies to treat illnesses such as the common cold. Unfortunately, medicine in the United States has a different approach to herbs. In most medical schools in this country, the herbal remedies of Asian and European societies are simply not taught.

For example, the only medicinal herbs I learned about in medical school were the flowering foxglove plant, which is a source of the heart medication digitalis, and rauwolfia, the source of a medication used to control high blood pressure. Most other medicinal herbs were not given any credibility, despite the fact that many common pharmaceuticals originated from plants and barks. Herbal treatment was belittled and even scorned. Nevertheless, as my comfort level with botanicals grew, I decided to use them in my practice.

There is a large volume of literature on the medicinal properties of plants and herbs. My purpose in this brief section is to raise your awareness about how to use botanicals as an alternative or adjunctive path in health and healing. I will discuss the healing properties of two other botanicals: onions and garlic, in chapter fourteen, entitled "Nutritional Healing for the Year 2001."

Ginger

Since my youngest son is often plagued with motion sickness, I tried countless cures for nausea in an attempt to relieve his symptoms. Eventually I found ginger to be the most effective remedy. This discovery has also helped my patients. Many of them suffer from nausea and vomiting as a result of heart attacks, coronary artery bypass surgery, or medications.

I have used ginger tea in coronary care units, my office, and my home. Creating a tea infusion is perhaps the oldest form of preparing herbal remedies. The recipe for ginger tea is quite simple. You can buy ginger root in any supermarket. Take about a one-inch segment of the root and slice it into thin pieces and add boiling water. Let it steep for approximately half an hour and add some honey and freshly squeezed lemon. You will be amazed how your nausea, indigestion, and even vomiting will cease after a few cups of tea.

In addition to its use for digestive disorders, ginger has long been touted as an immune system stimulant. It also thins the blood, relieves symptoms of PMS, and may have favorable impact on cholesterol as well.

Cayenne

Cayenne, or capsicum, comes from the fruit of the red pepper plant. Cayenne is cultivated all over the world. My first exposure to the medicinal use of cayenne was its role in preventing the oxidation of harmful LDL.

In addition to having a favorable impact on cholesterol, capsicum will also increase one's energy and has proven quite effective in relieving the symptoms of arthritis. In both my cholesterol-lowering program and my natural healing program for arthritis, I include cayenne as a phytonutrient. This botanical also contains valuable vitamins and minerals such as vitamin C, beta carotene, and sulfur.

I use cayenne externally as an effective painkiller. Patients with herpes zoster, a viral neuromuscular affliction that causes terrible discomfort, often benefit from the external use of cayenne. Patients may report irritation and pain at the site of application, but prolonged exposure deadens the nerves to pain and provides significant relief. Therefore, I always tell my patients that capsicum will at first stimulate and then inhibit the flow of pain from the skin and membranes. Capsaicin ointment can be obtained from pharmacies in various strengths. Begin at the lowest (.025 percent), and increase if needed to the .075 dose.

It is important to note that taking cayenne internally (40,000 heat units) may cause stomach irritation. The remedy for such an occurrence, either from food or from supplementation, is to eat bread or other starches.

Gotu Kola

Gotu kola is a quick-acting herb that comes from a medicinal plant popular in Pakistan, India, and Ceylon and is used for the treatment of fatigue. In Ceylon it is considered a brain food and is reported to stimulate the memory. I once sat on a plane next to an anesthesiologist from India. He saw me reading about gotu kola and told me that this plant is often used as a tea in his country, primarily for enhancing memory and rejuvenating energy. Gotu kola contains no caffeine.

Studies have also demonstrated that gotu kola is effective in treating inflammation and in stimulating the immune system. Gotu kola contains chemicals called saponins, which inhibit the growth of harmful bacteria.

Consequently, gotu kola has been an important remedy in the ancient Indian medicinal tradition called ayurveda and today is held in high esteem by herbalist physicians all over the world.

Ginseng

Over the years I have become more comfortable with the medicinal use of ginseng. Ginseng is a small leafy plant with a taproot system. The roots of both wild and cultivated plants contain the ginsenosides—the active ingredients that contain medicinal properties. As ginseng is cultivated all over the world, including the United States and Asia, there has been much confusion about its many varieties. For example, Siberian ginseng (*Eleutherococcus senticosus*) grows abundantly in parts of Russia, Korea, China, and Japan. Its distribution is actually far greater than its cousin, *Panax schinseng,* which is also referred to as Korean or Chinese ginseng. *Panax schinseng* is also related to the American ginseng, *Panax quinquefolius.* American ginseng (white) is considered less stimulating than the Asian varieties (red). The chemical constituents of Panax schinseng have been known to stimulate the immune system, leading to improved resistance to infections. Its biological name, *Panax schinseng,* is appropriate, since it originates from the word "panacea," which comes from the Greek words "pan" and "akos," or cure-all.

Both *Panax schinseng* and Siberian ginseng are believed to function as adaptogens. The Russian pharmacologist Brekman stated that an adaptogen is an innocuous substance that has nonspecific action and increases resistance to adverse forces on the body. It has been used for centuries as a general body tonic to alleviate physical and mental exhaustion. Chinese folklore also indicates that ginseng helps to restore sexual vitality by replacing lost life energy, or "chi." The Chinese believe that the regular use of Siberian ginseng will improve the general health of humans by improving circulatory and kidney function as well as lowering serum cholesterol. Ginseng has also been used to regulate blood pressure; however, some paradoxical effects have been observed when dosage is varied.

Since there is no quality control on ginseng products marketed in the United States, there can be considerable variation in their chemical constituents, that is, the ginsenosides. This may result in almost no medicinal effect or even a toxic reaction. Other ginseng products are also marketed with nutrients such as germanium. I would not take this combination product, as toxicity has been reported with it. Ginseng toxicity may result in insomnia, diarrhea, high blood pressure, and nervousness. Thus, when taking ginseng you must exercise some caution. Report any side effects to your physician. Do not drink coffee or tea when taking ginseng. Like echinacea extract, ginseng should not be taken on a continuous basis but rather on an on-off basis, such as two weeks on and two weeks off. Ginseng preparations can be purchased in most health food stores.

Wild Yam Extract

Another agent with the potential to enhance libido and psychological well-being is wild yam extract (*Dioscorea villosa*). Wild yam extract is a precursor of DHEA (dehydroepiandrosterone), the "mother" steroid of the body. The use of DHEA has been gaining increasing popularity recently. Current studies have demonstrated that low DHEA levels in younger men may be an indicator of myocardial risk. Evidence in the cardiological literature has demonstrated an increased risk of heart attacks in men with low DHEA levels. This suggests that higher levels of DHEA may offer protection against heart disease. Although it requires a medical research license to prescribe DHEA in this country, wild yam extract is a form of DHEA that can be purchased without a prescription in most health food stores. Usually 500 mg of wild yam extract is the equivalent of 5 mg of DHEA.

The use of wild yams for medicinal purposes dates back to ancient times. Natives in New Guinea, for example, celebrated the wild yam harvest. Prestige and authority were bestowed upon tribesmen who grew the largest yams. These tribesmen practiced visualization techniques to increase the size of their yams and even used magic to cause rival tribesmen's yams to shrivel!

Hawthorn Berry

Hawthorn berry is another herb that I frequently use in my cardiology practice. Although hawthorn has been used medicinally for centuries, in the last one hundred years it has become increasingly popular as a remedy for various cardiac problems. In fact, European physicians often prescribe hawthorn as a substitute for digitalis, perhaps the most popular medicine in the United States for enhancing the contractility of a weakened heart. However, the herbal properties of hawthorn far exceed this indication.

Hawthorn is a shrub that is often grown as a hedge. Its leaves, berries, and blossoms contain powerful flavonoids and proanthocyanidins as well as a host of other phytonutrients with health-promoting effects. Its chemical nature is very complex, so for this discussion I will focus on the flavonoid components' contribution to health. Remember, flavonoids are a group of flavone-containing compounds that include many of the colorful plant pigments that are found widely in nature. Plant pigments such as bioflavonols, proanthocyanidins, and anthoxanthins are but a few of the compounds that are included in the flavonoid group. These chemical plant pigments can exert a wide variety of physiological and medicinal effects on the human body. They also possess tremendous free-radical scavenging activity that protects the heart and the rest of the vascular system from the harmful effects of free radicals.

The cardiovascular benefit of hawthorn is especially noteworthy. Studies have indicated that hawthorn exhibits vasodilatory reaction, which means that it increases blood flow in the blood vessels. Thus, hawthorn may be helpful in preventing the cramping sensation in the chest that cardiologists frequently refer to as angina.

The mechanism of action of hawthorn is complex. It acts like the class of blood pressure medications known as ACE inhibitors that doctors frequently prescribe. It is the bioflavonoid activity of hawthorn that can inhibit angiotensin-converting enzymes (ACE)—the enzymes responsible for creating angiotensin 2, which is a very potent constrictor of blood vessels (causing an increase in blood pressure). Some studies have shown that the proanthocyanidins found in hawthorn are similar to the drug called captopril (Capoten), a popular medication prescribed by many cardiologists to lower blood pressure. Since hawthorn acts as an ACE inhibitor, its natural blood-pressure-lowering ability is quite unique.

Since hawthorn extracts contain proanthocyanidins comparable to grapeseed or pine bark extract, a variety of additional health benefits arise from its use; for example, it interferes with the oxidation of LDL, thereby impacting cholesterol effects. Hawthorn has also had a long history of being a particularly useful agent in the treatment of congestive heart failure.

In summary, hawthorn has many clinical applications that include the treatment of atrial fibrillation, digitalis enhancement, blood pressure reduction, atherosclerosis prevention, and heart failure improvement. It has been used widely and successfully in Europe for the last hundred years.

Hawthorn can be taken as a tea, in a tincture, or in capsule/tablet form. The dose I usually use is one 500 mg capsule one to three times per day. Since hawthorn has wide applicability and no major adverse side effects, this herb should be considered by more cardiologists. Small doses should be administered when using the herb with digitalis, since it can enhance the action of this drug. In hawthorn's long clinical history, there have been no reported toxic reactions. Similarly, in the animal literature, hawthorn has not demonstrated any significant toxicity.

Ginkgo

In western Europe ginkgo is perhaps the most popular herbal medication on the market, with doctors writing millions of prescriptions annually. The leaves of the ginkgo tree have been used for medicinal purposes for the last five thousand years. European studies demonstrate that ginkgo not only improves memory, but also enhances mental alertness. I use it to help patients who suffer from memory loss, depression, and ringing in the ears. The active compounds in ginkgo include kaempferol, bilobalide, and quercetin.

Ginkgo biloba increases blood flow in deprived areas, particularly the inner ear and the macula, where it may have an effect on macular degeneration. In addition to its ability to counteract free-radical damage and inhibit blood clotting, ginkgo may have some ability to assuage Alzheimer's disease, although there have been no definitive studies demonstrating this effect. No toxicity from ginkgo has been reported in the literature, even after prolonged treatment.

Echinacea

Echinacea is another herb I frequently recommend. Echinacea is one of the many coneflowers, a group of native American wildflowers in the sunflower family. There are nine species, but *Echinacea angustifolia, Echinacea purpurea,* and *Echinacea pallida* are the most commonly used. Since it provides the most active range of medicinal chemical compounds, *Echinacea purpurea* is used more often than the other two species mentioned above.

Used widely by Native Americans to treat a host of ailments, echinacea has a reputation for healing venomous bites from both spiders and snakes. When combined with the herb goldenseal, echinacea has been very effective in stimulating the immune response. Both of these herbs can increase the number of T cells in the body, thus bolstering the immune system.

I have found echinacea, goldenseal, and garlic, as well as other botanicals, quite helpful in enhancing immunity. Echinacea is the perfect choice for colds and flu because it assists the body in the production of white blood cells and interferon, two substances capable of increasing the body's defenses to infection. I use echinacea myself and have given it to my children when they had infections and flu-like illnesses. European studies have demonstrated that doses of up to 900 mg of echinacea significantly relieve cold and flu-like symptoms. A combination of echinacea and other botanicals also relieves inflammation. Although prednisone and other corticosteroids effectively reduce inflammation following coronary artery bypass surgery, they can also cause considerable side effects when used for several weeks; to avoid these side effects, I prefer to treat chest cavity inflammation with a combination of botanical agents and occasionally add a low dose of prednisone.

Echinacea is most potent when taken for limited periods of time. Because its immune-enhancing effect may diminish after prolonged use, it should not be used daily or on a long-term basis. It is important to give the body a "rest period." The usual recommended time frame is six to eight weeks followed by one to two weeks off. For more progressive systemic diseases such as tuberculosis, and for autoimmune disorders such as lupus, severe rheumatoid arthritis, and multiple sclerosis, echinacea should probably not be used.

Astragalus
Astragalus is another ancient Chinese herb that is frequently combined with ginseng to strengthen the body's natural defenses, namely, the immune system. Astragalus has also shown some vasodilatory as well as anti-inflammatory action. Its anti-inflammatory effects occur, it seems, because it inhibits the release of histamines from mast cells. Quercetin, a polyphenol, works the same way. Consequently, astragalus could help relieve hay fever and other allergic conditions. I have personally used astragalus as a remedy for my seasonal hay fever.

In China, astragalus has also been used to treat cancer. It enhances the body's natural defense functions by stimulating the responsiveness of T cells.

Chamomile, Myrrh Gum, and Fenugreek
Three other botanicals I use are chamomile, myrrh gum, and fenugreek. Chamomile is heralded in Europe as a cure-all. Its gentle action makes it safe for use by both children and adults. It has calming, antispasmodic, and even anti-inflammatory effects. In my own household, when one of us has trouble sleeping, we drink a cup of chamomile tea. It may also be

used for indigestion and headache, or in a steam inhalation for sinusitis. Chamomile blossoms contain chamazulene, which is responsible for the herb's anti-inflammatory action. It has also been used topically and is an ingredient in many facial and hair-care preparations. Compresses of chamomile may bring relief in a variety of irritating skin conditions such as eczema, sunburn, and even diaper rash.

Myrrh gum, prized as a valuable herb since biblical times, was presented as a gift (along with gold and frankincense) by one of the wise men to the Christ child. It contains volatile oils ideally suited for promoting easier breathing during congestive colds and for clearing out mucus-clogged nasal passages. Long noted for its antiseptic and healing properties, myrrh gum was used in ancient Greece to treat wounds. It has also been used in oral preparations to tone the gums and to prevent tooth decay. Mixed with witch hazel, a tincture of myrrh may be applied to cold sores. It has even been mixed with water for an antiseptic douche.

Fenugreek may affect cholesterol in a manner similar to pectin. European cultures also use it as an important remedy in cases of diabetes. Traditionally, fenugreek has been widely used, particularly in the Middle East, to expel excess mucus from the respiratory and digestive systems.

ENZYME REPLACEMENT THERAPY

Enzyme replacement therapy can play an important role in your program for optimum health. Although there is much truth in the expression "You are what you eat," even truer is the statement "You are what you absorb."

For cells to absorb and distribute nutrients to the body, food must first be properly digested. Unfortunately, some of the compounds in food may not be digested well by the body's endogenous enzyme system. For example, the complex sugars (oligosaccharides) contained in beans or cruciferous vegetables may not be completely broken down in the body. These complex sugars pass down into the large intestine, where they are then acted upon by the normal endogenous, but not so friendly bacteria, *E. coli*. The metabolic by-products of this functional maldigestion/malabsorption are the gases carbon dioxide, hydrogen, and methane. Even eating only small quantities of these complex oligosaccharides may produce considerable waste gas. This may cause cramping, discomfort, and flatulence. It is no wonder, then, that beans, Brussels sprouts, broccoli, cabbage, cauliflower, and other vegetables are avoided by some individuals. In addition, bacterial action on undigested food in the colon may produce toxic metabolites that could even prove to be carcinogenic.

Fortunately, modern technology has developed enzyme systems that are able to convert the offending complex sugars into simple, more digestible sugars such as galactose, fructose, and glucose, which can be absorbed in the small intestine. Laboratory tests have shown that various enzymes can convert large, undigestible sugars into smaller sugars, resulting in better absorption and digestion. You can find compounds to break down carbohydrates (Carbozyme and Digezyme), as well as those that break down protein (Aminozyme), in health food stores.

OUR BACTERIAL BODIES

In addition to inefficient enzyme systems, there are many conditions that disturb the delicate workings of the gastrointestinal tract. Individuals complaining of long-standing constipation, diarrhea, or irritable bowel syndrome, or those with pancreatic disease, gallbladder disease, or inflammatory bowel conditions (with and without diverticulosis or hemorrhoids) may have disturbed gastrointestinal function. In addition, there are other factors that contribute to the maldigestion/malabsorption syndrome, including the use of antibiotics, birth control pills, corticosteroids, processed foods, and continuous overuse of the same foods. One way to enhance the health of the gastrointestinal tract is by supplementing it with "friendly bacteria." Regular use of friendly bacteria such as lactobacilli and bifidobacteria not only will improve digestive health, but also will protect against infections by fungi and other, less friendly bacteria. In addition, these bacteria can increase the absorption of calcium.

Increasing our body's supply of lactic bacteria is one important step toward optimum health. Lactic bacteria are single-cell organisms that may occur alone, in pairs, or in short chains. These organisms have the ability to transform sugar into lactic acid. They play a significant role in the production of fermented milk, yogurt, and some cheeses. By eating yogurt (particularly yogurt cultured with acidophilus), sourdough bread, and sauerkraut, you encourage the growth of lactic bacteria in the intestine. Supplements containing lactobacilli, acidophilus, and bifidobacteria could also be taken.

CHAPTER
Ten

Women and
Children First

Off the coast of Newfoundland on a cold and dark night, the
phrase "Women and children first" echoed through the frigid
night air. The *Titanic* was sinking. While most of the men on
board the luxury liner perished with the "unsinkable" ship, many women
and children survived, their lives placed above all other concerns in the
face of crisis. Sadly, in the 1990s, with many facing social and economic
crisis, women and children have not been made a priority when it comes
to health, nutrition, and overall welfare.

THE SPECIAL NUTRITIONAL NEEDS
OF CHILDREN

Children are extremely vulnerable to nutritional deficiencies, especially
during their years of most active growth. More and more children are
consuming unhealthy processed foods full of additives, preservatives, and
sweeteners. In addition, the fast-food industry has promoted eating habits
in children (and busy adults) that provide them with too much fat and too
few nutrients. Studies show that many schoolchildren, particularly of
elementary-school age, take in dangerously low levels of important nutrients, even less than the RDA.

In March 1995, the American Health Foundation reported alarming findings on the health of children between the grades of two through six. In this study, based on the results of questionnaires surveying 3,112 children, results showed that American adults are doing a disappointing job of educating youngsters in healthy ways of living. Of the children polled:

- Twenty-four percent had eaten no fruit and twenty-five percent had eaten no vegetables the day before the survey.
- Fifteen percent of the children believed cheese was a good source of fiber.
- Forty-eight percent believed apple juice was higher in fat than whole milk.
- Thirty-six percent of the children surveyed believed watermelon had more fat than American cheese.

This study confirms that bad habits as well as good ones may begin early. Education is the key to proper nutrition, for both parents and children.

There is growing concern that many children may be deficient in vitamins B, C, and E as well as iron, calcium, and zinc. A poor diet of fast food, canned or frozen foods (convenience foods), and microwaved meals, not simply the status quo of the financially challenged, but often prepared by busy career parents who would rather "pick something up on the way home," is conducive to such imbalance. In a report published in the *Journal of the American Diabetic Association,* children exhibited serious deficiencies in folic acid and vitamin B-6. Symptoms such as allergies, fatigue, low motivation, skin problems, short attention spans, and low social and academic interest in youths may be the product of vitamin and mineral deficiencies. The National Cancer Institute recommends at least five to nine servings of fresh fruits and vegetables daily, yet statistics have shown 40 percent of Americans—including children—do not get even one serving per day!

It is no secret that most children would stand firm on going to bed without supper rather than eat their spinach. As a result, physicians and researchers have suggested that a multiple vitamin is good insurance for growing children. Zinc, for example, is needed for growth and sexual development. Folic acid is crucial during the neonatal stages, as well as throughout adolescence. Iron is also important, with an estimated 5 percent of children between five and eight years old and 2.5 percent of adolescents (not to mention a tragic 25 percent of pregnant teenagers) affected by iron deficiency. Iron deficiency also occurs frequently in young female athletes. An increase in iron levels can be achieved by including foods high in vitamin C or consuming a glass of orange or tomato juice with every meal. Taking an iron supplement is of course helpful.

To meet the needs of a growing body, children should receive an ample supply of iron. Standard children's vitamin and mineral supplements often include small doses of iron. Caution is required, however, in dispensing iron to children, as several deaths have been attributed to iron overdose in young people. A typical overdose scenario involves a young child tampering with adult (especially women's formula) vitamins, which typically contain high levels of iron. Since only a few tablets can cause fatal shock in very young children, it is absolutely essential that parents keep any iron supplements as well as adult multivitamin and mineral preparations away from children. Also, children's chewable vitamins, made to resemble and taste like candy, have proven a dangerous temptation to small children.

Despite these concerns, parents can safely give their children vitamin and mineral supplements, providing that the formula does not contain more than the RDA of iron appropriate for the child's age. In addition to supplements, parents can certainly give their children foods naturally high in iron, such as prune juice, organic raisins, or juices like V-8 vegetable cocktail.

One way to improve a poor diet is through targeted nutritional supplements. For small children, I believe strongly in multivitamin and mineral preparations, preferably chewable and made without artificial colors, preservatives, sugars, or oils. Since young children often do not consume the amounts of fresh fruits and vegetables they need, vitamin preparations based on natural food sources, such as alfalfa, chlorella, green barley, wheat grass, carrots, spinach, and kale, are preferred. A varied diet, consisting of a balanced supply of protein, carbohydrates, and healthy fats, with minimal amounts of sugar, fast foods, and processed foods, will help provide a sound nutritional base for a growing child.

Many parents are unaware of the inadequate or even harmful eating habits of their children. For example, school-prepared lunches, which often contain significant amounts of cheese, other dairy products, and processed meats, perpetuate a junk-food lifestyle. Many schools have vending machines full of salty, fatty, and synthetic-filled snacks and sugary sodas, or sell ice cream and sweets like brownies or cakes as desserts.

Drinking too many carbonated beverages, high in phosphoric acid, can literally remove calcium from the bones. Since increasing sodas usually means skipping milk, children, especially females, run the increased risk of bone fractures.

In response to this information, many patients have asked me if their children need vitamin and mineral supplements, or even herbs for that matter. I would not hesitate to recommend ginger, garlic, and echinacea for children, nor do I have any reservations about giving children natural vitamin and mineral supplements. In addition to a healthy diet that includes fresh fruit and vegetables, it makes good sense to consider targeted nutritional supplementation for every growing child and their moms too.

WOMEN AND HEART DISEASE: SPECIAL RISKS AND SPECIAL NEEDS

I worry about the fact that most women do not get the type of care they need to prevent and treat heart disease. It has been established that in many large-scale clinical trials, women have been underrepresented. Data on the incidence and course of heart disease have been obtained from large groups of men and then applied to women. Why? Unfortunately, heart disease has not been regarded as a major health risk for women until recently.

The fact is, however, that cardiovascular disease is the leading killer of American women. Although most women fear breast cancer as their number one threat, death from heart disease occurs a staggering five times more often than death from breast cancer.

It is estimated that 50 percent of all American women will die of cardiovascular disease, such as a stroke or heart attack. Despite this high incidence of heart disease, data seem to indicate that misdiagnosis, underdiagnosis, and lack of effective treatment are major problems affecting women today. Recent research indicates that women differ from men not only in terms of risk assessment, but also in the treatment they receive for cardiovascular problems. Most cardiologists continue to treat women less effectively and aggressively than they treat men, sometimes with catastrophic results. Because heart disease is considered a male-oriented phenomenon, physicians have sometimes failed to diagnose coronary artery disease in female patients. However, since World War II, when women began to more and more assume the additional stresses of careers, strenuous labor, raising families while working, and the relaxation of society's views of women smoking and drinking, the statistics for heart disease and hypertension for women have increased with each decade.

For example, if a forty-five-year-old woman was brought to an emergency room with chest pains, and a forty-five-year-old man came in with similar complaints, most physicians would admit the male and presume he was experiencing cardiac distress but presume the woman's problem was caused by stress and anxiety. Many physicians have been trained to regard cardiovascular disease as a low probability for women. However, in the perimenopausal and postmenopausal woman, nothing is further from the truth: The number of coronary events quadruples as women approach middle age.

Studies also indicate that women who are hospitalized with coronary artery disease are given fewer diagnostic and therapeutic procedures than their male peers. Women also experience higher rates of complication. Even before surgery takes place, women undergoing coronary bypass surgery may be at a disadvantage due to delayed diagnosis, causing the postoperative mortality rate for female bypass surgery patients to be almost twice that of men. Postoperatively, women also experience higher instances of congestive heart failure, psychosocial impairment, and lower symptomatic relief.

Because of the smaller size of their coronary vessels, women also endure more complications with coronary artery angioplasty. These are only some of the many significant clinical differences between male and female cardiac patients. If equal diagnostic criteria and evaluation procedures were applied to both female and male patients, there could be lowered risks of misdiagnostic or late diagnostic complications.

In preventive cardiology, risk factor modifications also differ according to sex. Consider the following:

1. Risks from diabetes are higher for women than they are for men.
2. Risks from being overweight are higher for women than they are for men.
3. Women have a higher risk than men if they have high triglycerides.
4. Women have a higher risk than men if they have low levels of HDL.

Clinical research has shown that the incidence of diabetes and its complications is much higher in women. Diabetes increases the risk of heart disease five to seven times in women, compared to only two to three times in men. This simple fact alone should raise the eyebrows of any reputable cardiologist evaluating suspected heart disease in diabetic women.

ONLY YOU CAN PREVENT HEART DISEASE

How can a woman prevent the onset of heart disease? For all women, proper heartsense includes reducing the risk of diabetes by increasing physical activity and maintaining ideal body weight. Recent studies report that being a mere twenty pounds overweight correlates with a two-fold increase in risk of heart disease in women. It is absolutely essential for women to understand the potentially dangerous combination of risk factors that render them vulnerable to heart disease: being slightly to severely overweight and having low HDL and high triglyceride levels.

High triglyceride levels appear to be a more significant risk factor in women than in men. Among diabetics, as triglyceride levels rise, cardiovascular risks increase approximately three times in men but an alarming two hundred times in women. The interpretation of other cholesterol fractions also requires gender-specific consideration.

Cholesterol levels have been a major issue of interest among cardiologists in treating and preventing cardiovascular disease. Much of the research has focused on high levels of LDL (low-density lipoprotein) as a major risk factor in coronary artery disease. LDL is a risk factor because of its tendency to become oxidized in the blood. Oxidized LDL is injurious to blood vessels; it results in plaque formation and a decreased diameter of blood vessels, leading to the symptoms of heart disease, or ultimately, heart attack. From research conducted on male patients, high LDL has been proven to be a powerful risk factor for heart disease. In women, however, it appears that low levels of HDL (high-density lipoprotein) is a much stronger risk factor. HDL functions as a scavenger lipoprotein that helps prevent LDL from doing its damage.

It is important for your physician to know these differences concerning HDL and LDL in women. Why? Because the cholesterol-lowering strategies of many pharmacologic therapeutic agents on the market have different interactions and certainly different implications in women. Heartsense strategies in women should focus not only on lowering LDL, but also on enhancing other means of raising HDL, such as exercising and maintaining ideal body weight.

Hormone Replacement Therapy (HRT)

Another important risk-reducing strategy to consider is hormone re-placement therapy (HRT). This has become a highly controversial and important topic for women in the 1990s. For the first time in history, large numbers of women are living into their eighties and nineties. This means that for many, one third to one half of their lifetime will be spent without functioning ovaries and the hormones they produce. To take or not to take HRT may be one of the most important health care choices that women face. HRT's long-term preventive benefits against osteo-porosis and coronary artery disease must be weighed against present qual-ity of life and the potentially increased risk of uterine and breast cancer. Although there is much we still have to learn, the data we already have can leave many women confused.

Even the physicians who care for these women often have mixed feelings about recommending HRT for the peri- and postmenopausal years (usually between the ages of forty and eighty-five). The decision is complicated even further by the inescapable fact that each woman has individual needs and unique balances, making it impossible to standardize an algorithm for HRT. Before embarking on a course of HRT, a woman and her physician need to consider her personal and familial medical history, lifestyle, the short- and long-term risks and benefits and the expectations regarding her quality of life.

Let's explore some of the pluses and minuses of this hotly debated treatment option.

One of the primary uses of HRT is to ease the physical and mental discomfort of menopause, which can be extreme. Most physicians are aware of the most common symptoms, such as hot flashes, night sweats, chills, insomnia, mood swings, and irregular bleeding. As a cardiologist, I see many women with the less often acknowledged "hot flash equivalents"—palpitations, dizziness, and tingling or numbness in the hands or arms. All of these symptoms are manifestations of vasomotor instability and are triggered by declining estrogen levels.

Such symptoms are not only uncomfortable; they can also be alarm-ing. At times, the anxiety these women experience from believing some-thing is wrong with their heart is more incapacitating than the physical discomfort itself. I have even met some women who said their menopausal symptoms had actually taken control of their lives. They felt exhausted, depressed, miserable, disconnected, and out of control. Fortunately, hormone replacement with estrogen works quite well to alleviate these problems, and most women can tolerate the hormone. The common side effects, such as headache and breast tenderness, usually disappear within the first three months. And there is certainly room for adjustment in medication, brand, dosage, and dosing regimen. For women who are truly uncomfortable and/or suffering during menopause, quality of life itself is a valid reason to initiate HRT.

But what if your quality of life is not so bad? Are there other advantages to HRT? Definitely. Estrogen helps to maintain the integrity of the skin, hair, and nails, as well as the cellular lining of the vagina and urethra. Of greater significance is the protective effect it has on the structure of women's bones. Osteoporosis is a notorious crippler. While some bone loss is a normal part of aging, it is estimated that 25 to 35 percent of all postmenopausal women will develop severe skeletal problems. Approximately 93 percent of all women who do not take estrogen will suffer a fracture of the hip, spine, pelvis, or forearm before reaching the age of eighty-five. Patients of mine have even suffered stress fractures while opening windows, lifting babies, or running to pick up the phone.

When weighing the risks and rewards of taking estrogen, keep this in mind: More women die each year from complications of fractures brought on by osteoporosis than die from cancer of the breast and uterus combined. Estrogen replacement has clearly been shown to delay the onset of age-related bone loss and, in combination with calcium, is critical in the prevention and treatment of osteoporosis.

The National Institutes of Health has recommended up to 1,500 mg of calcium per day for postmenopausal women, especially for those over the age of sixty-five. Unfortunately, calcium intake of less than 600 mg per day is common for both men and women after reaching fifty. A related concern is insufficient intake of vitamin D. Essential for the development of bone, vitamin D becomes low in elderly populations due to dietary restriction or reduced exposure to sunlight, which may keep them indoors. Few of us at any age have a significant intake of the trace minerals silica and boron, which help calcium bond and strengthen existing bone.

In addition to these nutrients, exercise is still of critical importance.

Aside from contributing to a body's overall well-being and cardiovascular fitness, weight-bearing joints benefit from strengthening exercises.

My primary interest in recommending HRT centers on its cardio-protective functions. Estrogen produces favorable alterations in the cholesterol risk profile. By raising favorable HDL levels and lowering unfavorable LDL levels, estrogen decreases the possibility of cholesterol plaque depositing in blood vessels. Estrogen's dilating effect on blood vessels also promotes optimum blood flow and stimulates endothelial cell releasing factor, thereby preventing accumulations of harmful LDL within the vessels. There is also some evidence to show that the cardioprotective effect of estrogen may be related to increased utilization of insulin, as well as improvement of the balance between blood coagulation and blood thinning. All these actions of estrogen may improve blood flow and re-duce myocardial insufficiency. Finally, HRT is known to promote some beneficial antioxidant activity as well. Despite these advantages, a woman and her physician must balance the benefits of HRT with its potential risks.

Previously, I stated that most women fear developing breast cancer, even though cardiovascular disease is still the leading cause of death for women. While it is true that there is an HRT-related increase in the chances of death from breast or uterine cancer, the risk of cardiovascular disease is so great in older women that if a woman has a family history of heart disease, or at least two or more of the cardiac risk factors, then it is extremely important to consider estrogen replacement therapy.

In one hypothetical cohort study of 10,000 women assumed to be at least fifty years of age, health outcomes were plotted through the age of seventy-five. The risks and benefits of estrogen replacement were ex-amined based on studies reported in the literature. The outcome looked something like this: For women of approximately fifty years of age who take estrogen for the next twenty-five years, there would be a decrease in the number of fatal coronary artery disease events by 48 percent, and deaths relative to hip fracture would drop by 49 percent. Unfortunately, deaths relative to breast cancer would increase by 21 percent, and uterine cancer deaths would increase 207 percent if unopposed estrogen (not supplemented with progesterone) was applied.

What this means in actual numbers is that over a course of twenty-five years of estrogen replacement therapy, approximately 574 deaths per 10,000 women could realistically be prevented. In an earlier study, crude estimates showed that approximately 5,250 women per 100,000 could be saved through HRT treatment. Thus in the hypothetical, population-based evaluations, it appears that the health benefits of HRT in the post-menopausal woman exceed the health risks.

The greatest and most frequently invoked fear on the part of both women and physicians in regard to HRT, as I mentioned, is of breast and uterine cancer, with numerous studies offering contradictory findings. It is important to mention much of the data showing danger from HRT come from research using doses or types of estrogen not used and not approved for use in the United States. Additionally, many studies, and particularly a 1995 study documented in the *New England Journal of Medicine,* showed a significant increase in breast cancer in women over fifty-five who had taken HRT for five years or more. This same study showed that in women over fifty-five some 300 of 100,000 will develop breast cancer without any hormone use. Women using HRT in that age group for the specified five-year period increased the figures to 600 of 100,000 per year, though the study unfortunately did not cross-reference to show how many of those women studied had been saved from fatal heart disease.

As previously mentioned, estrogen does promote growth of the uterine lining, or endometrial tissue. If growth of this tissue continues unchecked, endometrial hyperplasia (overgrowth) may develop. To modify this effect, physicians often prescribe doses of complementing progesterone to prevent estrogen dominance in women with intact uteruses. The progesterone may be used for part of each month or at lower doses on a daily basis. This practice virtually eliminates the risk of endometrial or uterine cancer. For those women who cannot tolerate progesterone, estrogen may be used alone, but the patient must then undergo regular endometrial biopsies.

Another consideration in HRT is fibroid tumors, which are benign tumors developing on the uterine muscle. Fibroid tumors are believed to occur in circumstances of estrogen dominance caused by a woman's own naturally occurring body chemistry or as a side effect of HRT. Though estrogen may cause these noncancerous growths to enlarge, the hormone itself does not cause them. Common (maintenance) doses of estrogen may be sufficiently low as to not affect fibroid growth at all.

Given the number of life-enhancing health benefits and low level of proven risk for the majority of women, HRT can be quite beneficial.

However, there are women who are not sound candidates for HRT, who cannot or will not tolerate its side effects, or who for various reasons reject HRT. What are the options for these women? A woman may choose dietary modification, vitamin and mineral supplementation, or herbal preparations to smooth the menopausal transition and pave the way for optimum health during the postmenopausal years.

Alternatives to HRT

Phytoestrogens are compounds occurring naturally in plants. Many of these compounds come from soybeans or soy-based products. In women who prefer to avoid pharmaceutical preparations of estrogen, phytoestrogens can be an alternative therapeutic agent. These phytoestrogens are even good for the heart. Studies conducted in China and Japan have shown that people who consume large quantities of phytoestrogen-containing plants have a low incidence of heart attack. Soy products like miso, tofu, and soy milk are traditional in the Japanese diet, and Japanese women experience virtually no menopausal symptoms. Bioflavonoids, concentrated in citrus fruits (especially in the pulp and white of the rind), also have estrogenic properties and have been helpful in controlling hot flashes, anxiety, and mood swings in some women.

Certain dietary restrictions may be beneficial to women undergoing the transition of menopause. These guidelines may also help young women coping with premenstrual syndrome. Foods with a high fat content, refined sugars, and chemical additives disrupt hormone production. The chocolate frequently craved during PMS can increase breast sensitivity, sleeplessness in caffeine-sensitive women, water retention, and mood swings. Members of the nightshade family, such as peppers, tomatoes, potatoes, and eggplant can also heighten the symptoms of PMS, as can overuse of alcohol or caffeine, and sodium. These substances also deplete the body of usable levels of B vitamins, minerals, and calcium. Vitamins C and B are also important supplements for menopausal women in treating irritability and fatigue.

Women in HRT, whether using phytoestrogen or pharmaceutical estrogens, should take additional B vitamins, as HRT can negatively affect nutritional status. Weight gain has also been a frequent complaint of women on estrogen therapy, as are headaches, abdominal cramps, diarrhea, and nausea similar to morning sickness. Calcium needs should also be monitored during HRT. Iron levels in menopausal women are in general higher than in menstruating women, so iron supplementation may not prove an additional necessity. To alleviate hot flashes, anxiety, and the irritability that accompany menopause, some women may use vitamin E as an estrogen substitute. Vitamin E may be taken orally or applied directly to the vaginal tissue. It is also used to reduce the size of breast cysts and, when combined with magnesium and vitamin B-6, may ease PMS.

Menopause and Options

It is a very common practice for middle-aged women to cut back on fats as a way of controlling their weight. Menopause, however, is an unwise time for reducing intake of fatty acids. Linoleic and linolenic acids are useful in preventing dryness in skin, hair, and vaginal tissue. Herbal preparations like evening primrose oil, borage oil, or black currant oil can regulate prostaglandin levels, positively affecting the hormonal shifts of menopause and PMS. EFAs (essential fatty acids) also alleviate many such hormonal changes, and are commonly found in nuts and seeds, wheat germ, and oatmeal.

In addition to vitamin and mineral supplements, many herbs are extremely useful in helping to manage specific menopausal symptoms. Hot flashes may be subdued by wild yam root, dong quai, and black cohosh root. Blue cohosh root is also useful as an antispasmodic and tonic, but can be powerful in initiating the sloughing of the uterine lining. It should be avoided by young women experiencing PMS-like symptoms that may actually be early signs of pregnancy.

Dong quai is a favorite Asian herb long prescribed by traditional Chinese and Indian herbalists to balance the vital energy of the body. Dong quai is frequently used in the West to moderate PMS symptoms and menopausal hormone imbalances. Dong quai is a vasodilator; it also reduces cramps and muscle spasms. This herb also is high in phytoestrogenic properties, and additionally alleviates vaginal dryness. As a uterine relaxer, it should be avoided during pregnancy and may cause sun sensitivity. This herb is commonly available in many health food shops and in pharmacies in urban areas.

Fatigue, another major menopausal symptom, may be aided by ginseng, ginger, or cayenne pepper, while anxiety, irritability, and insomnia can be soothed with chamomile, hops, valerian root, or passionflower. (Passionflower is gentle enough to treat hyperactive children and can be used for the elderly who suffer from sleep disorders as well.) Alfalfa and licorice root are also calming herbs; all of these natural remedies are available commonly in forms ranging from teas and prepared tinctures to capsules. The form you take is a matter of choice and usually does not alter the efficacy of the herb, though they should all be stored away from sunlight in a cool dry place and discarded after the manufacturer's specified expiration date, as with any medication. Keep in mind that alcohol use, caffeine, and poor diet can hinder the herb's ability to be absorbed by the body and be effective.

Aside from herbal or pharmaceutical intervention, exercise and even mental imagery can also greatly assist women who experience hormonal symptoms from PMS or menopause. Acupuncture, yoga, and other therapies focusing on the body's energy centers have also proved effective in assuaging the physical and psychological symptoms that often occur as a consequence of these hormonal swings.

As I have mentioned, today's menopausal woman has an abundance of options. Begin by selecting a physician who will work as your partner. Then read, experiment, and talk to other women. Do whatever is necessary during this important transitional time in your life to maximize your health and well-being.

Preventive Strategies for Women

If you are a woman, you are probably wondering if there is an easy self-help program for optimum health. There really is. First of all, don't smoke. In addition to causing heart disease and cancer, smoking is a contributing demon to the bone loss of osteoporosis. Smoking also pollutes the blood with heavy metals and toxic chemicals that raise havoc with the immune system. It contributes to many symptoms, ranging from the common cold and bronchitis to cardiac irregularities and even rare instances of sudden cardiac death.

In the previous analysis, I told you how risk factor profiles for heart disease differ greatly according to gender. For women, the major risk factors include diabetes, being overweight (by as little as twenty pounds), low HDL, and high triglyceride levels. If, however, a woman has high blood pressure or smokes, the risk increases considerably, and in post-menopausal women the risk becomes higher still. Thus it makes heart-sense for women to become more proactive in reducing their risk of cardiovascular disease by consuming a healthy diet, getting enough exercise, taking nutritional supplementation, and possibly considering HRT.

Eating a high-fiber, healthy-fat diet and consuming generous amounts of fresh fruits and vegetables will provide the necessary flavonoids and carotenoids to combat cancer and heart disease—and will also protect you from breast cancer, according to current research. Other studies report that the saturated fat commonly found in meats and full-fat dairy products increases a woman's risk of ovarian cancer by an average of 20 percent.

Regular daily exercise, as previously mentioned, is extremely beneficial, especially for cardiovascular health. In addition, recent studies show that women who exercise three or more hours a week in the decade following the onset of menstruation (approximately age twelve) can lower their risk of breast cancer. If a woman continues to exercise moderately, incorporating four hours a week into her lifestyle, she can reduce her risk of breast cancer by almost 60 percent as she approaches middle age.

Targeted nutritional supplements also support health and help patients prevent many of the most serious health problems women face, such as birth defects, heart disease, cancer, and osteoporosis. I emphasize that adequate folic acid should be consumed by every woman on the planet. In women of childbearing age, it helps prevent neural tube defects such as spina bifida in the fetus. In women of all ages, it helps prevent accelerated cardiovascular aging if high homocysteine levels are found in the blood, and it protects against cervical cancer in both younger and older women.

In addition to vitamins, minerals, and herbs, there are other particular targeted nutrients that are instrumental in protecting a woman's health. Consider coenzyme Q_{10}, which I have already discussed at length in an earlier chapter. For women, it has been tremendously successful in alleviating congestive heart failure and improving the heart's ability to contract. In cases of cancer, it has also proved to be life-saving: Recent research confirms that treatment with high doses of coenzyme Q_{10} (up to 390 mg daily) encourages cancer regression. Another nutrient that has been particularly helpful is L-arginine, an amino acid.

Several studies have documented L-arginine's role in improving wound healing, the immune response, vasodilatory activity, blood clotting, and cholesterol levels. Dietary L-arginine is found mainly in plant proteins, pumpkin seeds, and peanuts. In lower concentrations, it is found in animal proteins such as beef and in fish such as halibut. Since L-arginine has been shown to cause tumor regression in animal studies and in clinical studies of women with breast cancer, the use of L-arginine may have a unique role in promoting and maintaining the health of women.

As trite as it sounds, prevention is easier than cure. This is particularly true in promoting the health of women and children, who have specific needs and vulnerabilities. Given the array of available resources reviewed in this chapter, women and children today can place health first by implementing these simple approaches for achieving optimum health.

Eleven

Emotional Healing

This book is designed to give you valuable tools to effectively and permanently transform your relationship with your body. Of course, one of the benefits is that you will have a trimmer, more physically fit, healthier body. But the deeper, more profound transformation concerns your relationship with yourself. This requires a physical, mental, and emotional shift. If you now find yourself criticizing your body, condemning yourself, hating yourself, or hurting yourself, working through these core emotional issues and getting to the heart of the matter will free you.

Weight loss is one of the positive outcomes of healing the relationship between the mind and the body. Other results of healing your inner conflicts are self-acceptance, self-love, and a sense of truly honoring your body. Using a holistic approach to weight loss prevents you from using dieting as yet another unhealthy, neurotic expression of an unresolved self. The vicious cycle of hating your body, going on a diet, losing weight, gaining the weight back, and hating yourself and your body must be interrupted and healed. These are habits disrespectful to the self and the body.

A holistic approach does not mean you have to go on a vegetarian diet or search for a guru. It simply means that the approach to a permanent body transformation is a multilevel one: emotional, behavioral, physical, and nutritional. In the overweight syndrome, we create negative feelings about ourselves and our bodies. Emotional factors such as depression, helplessness, guilt, loneliness, boredom, denial of anger, fear, and hopelessness are all enmeshed in this cycle.

IT'S TIME TO REFRAME

But let's reframe your attitude toward your body and weight loss. The concept of "reframing" involves reshaping negative attitudes and beliefs— some of which we learned as young children—and redirecting them in a more positive direction. Reframing results in seeing the positive aspect of any given situation or person, including ourselves. For example, let's reframe your attitude toward your body and weight loss. You can view your overweight condition as a gift because it is now the impetus that drives you to delve deeper into your psyche and into the blocks that have hampered your self-image and self-esteem. You can use it as a motivating force to heal deep emotional issues, become more alive, and live a more pleasurable, fulfilling life free of obsessive-compulsive behavior.

What a joy life can be when your thought process is free from its preoccupation with your body and/or your food. After all, what we think, we can internalize and begin to believe. What we believe, we become. If we *think* we have an unattractive body, for example, and think it often, we come to *believe* we are unattractive and thus may *act* in an unattractive manner. This negativity limits the vast possibilities of experience. If we reframe this view, we will consciously look at ourselves in a constructive, not destructive, way. In other words, we can now look at our beautiful hair or bright eyes and see ourselves as attractive. This does not mean that we should remain stuck in fat bodies but that we should use positive reframing as a tool to move past our unconscious blocks.

For people who are chronically overweight, food becomes a vehicle with which to block the emotions. In their book *Overcoming Overeating,* Jane R. Hirschmann and Carol H. Munter distinguish between "stomach hunger" and "mouth hunger." When you eat in order to fill your body because your stomach is hungry, you have a healthy relationship with food. If you find yourself wanting food out of mouth hunger, even when you are not really hungry, you are experiencing something emotional, an anxiety beneath the level of conscious awareness; that is, you are using food to try to assuage, hide, or substitute for the feeling. I agree with

Hirschmann and Munter's theory. For example, perhaps we are feeling deep despair or intense rage, but these emotions do not feel safe. We then feel anxiety about having these emotions. If we are not getting in touch with our true feelings and expressing them, overeating may be a futile attempt to sublimate whatever the true feeling is.

Another example of this type of sublimation might be love. Many of us can give love but cannot receive it. We may not be able to take in love, but we can take in food. Therefore, we use food as a substitute for emotional and spiritual satisfaction. Afterward we get upset and scold ourselves for overeating and being fat, though it is not the food that is the problem but what it represents. The question of what the food is replacing is one that people really *need* to ask themselves. Food may be used as a drug. As with alcohol, we may medicate ourselves with food, especially sugar, but it never cures the problem. It exacerbates it. It continues it. And the reality is that we physically feed ourselves to death while we emotionally starve ourselves to death.

The causes of eating disorders, addictive behavior, and obsessive-compulsive patterns may stem from a variety of painful childhood experiences, frequently combined with bad habits learned within the family system. Unless we are actively involved (through support groups and workshops, therapy, or a personal search) in uncovering the causes of these patterns of behavior, the core issues remain, although they remain unconscious. A powerful beginning is to get in touch with our own experience; that is, to bring out of the darkness and into the light our own unconscious motivations for overeating.

You may be thinking, "I don't need to do that. My body may be a problem, but not my mind. Why open a can of worms?" However, as a physician and psychotherapist, I know that the body speaks the truth even though the conscious mind can be deceived. I choose to trust the body. The body reacts to repressed emotions. Unfortunately, most parents do not teach children to honor or express their emotions. They send their children mixed messages about the very natural human aspects of their physical being. Children are told to stop crying when they are hurt and need to cry. They are told that anger is not ladylike or that men should not be afraid. Many people have been treated disrespectfully and abusively (physically or emotionally) through the years and have come to view this treatment as normal, acceptable, to be expected, even deserved. Some children would even get hit, emotionally abused, reprimanded, or abandoned when they expressed emotions such as anger, sadness, or fear. Alice

Miller, author of *The Drama of the Gifted Child,* tells us that parents unknowingly have the power either to form or deform the emotional and physical lives of their children.

We were all born with the natural ability to release emotion. If we watch a baby who is upset, we will see that he or she will cry or scream and that when finished, the body will relax and the baby will be peaceful and smiling again. However, if the baby is misdirected from its natural expression of emotions, this may result in a lifelong repression of feelings. Where does all this repressed emotional energy go? It becomes an unresolved memory in the unconscious. The energy actually gets stuck in the body, in the muscles and in the cells. This unreleased energy becomes the seat of dis-ease and disharmony inside us. For a deeper discussion of this repressed energy see my previous book, *Heartbreak and Heart Disease.*

DOWN MEMORY LANE

For you to begin to lose weight, it is very important to take an honest look at how your parents related to you in terms of food, diet, your emotional needs, and your self-image. This may be a painful look. Be aware that you might have some denial systems blocking you from seeing the truth, but it is worth a try. This is why support groups can be so helpful when one is attempting to lose weight. What feelings were you not allowed to have as a child? Were you told to stop crying when you were sad? Did you get punished? Were you taught to control yourself, control your feelings? Were your parents controlling about what you ate and how much you ate? Did they force you to eat everything on your plate, even if you were full?

Take some time to look back at their views on food and body size. Did your parents believe that "a fat baby is a healthy baby"? Were you ever given the message that if you didn't eat, you would get sick? Were there reward systems set up around food? If you were hungry and wanted to eat, did you ever hear the familiar phrase "Don't spoil your appetite"? What does that mean? How can anyone "spoil" an appetite by eating? Appetite is an internal signal; hunger pangs indicate a need for food. Eating satisfies, not spoils, an appetite. What parents really mean when they say this is that the child should stifle his or her appetite, or natural feelings of hunger, in order to please the parent. They mean, "Don't eat when and what you want to eat, but eat when and what I want you to eat."

A powerful way to heal the wounds that we carry from childhood is to be able to express now what we wanted to express back then but couldn't. This is best done in therapy or in some other safe environment. In this way, we will be able to diffuse the old feelings we have about past events and not apply them to current situations. In other words, once an old feeling is released, a new experience will no longer cause us to react in ways that contain the charge or the excess baggage of all the other past repressed feelings. Therefore, the present feeling will be more manageable, the anxiety lessened, and the need to turn to food considerably assuaged.

It is important to allow negative emotions to come up so they can be released, and yet it is also important to reframe them. This may sound like a contradiction. How do you know when to do what? The rule is to first *experience* the feeling without judgment or self-editorialization, and then to investigate it once it has been discharged. For example, let's say you constantly insult your body. You can feel how angry you really are at yourself. You have been having these particular feelings for quite some time, and the intense emotional charge must be expressed and released. Take some time privately or perhaps in a therapy session to vent this anger.

Once you do this (perhaps you will need to do this every so often for a while), you can eventually try to understand the roots of this behavior. It will then be easier to catch yourself saying or thinking something self-destructive and reframe it in a positive light. This process can be particularly effective in losing weight. When you find yourself reaching for food when you are not hungry, rather than eating right away, sit down with a pen and a pad and write down what you are feeling, or immediately express these feelings verbally. In this way, you detail the maladaptive motivation behind the mouth hunger.

TAKE SUCCESSFUL SMALL STEPS

It is important to point out here the need for patience. If you want to successfully change your patterns, it will take time, repetition, and a tremendous amount of patience. Realize that you are taking a totally new approach to reshaping your body. Let go of any sense of time and urgency. Relax. Pushing too hard and forcing the flow will create a destructive, frenetic energy that will not help this process. People want immediate results, quick cures, and instant gratification, but I am a firm believer in not driving ourselves beyond normal capacity. Healing unhealthy and destructive patterns requires focus, time, energy, and patience; lots of nurturing self-love and self-support are necessary here. It is healthful to let go of preconceived notions of how much weight you have to lose and how long it should take you to lose it. Expectations, after all, can lead to disappointments. They can trigger a sense of failure and a vicious cycle of obsessive eating.

A major pitfall in losing weight is creating an unattainable goal. Our society has placed tremendous pressure on us to be beautiful. The model of beauty we have been given is a thin body. But we must all get to a place where we feel a sense of peace and acceptance about our particular body type. There is indeed a danger in seeking total perfection, especially since it is truly unattainable. Perhaps you are bottom-heavy and overweight, but you begin to make changes in your lifestyle and you start to reduce. You are exercising, firming up, and looking much slimmer and much better. If you continue to focus on your heavy thighs, however, you create a counterproductive attitude. Instead of feeling and expressing a tremendous gratitude toward yourself for reshaping your body, an expression that will encourage your entire being to continue to change your patterns, you are busy putting yourself down for having "heavy thighs." This creates a futile, rebellious feeling inside. A part of you will be feeling, "Why bother? No matter what I do, it's never enough."

SEX

In this multilevel approach to creating and maintaining a new body, it is very important to establish a positive goal. If you want to change your body in order to have a healthy mind–body connection, your focus is in the right place. If your reasons for losing weight are that you think if you do so you will get love, or so-and-so will want you or envy you, or you'll get that job, or someone will pay attention to you, then you are setting yourself up to fail. What if you lose the weight and it doesn't happen? Or what if you lose the weight and it does happen, but you still feel unfulfilled? The way to protect yourself from these sorts of programmed failures is to set your sights on a beneficial intention: "When my lifestyle patterns change, when I have a healthier relationship with myself and my body, I will feel more alive and more at peace, and therefore I will experience more pleasure." If you can begin to see yourself in a healing process and feel a sense of hope and excitement about it, you can begin to enjoy the process rather than being caught up in the end result. Let go of the struggle, of the "I'll be happy when . . ." syndrome.

Liken your venture to reprogramming a computer. There are many circuits. Some circuits are emotional blocks, some are faulty belief systems, some are negative family patterns, some are your own destructive habits, and on and on. Where have you been short-circuited? What experiences have caused you to cut off from yourself? All this must be worked on in order to heal yourself and your unconscious obsession with food. The unconscious drives are stronger than the conscious drives, and it is frequently the unconscious desires that direct us. Thus, to begin to enjoy food and feel we have permission to eat, we must be at peace with ourselves emotionally.

There is often a direct correlation between anxiety and overeating. If understanding ourselves better and feeling that we are actively involved in our own healing reduces anxiety, it will have a positive effect on healing the eating compulsion. When we bring aspects of our unconscious into the light of awareness, they are no longer hidden forces, and we begin to have a greater ability to prevent them from controlling and harming us. If overeating is a negative way of coping with feelings, especially feelings of fear or powerlessness, then creating a better relationship with the emotional self will significantly support the healing of this compulsion.

This was probably the case with Roger, who must have had feelings of powerlessness, most likely rooted in his childhood. By becoming a successful businessman, he established the image of success, which gave him a sense of control. He obviously did not have this sense of control in his eating habits. The truth is, he was out of control. This is a typical scenario for many overweight individuals, male and female. With women, there may even be a greater risk of obesity because of social factors that discourage them from expressing themselves emotionally and physically, and particularly because of their feelings of vulnerability.

What I would like to help you get in touch with is the fearful side of weight loss. Both men and women have concerns about this deep core issue, which involves sexual vulnerability. To get in touch with your own feelings about this, write or say aloud the following, and take your time to fill in the blanks:

"If I lose weight, I'm afraid . . . will happen."

"If I lose weight, I'm afraid . . . will pull away from me."

"If I lose weight, I'm afraid I'll hurt . . ."

"By being overweight, I feel protected from . . ."

"By being overweight, I don't have to deal with . . ."

"If I have a sexier body, I'm afraid . . ."

While I was a therapist in the hospital-based weight loss program at Manchester Memorial Hospital, it became increasingly clear to me that the issue of sexuality was a major factor in the overweight syndrome. Many of my clients communicated their intense fears regarding losing weight. There were also love and relationship issues. For example, one of my clients said, "By eating, I will make myself so unlovable that I will never be hurt again." She had deep, painful issues involving love and sexuality. For some of my clients, losing weight was like shedding a suit of armor; the physical padding that being overweight provides can be viewed as an armor of protection. This maladaptive defense mechanism, unconsciously created to avoid pain, actually holds past pain deep inside your tissues.

Are you unconsciously or consciously holding on to the weight to protect yourself sexually? Do you use the weight to avoid other forms of intimacy? It is important to delve honestly into these possibilities, because unless they are uncovered and dealt with emotionally, it will be very difficult to reduce and keep the weight off. To shed the armor makes us vulnerable. It is this shedding of armor and the ensuing vulnerability that is for some a major cause of resistance in losing weight.

SEXUAL VIOLATION MAY CAUSE WEIGHT GAIN

One of the women in my program lost nearly forty pounds. She was quite intuitive about herself, particularly since she had been in psycho-therapy. After the miraculous weight loss, however, she became blocked and started to gain weight. She told us she was "sick of the diet." She was putting up tremendous resistance. I asked her if anything was wrong, and she said she had no problems. But there *was* a problem. The body told the truth, in that she started to put on weight. So I asked again what was going on with her. She told me she wanted to go back to her old manner of eating. Then I asked her what was going on with her relationship with her husband.

At that point she froze. She looked at me and started to cry. Then she said, "I'm very scared." She communicated to me that her husband was looking at her with a new energy. It was an energy that she did not feel comfortable with but did not know why. As he approached her with this new energy, she became more and more frightened; she was afraid of his sexual advances. She remembered those looks from when she was a little girl.

Although she had been in therapy before, she had not worked on sexual issues. For some reason both she and her therapist did not feel that this was important. Unfortunately, sexual issues are frequently avoided by the client as well as the therapist. Frequently in therapy there is a taboo on working on issues of sexuality. The therapist, experiencing some countertransference, may unconsciously move away from the real issues that both the therapist and client are confronted with.

In this case, this woman had been wounded as a child; she had a history of subtle sexual violation. Although this did not appear to be overt (that is, she did not appear to have recollected any childhood abuse or molestation), she did feel an uneasiness about a masculine drive and an energy suggesting sexual interest.

Previously I mentioned Alice Miller's work in discussing how parents unknowingly—and the key word here is *unknowingly*—cross a boundary that has a sexual connotation. A five-year-old child cannot distinguish between love and sexuality; for that child they are the same thing. When a child sits on her father's lap, for example, and enjoys the warmth and love of cuddling and then wants to leave, she satisfies her need for simple contact and then her need for separation. This is a common phenomenon in children. However, if the father frequently uses his daughter as an object for his own need for contact, he crosses a boundary. The child feels this intrusion energetically, which is also transferred into the unconscious and later experienced as a sexual taboo or a fear of subsequent sexual contact. But where does one leave off and the other begin? Aren't fathers naturally loving toward their children, some more enthusiastically than others?

This crossing of boundaries can be very subtle, and in most cases unconscious. Feeling and expressing genuine love and affection for a child are natural. The trap for both parents and children occurs when the unfulfilled need for contact in the adult is acted out on the child rather than in the parents' relationships with other adults.

Of course, there are also more overt cases of sexual abuse that include not only seduction but molestation, incest, and rape. While not all overweight people have been sexually abused as children, abundant medical literature indicates that eating disorders are a frequent result of sexual abuse. Symptoms found in incest and rape victims include fear and sleeping and eating disturbances, as well as sexual dysfunction. Obesity and compulsive eating are ways that survivors of childhood abuse protect themselves. Overeating and putting on weight as body armor can be a way to avoid unwanted sexual advances and thus become less vulnerable.

Although many clients in psychotherapy do not remember overt or covert sexual abuse, the body does remember. For example, a female colleague of mine told me that several years ago she had a severe weight problem. While today she is an attractive woman who is five feet seven inches tall and weighs approximately 125 pounds, she used to weigh 180 pounds. She communicated to me that in her college days and particularly in graduate school, when she was training to become a massage therapist, she was very heavy and heavily armored. She did not know why. She had an obsession with food that she did not understand. She also related to me that she had the feeling that she was molested as a child, although she didn't know how, nor could she remember the circumstances.

When she was working on her own body, the memories began to come back. She saw a counselor and reconstructed some of the forgotten memories of her childhood. Although she could not put it together completely, she said that she recalled a feeling of aggressive male energy that was sexual in nature from when she was a young girl. When she went to college, she got involved in a very passionate relationship, and this brought up the previous unpleasant experience of male energy coming toward her as a defenseless young child. At that point she started to put on weight. She gained approximately fifty pounds, becoming less attractive. After she heightened her insight and the awareness that her sexuality was the key to her obesity, she began to cry and cry and cry. She grieved for months. She knew how important crying was and used it as a tool in her own healing process. After this long process of grieving, she got in touch with her true self and began to lose the weight easily. She now is able to help others who have been in similar situations.

In addition to sadness and anger, unrecognized fear creates forces in our personality that unconsciously compel us to eat. It is not uncommon to find that the root of an individual's weight problem is prior sexual abuse, which may be obvious in some and not so obvious in others.

It is also a simple fact that some people just like to eat. Not everyone has a hidden sexual issue as the origin of their weight problem. As a matter of fact, the converse was true in another of my clients. Jean had a strong sexual desire that she felt was imprisoned in her overweight body. After losing approximately forty pounds, however, she developed a feeling of freedom about her sexuality. This realization occurred in one of her dreams. She dreamed that her whole body was encased in an orthopedic cast. It suddenly started to crack from the front to the back. As her body armor was falling apart, she found herself in the bathroom with a naked man—a symbol of sexuality. She communicated to me that she had good feelings in the dream. She in fact liked the dream. She did not experience fear. What she did experience was a new emergence of feelings of vitality. She was excited about her new body and the way she looked. Her self-image was improving, and she was looking forward to experiencing her new awareness of sexuality. Jean's dream was indeed a sign of emotional healing.

The need for emotional healing is a global one. In our society, we often are not given tools with which to understand our emotions. On the contrary, our society has negated the value of emotions and judged certain emotions as weak or inappropriate. It considers strength to be holding yourself up. But true strength is not just acting strong while we don't feel strong. People have become afraid of emotions and tend to feel uncomfortable when around someone who is crying deeply. It is felt as dangerous and threatening. We have all been taught to cut ourselves off from and repress our feelings, and we have not been given healthy ways to release pent-up emotional energy. The following are a few good tools that will help bring about the emotional healing that will aid in developing greater self-esteem and subsequent weight loss.

BREATHING

When we are afraid, anxious, or nervous, we hold our breath. Because of the high level of stress in modern life, most people, unfortunately, don't breathe deeply enough. Faced with a situation that arouses the fight-or-flight instinct, a simple deep breath can sometimes save lives. It brings our focus of attention back to the immediate moment and grounds us in our bodies. The best way to become aware of our own need to breathe is to watch for signs of anxiety. Wanting to eat, even though we are not hungry, may be an overt sign of an unconscious motivation that deep breathing could assuage. Some of us may reach for a cigarette or an alcoholic beverage. Again, deep breathing can sometimes get us past the crucial point when we are about to do something self-destructive. A more prolonged form of self-aware breathing is meditation. If you are not ready to meditate or don't feel it is for you, however, you will benefit by simply taking time out of each day to sit quietly and breathe deeply and slowly. Making contact with your body through breath is an important part of reconnecting with yourself.

MEDITATION

Meditation is easy to learn. The most difficult part may be finding the time. But creating the time, whether it be every day or three times a week, can be rewarding, offering you growth and insight. You might feel tremendous resistance or fear of doing it incorrectly, but there is no set way to meditate. Often the biggest obstacle is our own judgment that we are not really in a meditative state. The mere fact that we have taken five minutes or fifteen minutes to sit or lie quietly and breathe, however, is meditative in itself. Don't compare your experience to others' accounts of their meditations. If your quiet time doesn't measure up to how you perceive meditation to be, you run the risk of thinking you failed. As you practice it more and more, you will find that your body quiets down more easily.

In order to do this, you must find a spot where you won't be interrupted. Put the answering machine on. Sit in a comfortable chair or lie down on a carpet or mat with a small pillow (optional) under your head. If this is the first time you are attempting to meditate, your body may find five reasons why you have to pop up and do something. You might lie down and feel very fidgety. Close your eyes. Start by taking five slow breaths in and out through the mouth. Tell yourself to relax. Continue to breathe slowly and deeply, either in through the nose and out the mouth, or in and out through the nose, whichever is more comfortable. Feel your body. Put your consciousness in your head and, slowly, as you breathe, run your consciousness down your body. If you are having trouble relaxing, tell each part of your body to relax by saying, "My head is relaxed . . . my legs are relaxed . . ." and so on.

Many thoughts may run through your head. Don't resist them, but don't focus on them either. Merely note them and let them pass. You may imagine opening a door and saying to all these thoughts, "I know you're there, but I don't want to let you in." See or feel these thoughts going out the door and close the door behind them. You may need to do this a few times.

When you feel you are relaxed enough, you will begin breathing naturally. Take in slow, deep breaths every so often, and remember to let the air out slowly. Imagine that you have an inner physician. This inner healer is very wise and loving and may be called upon for a vast supply of ideas and information. Tell it all about your pain, particularly about your body. Let yourself flow with this process. See what you need to express to this inner healer and then ask it for help or guidance. State, for example, that you want to attract the perfect support system. Know that you have a right to ask for this. If you feel sadness, let yourself cry. Whatever you feel, allow it completely. Stay open to receive insights, but don't struggle. Just trust that guidance will come in various ways. Follow whatever instincts you may have. When you feel complete, take a few more breaths. Slowly open your eyes.

You can also use meditation to reframe your self-image. If you have been overweight for many years, you may be holding on to a self-defeating attitude that you are a "fat person" who is doomed to a lifetime of being fat and/or struggling with fat. Go into a state of deep relaxation and remember to breathe deeply and take your time. When you are deeply relaxed, start to ask yourself to bring forth all your fears about your own body image. For example, you may fear that you will never have the pleasure of a thinner body. But affirm to yourself that you will by saying, "I am becoming thin." Take deep breaths as you do this. When you feel complete, start to work on the self-image you would like to have.

Tell yourself that you can indeed change your body. You can change destructive patterns. Remind yourself that other people have done it, and you can, too. Take some time to visualize yourself feeling healthier, lighter, stronger, and filled with vitality. Repetition is very important in shifting your belief systems and your attitude. Working your mind on a deep level will aid the momentum of this reprogramming process.

EMOTIONAL EXERCISES

Another essential process is getting in touch with various unconscious conflicts you may be experiencing about having a trimmer body. You can do this either by sitting down with paper and pen or by releasing them verbally or physically, as I will describe. There are many different exercises you can do. For example, when you feel very sad, try to lie down, tilt your head back, and let yourself down into the feelings. Get deep into sobbing. The more you cry from your abdomen, the better the release. As you are in this state, try to get in touch with your grief. Crying is the most healing of all the emotions. Crying will release the heartbreak, which will help prevent the possibility of real heart disease.

If you feel angry, however, or enraged, try yelling or screaming while in your car. Remember to roll up the windows so you feel private and safe. Or go out to the woods or a secluded beach and scream at the person at whom you are feeling angry. Get it all out. Say everything you feel, without editing your language. Because he or she is not present, this is your opportunity to release the energy. You could also take a tennis racket and physically hit your bed and scream.

Another good exercise is to lie on your bed and just kick. By kicking and screaming and shaking your head, you can simulate a temper tantrum. Other forms of anger-release work include making a fist and jutting out your jaw in defiance or protest. Another way is to twist a towel and release a sound while you are doing it. There are forms of therapy that teach you how to release your negative emotions using safe, private, effective, and beneficial techniques.

Getting in touch with your negativity and learning about your "dark side" can be the most healing aspect of therapy. For example, in our Healing the Heart workshops, exploring the dark side is absolutely essential and crucial in the healing process. This is particularly important for those with heart disease who have obvious issues centering on heartbreak, taking in love, and expressing intimacy and sexuality. Many people may find it difficult, however, to start to release the years of pent-up emotional energy.

It is a sign of great strength to realize you want to help yourself. This may include doing emotion-release work alone at home or in a safe place such as a therapist's office. It is important to release the core of your sadness, your anger, and your fears one way or another. When this happens, we begin to get in touch with our true needs and really experience our true selves. This is a significant step in the right direction and a profound step toward optimum health.

Twelve

Move!

BUT DON'T OVERDO IT!

No pain, no gain is a myth. Nowadays there is lots of confusion about exercise. For example, we really don't have to exercise strenuously to lose weight or to be in optimum health. Many cardiologists, myself included, do not recommend jogging or running. We have all heard of healthy people having accidents while jogging. Such occurrences may include strained muscles, tendonitis, back injuries, knee sprains, and even the rare occurrence of aortic rupture and sudden death. Excessive running has been reported to cause delayed menstruation and amenorrhea (absence or stopping of menstruation) in women. Jogging in polluted environments, such as on roadways with excessive exhaust fumes, is as unhealthy as jogging in very hot or very cold weather, which may result in heat exhaustion or frostbite. Okay, enough of this downside. What about the advantages of mild to moderate exercise?

Scientific evidence has consistently linked regular physical activity to a wide range of physical and mental health benefits, as well as the alleviation of occupational stress. Exercise training has been shown to benefit patients suffering from congestive heart failure as well. Regular exercise has been reported to have positive psychological effects that include improved self-esteem and lower levels of anxiety and depression.

In one study, we examined the physiological and psychological profiles of middle-aged dedicated runners. These subjects indicated that they ran an average of thirty miles per week. Fifty-nine percent had participated in at least one marathon, and most reported having participated in an average of nine races in the previous year. Although these runners had high cardiovascular fitness, slept better, and had a heightened sense of well-being, my personal observations led me to suspect a superficial or cosmetic acceleration of the aging process.

The physical demands of committed running are extreme. Evidence of a runner's "wear and tear" can be seen in the loss of hair and premature wrinkling of the skin. Although averaging forty years of age, many of the participants in our study looked much older. I was personally struck by how much pain these committed runners endured when exercising at a high rate of speed on the treadmills. There was profound clenching of the jaw, distortion of the mouth, and intense wrinkling of the skin around the mouth and eyes. In short, some exercise is good, but too much can be bad.

Estimates indicate that between 45 and 65 percent of the almost twenty million runners in the United States injured each year are hurt seriously enough to require that they stop running for some period of time. This raises the question of how risky exercise is. Also, if regular exercise is beneficial, exactly how great is that benefit?

Although relatively few heart attacks occur during or immediately after exertion, heavy exercise does increase a person's immediate risk. However, this risk is not the same for everyone; it varies with how much and how often exercise is performed.

Two major studies addressed the issue of exercise risk, indicating that the frequency of exercise is related to the relative risk of heart attack. For those who engage in heavy exercise less than once a week, the relative risk increased 107 times in the hour after heavy exertion. The increase in risk was twenty times greater for people who performed exercise one or two times per week, and about ten times greater for those who performed exercise on a more regular basis of three or four times a week. But the risk increased only 2.4 times for people who engaged in relatively strenuous physical exertion five times a week (the equivalent of slow jogging, singles tennis, swimming, or heavy gardening).

The risk of heart attack after heavy exertion was similar for both men and women, but what is it about heavy exercise that can trigger a heart attack? Researchers speculate that sudden surges in blood pressure and heart rate may cause atherosclerotic plaque in coronary arteries to rupture, thus initiating the cascade of clotting and eventual myocardial insufficiency. Although regular exercise has multiple health benefits, including control of blood pressure and cholesterol levels, one has to keep in mind that the heart may be more vulnerable at certain times than at others.

Even though regular exercise has been shown to reduce the overall risk of heart attack, the minute-to-minute risk is greater during or just after physical exertion. So perhaps the worst scenario is that of the inactive person who only occasionally engages in strenuous tasks. Obviously, most people will have moments in their lives when they must participate in heavy physical activity. However, during these times the rise of heart attack risk is certainly less for those who exercise regularly.

For this reason, as a clinical cardiologist, I recommend engaging in exercise at least every other day. Walking, dancing, and cycling, in my opinion, are still the most preferred types of exercise. Jogging, running, and other varieties of strenuous exercise may have negative trade-offs, particularly for the "weekend warrior" type. We must also be mindful of our increased need for nutritional support when we do such high-level exercise.

NUTRITION AND EXERCISE

There is direct evidence that the increased oxygen consumption that occurs during exercise leads to the production of free radicals and the oxidation of LDL, which is damaging to the blood vessels. We can measure this process by measuring levels of malondialdehyde (MDA) in the blood and the level of a gas called pentane in the breath.

Clinical research has suggested that the daily ingestion of beta carotene, vitamin E, and vitamin C results in a significant reduction in pentane and MDA levels, both at rest and after moderate and heavy activity. Since the natural antioxidant defenses of the body can be overwhelmed during strenuous physical activity, free-radical scavengers such as glutathione, vitamins C and E, beta carotene, coenzyme Q_{10}, and magnesium may be protective against free-radical damage. A healthy diet and targeted nutritional supplementation, then, can be a useful adjunct to a regular exercise program.

Glutathione, a polypeptide amino acid, is also a powerful free-radical scavenger and antioxidant. In a study of rats, supplementation with glutathione protected muscular membranes and smaller blood vessels against free radicals. Thus glutathione may be effective in reducing an individual's vulnerability to free-radical oxidative stress while exercising.

Vitamin E is a fat-soluble antioxidant. Vitamin C and beta carotene can also help protect tissues against damage by trapping free radicals. Since the levels of vitamin E found in muscles decrease in individuals pursuing endurance training, it may be reasonable to consider vitamin E supplementation in the well-trained athlete. Vitamin E supplementation in activity at increased altitudes, such as mountain climbing, may be useful as well. I recommend 200–400 IU of natural vitamin E daily. Since the oxidized form of vitamin E can be reduced by coenzyme Q_{10}, it can be helpful to take the two in conjunction, especially by those engaged in very demanding aerobic exercise.

Coenzyme Q_{10} has its own benefits as well. In another study of rats, animals receiving coenzyme Q_{10} showed a decrease in the initial release of muscle breakdown products, suggesting that coenzyme Q_{10} combats membrane and tissue damage from free radicals.

Like coenzyme Q_{10}, magnesium plays a facilitating role in stabilizing cellular membranes, while supporting ATP in the mitochondria. However, clinical research has shown that magnesium stores are depleted over time with athletic training, as magnesium is required for stabilizing muscle contraction. This is why some athletes just don't have the strength and physical ability to perform at the end of the season. Sometimes we refer to this phenomenon as being in an "athletic slump."

The vigorous training pursued by competitive athletes renders them more prone to catabolic stress—a situation in which tissues are constantly broken down. Because many athletes also are on low-fat diets, a low dietary intake of antioxidants, combined with this overconsumption of catabolic stress, may lead to a syndrome of antioxidant insufficiency. Thus it makes sense for competitive athletes and others engaged in strenuous exercise to optimize dietary sources of antioxidants and to consider targeted supplementation to maximize the benefits of training. Although there are few conclusive studies demonstrating enhanced antioxidant levels and athletic performance, the supplemental use of glutathione, vitamins C and E, coenzyme Q_{10}, and magnesium seems reasonable. Some athletes, such as menstruating women, may also need iron supplementation.

MAY I HAVE THIS DANCE?

Exercise has been shown to moderate several cardiovascular risk factors, including obesity, high blood pressure, diabetes, and elevated blood levels of lipids. The benefits of exercise are many. In cardiovascular rehabilitation, people exercise after heart attacks and bypass surgery to improve physical endurance. Physical conditioning may result in more efficient cardiac oxygen utilization, thereby increasing the amount of exercise that can be done before developing chest pain (angina). We refer to this phenomenon as "increasing the anginal threshold."

Exercise can reduce body fat and increase muscle mass. Another important and beneficial metabolic result of exercise is an increase in serum HDL levels. High-endurance and aerobic exercises such as cross-country skiing are excellent for increasing HDL. Other biochemical benefits of exercise include a reduction in the stickiness of platelets, which may prevent the blood clots that cause heart attacks. Other favorable effects on insulin and glucose metabolism occur. In both men and women, exercise also protects against osteoporosis.

Perhaps the greatest benefit of exercise is the reduction of emotional stress. Exercise has been known to assuage the driven type-A behavior pattern and is also an outlet for high stress levels, thus sparing our precious heart muscle.

Although there is considerable debate about how much exercise is necessary to promote optimum physical and emotional well-being, it is my belief that any amount of activity is better than none. In our study of ninety-four women, it was found that any activity proved beneficial; even the passive-exercise toning tables appeared to be as beneficial as walking in terms of overall health and reports of well-being. Although walkers had better cardiovascular fitness, the women who utilized the toning tables had the same favorable metabolic and physical improvements in their health and well-being. When measured with calipers, both groups had lost the same amount of body fat as well. Therefore, for optimum health it really is not necessary to get involved in strenuous forms of exercise such as high-impact aerobics, running, or racing. The expression "no pain, no gain" is completely untrue. Any activity, active or passive, will have some beneficial effect on health and well-being.

As we shall see, dancing and walking are the best forms of exercise. Even as simple everyday activities, they can make a difference in your overall cardiovascular health. Walking and dancing are forms of aerobic exercise that strengthen the heart and improve circulation. In aerobic exercise we move our bodies freely, as opposed to isometric exercise, in which we push against resistance.

Isometric exercises, such as weight lifting and resistance exercises (including water skiing), do not improve the conditioning of the heart. Rather, these types of exercise may increase strength and perhaps add extra muscle or provide additional bulk to the body. It is aerobic exercise that causes us to breathe deeply, expanding the chest and thereby providing more oxygen to the heart and the rest of the body. Cardioprotective types of aerobic exercise include dancing, brisk walking, swimming, cycling, skiing, and some calisthenics.

If you wish to consider an exercise program more advanced than walking the dog, I recommend that you see your physician before beginning. If you are over forty, your physician may recommend an exercise stress test to determine the possibility of any cardiovascular risk. For those who wish to exercise strenuously enough to raise their pulse rate to greater than 120 beats per minute, an exercise evaluation is an excellent screening tool for assessing your risk. However, if you do not wish to involve yourself in a formal exercise program, you may wish to perform daily leisure exercise. Such exercise is accomplished simply by adding more exercise to your normal daily activities. Walking to the train or bus station, parking the car farther away from the entrance of your place of employment, using the stairs instead of the elevator, taking a walk during your lunch hour, and throwing away your television remote control are all suitable ways to include leisure exercise in your life.

For those who do wish to involve themselves in structured routine, the following are tips to make your fitness and exercise program more enjoyable:

1. Find a convenient time and place to exercise—before breakfast, during your lunch break, or after work.
2. Try to avoid the heat of the day or exercising at night. Too much exercise late in the evening may cause sleep problems.
3. Set a definite goal, such as walking one mile or cycling twenty minutes three times a week.
4. If you miss an exercise session, make an agreement with yourself that you will make it up at a later time.
5. After you have lost two pounds or a half an inch from your waist-

line, reward yourself by treating yourself to something like a movie, a haircut, or a sports event.

6. Keep your exercise program enjoyable and varied.

BETTER WARM UP FIRST

If you feel motivated, and I hope you do, and wish to engage in brisker aerobic forms of exercise, you will need to consider a warm-up period of stretching and breathing. These warm-ups will take only about five minutes. They are excellent exercises to stimulate breathing and stretch the legs, abdomen, chest, and lower spine.

Exercise 1

This exercise involves abdominal breathing. Lie on the floor and bend your knees, keeping your feet on the floor. With your eyes closed and your hands over your navel, breathe in and out through your nose. Feel your abdomen push against your hands. This form of breathing can be practiced prior to any exercise session or meditation.

Exercise 2

Lie on the floor with the pelvis extended and the knees bent. Put a rolled-up blanket or towel under the small of the back and place your feet flat on the floor. You will feel a sensation of stretching in the abdominal area that will allow fuller and deeper breathing. This is also a good stretch for the lower back. You may wish to push your buttocks against the floor to enhance the stretch.

Exercise 3

This is a back exercise. Lie on the floor. Bring your knees to your chest and then swing them to the right and then to the left. This frees up the lower muscles of your back. While keeping your lower back on the floor, gently rock yourself forward and backward several times so that you are rocking on your lower spine. Remember not to strain yourself. Repeat six or seven times, and rise slowly.

Exercise 4

For this exercise, assume a standing position. Place your hands on your hips and bend at the waist, bringing your torso down toward your knees. Bend as far as possible without straining. While keeping your hands on your hips, you may feel a mild stretching in your lower back and then in your hamstring muscles and the backs of the calves. Now slowly return to an upright position. Spread your legs as widely as possible, pointing your toes inward. Place the backs of your hands on the base of the spine, and lean as far back as possible. Additionally, open the throat by releasing a sound (a long "aah" for example). This will also stretch the chest muscles, diaphragm, and neck. Do not strain yourself! Repeat this five to ten times.

A PRESCRIPTION FOR EXERCISE

After you have warmed up, you may then choose to exercise as you like. In selecting your exercise, consider the following:

1. The type of activity
2. Duration of activity
3. Frequency
4. Intensity
5. Progression

Fitness experts, such as doctors in the American College of Sports Medicine, of which I am a member, have established the following recommendations for the quantity and quality of exercise required for the development and maintenance of both body composition and cardiovascular fitness:

Type of Activity

Aerobic exercise is preferable for fitness. Aerobic activity stimulates breathing by using large muscle groups in a continuous and rhythmical manner. Such exercises include jogging, running, walking, hiking, dancing, swimming, skating, rowing, cross-country skiing, jumping rope, and bicycling.

Duration of Activity

Fifteen to sixty minutes of continuous or discontinuous aerobic activity is required for health and fitness. For example, to perform fifteen minutes of continuous rope skipping would be difficult. Perform this type of activity for three to five minutes, however, take a short rest, and then continue for a total of twenty minutes. In this way the activity becomes manageable and effective. Brisk walking can be performed for a twenty-minute stretch. Since walking is not as intense as rope skipping, it does not need to be discontinuous, though both are aerobic.

Frequency

Three to five times a week is considered by most sports experts to be an appropriate frequency of exercise.

Intensity

The intensity of activity can vary. Most fitness experts are in agreement that *between 70 and 85 percent of one's predicted maximal heart rate* is a good reliable index of intensity. For example, suppose you had an exercise stress test with your physician, and your maximal heart rate obtained during the evaluation was 150 beats per minute. If you take 70 percent of this, you arrive at 105. Eighty-five percent of 150 equals 127.5. Therefore, if you exercise in an aerobic activity and wish to enhance your cardiovascular fitness, your exercise target heart rate should be between 105 and 128. Although there are other formulas that have been advocated, this is the easiest for developing an exercise prescription. For the unfit or overweight individual, this exercise prescription is perhaps the safest. If you are in this category, an exercise program should be utilized only under the advice of your physician.

Progression

In the unfit or overweight individual, little progression or increase is advisable. If, however, you have begun to notice improved fitness and a reduction in weight, you may *increase your total work effort by perhaps 10 percent per month*. However, recommended rates of progression vary with individuals, so be sure to consult your physician concerning any increase. It is usually best to progress slowly and increase gradually in a spirit of keeping your motivation and interest intact and not torturing yourself.

THE EXERCISE SESSION

To safely undergo an exercise program, it is necessary to include at least three phases: warm-up, workout, and cool down. Each phase has a particular purpose.

The warm-up phase usually includes the stretching and breathing exercises that I have already mentioned in this chapter. This phase may last from five to ten minutes, with the purpose of increasing the body temperature, loosening the joints and ligaments, and preventing any undue strain or soreness. A slight elevation in heart rate is also a benefit of the warm-up phase. In general, the older or more overweight the individual, the longer the warm-up should be.

The workout phase usually lasts from fifteen to sixty minutes, with an ideal period of approximately twenty minutes. To improve cardiovascular fitness and body composition, as well as to lose weight, continuous aerobic activities of low to moderate intensity are recommended.

The cool-down phase, which should last from five to ten minutes, brings the physiological system back toward the resting level at a gradual pace. After a vigorous workout, cardiac output may be considerably elevated, perhaps two to three times the resting level for an individual. Thus, it is important to cool down to permit a gradual readaptation of the body system. One of the best cooling-down exercises, again, is slow walking. After a workout such as running, jogging, or rope skipping, a walking cool-down period is usually all that is required. In structured rehabilitative-type exercise programs, such as our hospital's cardiovascular rehabilitation program, the cool-down period usually includes relaxation techniques. For example, after clients in our program have completed their workout phase, they will walk around the room. After a brief walk, we ask them to lie down and focus on their breathing; we then lead them into a meditation to help them get in touch with their feelings about their bodies. These procedures have been extremely helpful in relieving tension and stress on the cardiovascular system.

With many different types of exercise available to you, which of them is right for you? Let me begin this discussion with two of my favorite forms of exercise: dancing and walking.

DANCING

Dancing is without a doubt the best form of exercise, as it incorporates the whole body. The benefits from dancing are enormous. Have you ever seen people put their whole heart into dancing? Their bodies become graceful. Their movements become integrated with the music. Their hips, torsos, legs, and arms move in rhythm with the music. My patients often ask me what types of dancing are best. Any form will do, whether it is square dancing, ballroom dancing, freestyle, or line dancing. All have one common factor: movement with music.

Dancing is also a great way to get over inhibitions and become more comfortable with our bodies. Dancing gives us permission to use the pelvis, which many of us may feel is a socially taboo activity. The pelvic region is a major center of energy in the body. By rotating this area (remember how Elvis did it?), we move the entire body.

Have you ever been listening to the radio and found yourself swaying to a favorite song? Next time, get up and dance! Don't stop yourself from feeling the music and moving. When you see couples close their eyes while slow dancing, do you get a feeling of tranquility and connected-ness? Any exercise into which we put our feelings, particularly positive feelings, enhances not only the spirit but the core of our being.

By the same token, I feel that anyone who has negative energy, such as anger or rage, should not use strenuous physical exercise to work it out. Instead I would recommend the emotion-releasing exercises described earlier, such as kicking the feet on a bed or verbalizing feelings in a stationary car. Contrary to popular belief, trying to work out anger through exercise could perhaps do a disservice to the body. When we are enraged, our adrenaline level soars. Strenuous exercise can only over-charge an already overstimulated heart. It's like putting out a fire with gasoline or overdosing on our own hormones. For example, I resuscitated two victims of sudden death in the emergency room who both indicated that they had been very angry and had been using exercise as a way of venting their anger. They both had forced themselves to "exercise off" these highly charged emotions, thus making exercise an obligation and not a pleasure. Exercise will not take away anger; it merely burns off some of the excess energy associated with it. The way to get rid of anger is to own it and express it in a clear and straightforward manner.

WALKING

Walking is also an excellent exercise for all age groups. Young and old love to walk. I encourage walking in my older patients because of its safety. Rarely have I heard of people hurting their legs, ligaments, or knees while walking. Try to take in the surroundings while you walk, and don't worry about the pace. Most exercise enthusiasts believe that we have to walk very fast in order to burn calories. This is not the case. In fact, a mile of walking burns off as many calories as a mile of running. Enjoy this activity. Take time for yourself. Move your entire body and get into a natural rhythmic motion. Feel your body. Feel each step. It can be very enjoyable.

I would recommend a minimum of at least twenty minutes of walking at least once a day. After you have progressed and feel more comfortable about walking one mile, try more, or better yet, walk twenty minutes twice a day. Again, this should be both fun and leisurely. Remember, it costs nothing and you can do it alone, though walking with someone else or perhaps in a group offers an excellent support system.

Many of my patients have commented that walking can sometimes be boring when done day after day. This may be true if you always take the same route, so be creative. Go hiking in the woods, in the mountains, or on the beach, for that matter. I am an avid fly fisherman, and I frequently need to walk up and down riverbanks and through fields to get to my favorite fishing spot. Thus, I am both relaxing and getting health benefits from an activity I enjoy.

Another way to incorporate walking into our life is by playing golf. Again, this is an activity that is good for both young and old. In a cardiovascular sense, the amount of exercise is minimal; however, golf still requires considerable walking. If you choose to carry your own clubs or pull your own cart, you will burn up even more calories. Although many exercise specialists speak disparagingly of golf or even tennis, I feel these are excellent activities for both the mind and the body.

OTHER EXERCISES

Skiing, both cross-country and downhill, is another type of recreational activity that is also an excellent form of exercise. Cross-country skiing gives all the benefits of running without causing problems such as shin splints or ankle, knee, or hip injuries. Instead of pounding on a hard surface, the cross-country skier uses rhythmic movements to gently glide across the snow. Downhill skiing is another form of exercise that utilizes walking. Although most of us use chairlifts, many downhill skiers do lots of walking. Unfortunately, it usually occurs after losing a ski or while retrieving lost equipment.

Other activities I endorse are swimming and cycling. These two non-weight-bearing activities are especially good for the overweight or elderly person. Stationary cycling is preferred over outdoor cycling for the elderly or during inclement weather. I frequently tell my patients to cycle for approximately five to fifteen minutes. If you get bored, listen to the news or turn on the television; some patients even read while stationary cycling. My own recommendation is to let your mind go and just focus on the rhythmic activity of your legs.

Other indoor activities could include climbing stairs or using a rowing machine. A good rowing machine will exercise almost all the major muscles of the body, particularly the abdomen, arms, and lower back. Rowing also creates a rhythmic activity that many find enjoyable. Rowing to music can enhance your enjoyment. Try rowing to relaxing music with your eyes closed; you may forget you are exercising.

A treadmill is another form of exercise I recommend. My suggestion here is to just use a motorized treadmill as a walking machine, not another stress test. It is not necessary to increase the speed or raise the incline. For starters, it is best to start with the machine at 1.7 miles an hour, with perhaps a 5 percent grade for perhaps fifteen to twenty minutes. Walking on a treadmill is not as good as walking outside because variations in terrain allow different muscles to be worked. But this can be done as an alternative, particularly when weather conditions are not favorable for outdoor walking. Indoor exercise allows you to fit a program to your schedule as time permits, but it doesn't have the benefit of freedom and change of scenery that outdoor exercise programs can offer. Both indoor and outdoor exercise will offer an opportunity for supportive environments.

I can recall an example of how an exercise support group was helpful in bringing one of my patients out of a low-grade depression. The man had recently lost his wife to a sudden heart attack and had become very depressed. Also a victim of heart disease, he sustained a massive heart attack only nine months prior to his wife's death. After recovering from his heart attack, he had gained a new sense of self, only to lose his will to live when his wife died.

Although this was a very fragile man in his seventies with severe coronary artery disease, I advocated an exercise program as a way for him to strengthen his heart and develop a new vital connection. In our cardiovascular rehabilitation program, he indeed made many such connections and new friendships. He quickly became an exercise enthusiast, attending the program three times a week, walking and talking with almost everyone. Exercise not only increased his cardiovascular strength, but also gave him a new interest in life. Establishing new and vital connections after the loss of a significant other can truly be rewarding and life-sustaining.

Another indoor exercise I would recommend is repetitive light weight lifting. This form of exercise can be performed in the home or at a gymnasium. I am suggesting it more and more to my patients, even those advancing in age. As we age, the average person loses lean muscle mass, which is replaced by fat. This is especially true after the age of forty. Since aging is inevitable, it seems logical to exercise various muscle groups with light weights. If you prefer to exercise at home, you need not purchase fancy weight-lifting equipment. Objects such as heavy books will do. Repetitive light weight training is one of the most effective ways to improve and maintain muscle tone, reduce your body-fat ratio, and burn calories. To obtain maximum benefits from any weight lifting, it is important to take a deep breath before you exert, then exhale during the exertion. Avoid "holding your breath" while lifting. Never allow yourself to feel strained or pained during such a workout; it is not the amount of weight, but the number of "reps," or repetitions of lifts, that makes this form of exercise effective.

Sit-ups, with the legs elevated on, for example, a bed or a chair, are another good activity that can be used in conjunction with weight lifting. Sit-ups, like rowing, strengthen the abdominal muscles. Many of us have chronic back problems; simple toning of the abdominal wall may alleviate many lower back ailments. This was the most important aspect in rehabilitating my own lower back problems.

Push-ups are another choice. But individuals with hypertension or severe heart disease must be cautious about both push-ups and weight lifting. A stress test may be in order before adding these activities to an exercise program for such patients, since this exercise requires an individual to repeatedly lift most of his or her own weight.

Jumping rope is another favorite for at-home exercisers, requiring only athletic shoes and a jump rope. Remember that if you jump rope, do not allow both feet to leave the ground at once, but rather alternate your foot movement in a skipping manner. Five minutes of jumping rope can be quite exhausting and is the workout equivalent of perhaps ten to fifteen minutes of cycling or rowing.

HAVE FUN!

Exercise is a cardinal ingredient in weight reduction and can help you attain optimum health. Exercise not only increases muscle tone, but also alters the metabolic rate in our bodies; a fit individual will burn more calories than a less fit one, even at rest. If you wish to get involved in strenuous aerobic activity, I recommend that you get an exercise prescription from your doctor. Remember that exercise can be regarded as therapy having tremendous benefits; but it also has some hazards.

You may be wondering why I have not discussed taking a pulse reading during activities like walking or dancing. Since these are more relaxing and pleasurable forms of exercise, I feel that constant interruptions for such monitoring take the fun out of them! You can tell when you are overdoing it. You should not be gasping for breath or dizzy. Listen to your body and nurture it, don't torture it. Exercise should be safe as well as enjoyable.

However, if you are trying to achieve fitness in a high-level aerobic program, or if you are following a physician's prescribed exercise program, you will need to know if your pulse rate is within recommended guidelines. There are many devices on the market today that digitally display the user's heart rate at a glance. I feel these devices are preferable to pulse-taking because they do not take the individual's attention away from the relaxing aspect of their activity by requiring computations of heart rate. They permit a quick and accurate check to ensure that exercise is within safe cardiovascular parameters.

Exercise need not be a struggle. If you make it fun by choosing an activity you enjoy, you will more easily incorporate it into your daily life and more rapidly enjoy the numerous physiological, psychological, and biochemical benefits of exercise. To avoid boredom, you may wish to vary your daily routine. For example, walk one day, cycle another, and perhaps swim on another. If walking is the core of your routine, you can supplement it with recreational activities such as golf or tennis. The point is to try to do some light exercise every day.

CHAPTER
Thirteen

Foods That Heal

A prudent diet is your best asset in weight reduction and your best defense against illness. According to the old saying "You are what you eat," nutritional healing utilizes a diet that makes you feel better both in mind and body.

This chapter is designed to examine foods that enhance and nourish your body. We have previously discussed the advantages of the Mediterranean diet, the importance of water, the benefits of various vitamins and minerals, and the negative aspects of both caffeine and alcohol. This chapter is about experiencing a new array of foods. In the spirit of nondeprivation, and with a slow and patient approach, we can learn to consume less of certain foods and utilize new, equally enjoyable ones.

Changing your eating habits may not be easy. Since you have been building these habits all your life, it may be difficult to substitute one type of food for another. But if you have an open mind, it doesn't have to be painful. On the contrary, experimenting with new recipes and foodstuffs can be fun. For example, for years I loved red meat. I then switched to chicken and fish for most of my animal protein, and now I enjoy food as much as ever. I am even eating less animal protein. The transition to a healthier diet may take some time; however, my first exposure to seaweed was a disaster, for example. It tasted too fishy, and I didn't like it. Gradually it became palatable, and now I find it most enjoyable.

185

To make your transition to a new way of eating easier, I have listed below twelve foods that are both nutritious and heart healthy:

Twelve Heart-Healing Foods

1. *Onions and garlic* contain allicin, which helps lower cholesterol levels. Onions also contain quercetin, which is a powerful bioflavonoid that prevents LDL from clogging your arteries.

2. *Spinach and collard greens* contain vitamin E and lutein. Lutein helps protect blood vessels, especially those in the eyes, and helps prevent macular degeneration. Vitamin E prevents cholesterol from sticking to the inside of your arteries.

3. *Yams, cantaloupe, and summer squash* contain beta carotene, which helps protect the heart and blood vessels.

4. *Cabbage, broccoli, kale, and cauliflower* contain calcium, vitamin E, potassium, and folic acid, along with phytonutrients that help protect against cancer. Calcium helps lower blood pressure; vitamin E and folic acid help prevent atherosclerosis; and potassium helps decrease blood pressure and generally protects the heart.

5. *Asparagus* contains alpha-linolenic acid and folic acid, which help reduce hardening of the arteries.

6. *Soy foods (tofu, tempeh, soybeans, and other soy products) and sea vegetables (seaweed)* contain magnesium and linolenic acid. Magnesium helps protect against cardiac arrhythmia, and linolenic acid is an essential fatty acid necessary for cardiovascular health.

7. *Mackerel, sardines, salmon, and anchovies* contain coenzyme Q_{10}, and anchovies and sardines contain DMAE (dimethylaminoethanol). Coenzyme Q_{10} is essential for the production of cellular energy and has been shown to strengthen weak heart muscle. DMAE increases the level of choline in the brain, which enhances memory.

8. *Legumes, such as chickpeas and lentils,* contain folic acid and lower insulin levels.

9. *Miso* (an inexpensive dried Japanese soup mix made from soy, barley, and other nutritious ingredients) contains many vitamins and minerals and lots of linolenic acid, which helps lower cholesterol. You can find miso in health food stores, Asian markets, and some supermarkets.

10. *Fresh grapefruit, strawberries, peaches, cherries, raspberries, and kiwi* contain pectin and vitamin C and have a low glycemic index as

well. Pectin helps lower cholesterol, and vitamin C helps protect the vascular system.

11. *Almonds, macadamia nuts, walnuts, pumpkin seeds, and sesame seeds* contain essential fatty acids, potassium, calcium, and magnesium.
12. *Eggs* contain sulfur and magnesium.

WHOLE GRAINS

Most expert nutritionists and some physicians, particularly those interested in a macrobiotic approach, feel that an optimal diet should include a variety of whole grains. Whole grains (wheat, corn, rice, oats, millet, rye, barley, and buckwheat) are those that are not highly processed; they are exceedingly nutritious. They contain more vitamins, minerals, and fiber than their lighter, whiter, and fluffier counterparts found in commercially packaged goods. In their whole form, grains contain a seed and a covering to protect the seed. With the advent of the Industrial Revolution and modern processing, it became easier to remove the germ and bran layers, making available to the general public white flour that had once been reserved only for the wealthy. Unfortunately, these discarded portions of the grain contain virtually all the fiber and the vast majority of the B complex vitamins, as well as the vitamins E and A and the minerals magnesium, potassium, zinc, iron, and selenium. In refining grains, the flour is commonly bleached, giving it a lighter, seemingly more presentable appearance and a softer texture. Additionally, these refined grains are frequently laced with additives and preservatives. White flour contains many empty calories, simple carbohydrates, and little fiber. This type of carbohydrate—with a high glycemic index—as mentioned in an earlier chapter, can be easily converted to glucose and stored as fat in the body.

Many people are now purchasing whole-grain breads. Many whole-grain and fiber-rich breads are now quite plentiful in supermarkets, but the best sources of vitamins, minerals, and fiber are the whole-grain bread products available at your local health food store. Since whole grains contain many nutrients, they are nutritious because they contain not only carbohydrates, but also a balanced amount of protein, multiple vitamins and minerals, and sufficient fiber; they are also low in fat.

Cultures that rely on whole grains as a staple of their diet have the lowest rates of cancer and heart disease. The fiber in whole grains, as discussed earlier, decreases transit time through the bowels. The complex sugars in whole grains are less quickly converted to glucose than the simple sugars found in refined products and therefore are less available for conversion to fat. It is important to consider some whole grains when planning your diet. Because barley, rye and wheat kernels, and spelt have a lower glycemic index than corn and millet, I'm more partial to these grains. Brown rice and buckwheat have a moderate glycemic index.

Brown rice may be obtained in short-, medium-, or long-grain varieties. It is also available in a sweet version called basmati. In addition to containing many vitamins and minerals, brown rice contains the mineral silicon, which is a necessary element for the body. Some investigators suggest that silicon can help prevent burnout in high-performance individuals who drive themselves excessively in both their personal and professional lives. To cook brown rice, rinse the grains thoroughly and soak in water for several minutes, then rinse and drain. Add one cup of grain to two cups of water and a pinch of salt in a saucepan. Bring to a boil, then immediately cover the pot and turn down the heat to a simmer; do not lift the lid or stir until the water has been absorbed, approximately forty-five to fifty minutes. When brown rice is used in combination with beans, fish, or meat, it provides a well-balanced source of protein in the diet.

Barley is grown throughout the world and is a popular grain in America. It is chewy with a nutty taste. Barley malt has been used as a natural sweetener and in making beer. It is an excellent grain to use in soup. It can also be mixed with brown rice and served as a side dish; add one-third cup of barley to one cup of brown rice and prepare in the same manner as brown rice.

Buckwheat is technically a seed rather than a true grain. It has a rich and somewhat bitter flavor. Eastern cultures grind buckwheat into flour to make noodles. Buckwheat flour is a good flour to use, particularly in pancakes. A pancake recipe is included in chapter fifteen.

Millet is a grain that has been used for centuries by the peoples of Africa and China. Millet can be boiled by itself or with a variety of vegetables. It goes especially well with broccoli or cauliflower and may be substituted for brown rice or barley.

Corn has been the staple grain of the Native American cultures for centuries. Corn can be ground coarsely into cornmeal or finely into flour. It can be used to make cereals, polenta, and tortillas. It also makes a delicious muffin. This is an excellent substitute for people allergic to wheat. Whole corn is a good source of fiber as well as vitamins and minerals, particularly beta carotene. Avoid overprocessed or canned corn; it causes an overly high insulin release.

Wheat is especially rich in B vitamins and vitamin E. In its refined form, it is lacking in many of the important nutrients, but in the form of whole-wheat flour or berries, it is an excellent source of vitamins and minerals. Wheat berries, when cooked, create a tasty and nutritious dish with a hearty, chewy texture.

BEANS

Beans are another highly nutritious food that I would recommend you consume on a daily basis. Although high in complex carbohydrates, beans are also high in calcium and contain a considerable amount of protein, comparable to meat or dairy products. When combined with grains, they provide all the necessary essential amino acids. Beans are really the best single vegetarian source of protein. Among my favorites are black-eyed peas, chickpeas, lentils, pinto beans, split peas, adzuki, and lima beans. Lentils are a particular favorite of mine, especially in soups. They are easy to digest as well as to prepare, and they also are an excellent source of iron as well as folic acid.

Boiling is the best method for cooking beans. Most beans should be soaked overnight. When preparing them, a pinch of salt and/or a piece of seaweed may be added.

Soybeans are perhaps the highest in protein and are a favorite in macrobiotic cooking. Tofu, tempeh, tamari, and miso are all made from soybeans and are easily found in health food stores. Miso is a particular favorite of mine, and in soup is highly recommended to virtually all clients in our weight-reducing program as well as many of my cardiac patients. Miso is made from fermented soybeans, grains, and sea salt and contains many of the enzymes that strengthen the body. In a major Japanese study, those who ate miso soup every day had a significantly lower risk of dying from cancer and heart disease compared to those who never consumed miso or did so only on occasion. This large study, involving over a quarter of a million people, demonstrates one of the best-kept secrets of Asian medicine: Sea vegetables and miso preparations do appear to enhance health and increase longevity.

SEA VEGETABLES

Sea vegetables not only are highly nutritious, but also help protect against radiation. Medical research has found that sea vegetables contain a substance called sodium alginate that helps eliminate from the body radioactive strontium, a breakdown product of uranium. Since we constantly take in minute amounts of radiation from sources as varied as the sun, X rays, and microwaves, sea vegetables are a good form of insurance.

Sea vegetables are extremely rich in vitamins, minerals (at least fifty!), and other nutrients. As a food group, sea vegetables contain a higher amount of magnesium, iron, iodine, and sodium than any other kind of food. Because of the high sodium content, it is recommended that individuals who have a history of congestive heart failure or high blood pressure consume sea vegetables only once a week. It is also important to soak sea vegetables for at least half an hour before preparation to reduce the sodium content.

As sea vegetables contain extremely high amounts of calcium and phosphorous, they are beneficial in situations in which calcium is needed in the body, such as in osteoporosis. Sea vegetables are also approximately 25 percent protein and 2 percent fat by weight. They are low in calories, which makes them extremely useful if one wishes to limit caloric intake, and are rich in many vitamins and trace elements as well. For example, they are high in beta carotene, vitamin B-12, niacin, pantothenic acid (vitamin B-5), and vitamins A, C, and E, as well as the mineral selenium. As previously noted, selenium, combined with vitamins A, C, and E and coenzyme Q_{10}, is extremely important in overall heart function.

In summary, many clinical studies indicate that sea vegetables are one of nature's best nutritional supplements. They contain virtually all of the vitamins and minerals that are useful in preventing the formation of free radicals. Additionally, sea vegetables have been used to treat cancer, to lower blood pressure, to thin the blood, and even to prevent ulcers. They are also known for their ability to dissolve fat deposits and eliminate heavy metal contaminants from the body. They are a dietary supplement that should be used by everyone; they are one of nature's wonders!

VEGETABLES

I believe that most vegetables are healthful for our bodies. My only reservations at this point are carrots and white potatoes, since these vegetables have a glycemic index that is quite high. I am not saying, however, that you should exclude carrots and white potatoes from your diet; you should just be aware of the greater insulin response that occurs when we consume these vegetables. Most vegetables provide abundant quantities of vitamins, including beta carotene, and should make up at least 20 percent of our caloric intake.

Root vegetables are rich in complex carbohydrates as well as vitamins and minerals. For example, daikon, a root vegetable resembling a long white radish, has a high calcium content and is extremely useful in healing. In general, most of the nonstarchy vegetables, from asparagus to zucchini, contain approximately two grams of protein and five grams of carbohydrate per half-cup serving. The more starchy vegetables, such as corn on the cob, carrots, or potatoes, have approximately fifteen grams of carbohydrate and two grams of protein per half-cup serving. Most vegetables have virtually no fat and are high in fiber. However, a word of caution: When consuming high-glycemic vegetables, try to limit yourself to small portions.

Green vegetables, including cabbage, kale, leeks, broccoli, watercress, Brussels sprouts, parsley, turnip greens, and bok choy, are tremendous sources of vitamins A and C. Kale is abundant in calcium, yielding approximately 300 mg per cup, which is comparable to the amount of calcium in a cup of milk.

Cabbage is a gift from the divine. Like broccoli, it is a cruciferous vegetable that contains major amounts of compounds called isothiocyanates. These compounds are particularly effective in preventing cancer. Cabbage also contains indole-3-carbinol, another anticarcinogen.

Vegetables can be cooked in many ways; they can be boiled, steamed, stir-fried, baked, pressure-cooked, or simmered in soups and stews. Raw vegetables are preferred when possible, especially with the skins intact.

Almost every vegetable is good for you. Some have particular advantages. Turnips are exceedingly high in chlorophyll and folic acid. As mentioned previously, in my opinion, asparagus is the best vegetable available in terms of overall nutrition. Chlorophyll, found in some vegetables, alfalfa sprouts, and green leaves, contains an abundance of iron and is a red-cell binder. Chlorophyll compounds such as chlorella, wheat grass, and green barley not only provide multiple vital nutrients and support one's energy, but also are quite helpful in the natural healing approach to arthritis. I also believe that these compounds, in general, possess antiaging properties. If you prefer lettuce, try leaf lettuce over iceberg lettuce. Leaf lettuce has almost a hundred times as much iron as iceberg.

You really can't go wrong by consuming as many vegetables as possible. The list is endless and far beyond the scope of this book, but generally speaking, try as many vegetables as you can. I do prefer organically grown vegetables, which are not cultivated with pesticides, herbicides, or chemical fertilizers.

FRUITS

Most fruits contain potassium and vitamin C. As a clinical cardiologist, I recommend that my patients include at least one or two servings of fruit a day as part of the recommended five to nine servings of fruit and vegetables, especially if they are on diuretics, which deplete potassium. Even though fruits are high in natural sugars that eventually turn into glucose, they are also a great source of fiber, as well as beta carotene and pectin. Grapefruit is the highest in pectin, and we know that pectin yields a favorable blood cholesterol profile. Animal research indicates that pectin not only reduces cholesterol, but also may lower the incidence of cancer. It was demonstrated that grapefruit pectin, even in the face of a high-fat diet, restricted the development of atherosclerosis. It is important to remember to eat fruits in their fresh state. Fruits grown locally and in season are the best. Dried fruits such as dates, currants, raisins, and figs, although high in magnesium, calcium, and fiber, are very high in natural sugar and will trigger insulin release.

Fruits and vegetables are an excellent source of bioflavonoids, carotenoids, and flavonoids. In addition to antioxidants, fresh fruits and vegetables may contain other vital nutrients such as polyphenols and quercetin (which we have already discussed). Carotenoids are the yellow and green pigments found in fresh fruits and vegetables and have been studied extensively in both heart disease and cancer. There are approximately six hundred carotenoids; some have greater antioxidant activity than others. Numerous studies report a reduced incidence of cancer in people eating fresh fruits and vegetables containing large amounts of flavonoids and carotenoids. Carrots are the primary source of the carotenoid beta carotene (which is converted to vitamin A in the body); tomatoes are the best source of the carotenoid lycopene. Lycopene has twice the antioxidant activity of beta carotene and has been touted to be particularly effective in treating pancreatic, prostate, and cervical cancer. Yet scientific research has focused more on beta carotene than lycopene. Several studies have shown that dietary intake of beta carotene is inversely related to risk of cardiovascular disease. In a recent study of 3,806 men with increased levels of cholesterol, participants with higher carotenoid levels in the blood had decreased risk of coronary artery disease. This finding was stronger among men who never smoked.

During the next several years, results from observational studies and randomized trials may permit specific public-health recommendations that go beyond eating a healthy diet of fresh fruits and vegetables. For now, it is a simple and established fact that the risk of heart disease can be modified by a healthy lifestyle that includes a high intake of fresh fruits and vegetables. So eat your spinach and kiwi!

SEEDS AND NUTS

Seeds and nuts are a crunchy and tasty part of the diet. While some contain high quantities of saturated fats, many nuts contain healthy fats and should be included in your diet. A study done among Seventh-Day Adventists, who eat a diet rich in seeds and nuts, has taught us that nuts can play a major role in preventing cardiovascular disease. I recommend macadamias, almonds, chestnuts, and walnuts as part of any nutritional plan. However, I'm sorry to say that peanut consumption should be restricted. It is my recommendation that peanut butter should be strictly avoided in all diets except those of growing children, since most of the calories in peanut butter are derived from saturated fat.

One of my patients, unbeknownst to me, was a peanut butter addict. George consumed approximately two jars of peanut butter a week, plus a jar or two of whole peanuts. He believed that peanut butter was a healthy food. After his first quadruple bypass operation ten years ago, I struggled with him to reduce his serum cholesterol.

He constantly told me that his diet was healthy—that he was consuming more fruits and vegetables and eating less meat and dairy products. After his second quadruple bypass when he was fifty-eight, I gave him my book *Lose to Win,* asking him to read it. He did, and was surprised to learn that peanut butter and peanuts were taboo. He did not realize that peanut butter and peanuts contain not only saturated fat, but other fats as well. If the peanut butter is hydrogenated, which it usually is, it contains cis-trans isomers, or trans-fatty acids. After George cut out the peanut butter, we were both amazed at how his cholesterol fell.

While walnuts also get approximately 80 percent of their calories from fat, they have a linolenic acid (favorable EFA) content of at least 7 percent. Almonds, on the other hand, are more favorable, and in some clinical studies have been shown to improve cholesterol levels. Chestnuts are the lowest in fat and are good raw or roasted. Sesame seeds, although containing some fat, are exceedingly high in vitamins C and E as well as calcium and protein. Tahini is a condiment made from ground sesame seeds; it can be used in salad dressings, soups, and can be combined with chickpeas, garlic, and lemon juice to make hummus, a Middle Eastern spread or dip. Tahini can be purchased at health food stores and in some supermarkets.

SOUPS AND SHIITAKE

Soups can be made with a wide variety of vegetables, beans, grains, and sea vegetables. Keep in mind that sea vegetables, especially kelp, are exceedingly abundant in magnesium and have 150 times more iodine than any of the commonly used land vegetables. Soups are also a way to incorporate shiitake mushrooms into our diet. These Japanese mushrooms have been used for centuries and are said to promote vitality and youth. Studies have shown that they help to build resistance to viruses and have been used to treat fatigue. They have a distinctive flavor and are an excellent source of protein. Dried shiitake can be purchased in health food stores and Asian markets and are found fresh in many supermarkets.

When preparing dried shiitake, it is best to cut them up into small pieces and add them to soups. One of my favorite recipes includes shiitake, garlic, and artichoke hearts. All you have to do is sauté freshly chopped garlic with a little olive oil, add fresh shiitake, and artichoke hearts from a jar. Add freshly chopped parsley, and you'll think you died and went to heaven.

SWEETENERS

As we have seen earlier, the use of table sugar should be strictly avoided in the diet. Other natural sweeteners are preferred. For example, barley malt and rice syrup make excellent sweeteners. Although I may be going out on a limb, I will recommend honey. Some of my colleagues may have difficulty with this recommendation, but after much research, I do feel this is an acceptable food that we need to consider in our diet. Since honey contains several amino acids and large amounts of B complex vitamins, as well as vitamins C, D, and E, and several minerals, honey is not considered an empty-calorie food like sugar. And because it is twice as sweet as most other sugars, smaller amounts can be used. However, keep in mind that honey has a very high glycemic index; minimal amounts will go a long way.

Honey, which comes from the nectar of flowers, is collected in the bee's honey sac. One tiny worker bee produces approximately half a teaspoon of honey during its lifetime. Honey is made up of water, dextrose, levulose, and other substances, including resins, gums, and pollen. The therapeutic uses of honey as a healing agent have been known by many civilizations over the ages. Honey is an outstanding energy food. It is also a far better sweetener than monosaccharides such as glucose, and it doesn't require additional metabolic energy to digest.

Honey has also been used as a remedy for hay fever, allergies, sleep disorders, sore throats, and colds. I am particularly impressed with Dr. D.C. Jarvis's book *Folk Medicine,* in which he discusses the therapeutic and healing effects of honey. I have tried some of his recommendations, such as his cold remedy of one tablespoon of honey and one tablespoon of apple cider vinegar with four ounces of warm water. I found it quite nurturing and healing. Since honey quickly enters the blood, however, it needs to be used with caution by diabetics. Because honey is a raw food, it should not be given to infants, since their immune systems are not fully developed.

Another food related to honey is bee pollen, which unlike honey is not a sweetener but like honey contains an abundance of vitamins and nutrients. The human consumption of bee pollen dates back to antiquity; it was frequently used in the Olympic games in ancient Greece. Today bee pollen is gaining increasing popularity as effective protection against many of the common pollutants in the environment, including carbon monoxide, lead, and mercury. Bee pollen is used to treat allergies, since it desensitizes the individual. There have also been studies showing that bee pollen strengthens the resistance of the immune system to both cancer and radiation. This is one particular product that may become more popular because of its high protein content and other nutritional benefits.

GARLIC AND ONIONS

Garlic and onions are considered by cardiologists to be two of the most healing foods. I have already discussed the healing properties of quercetin, found in onions. In addition, many clinical studies show that garlic and onions contain an active anticoagulant that acts very similarly to aspirin. Garlic has been known to lower blood pressure and inhibit platelet stickiness, thus reducing the possibility of blood clotting.

The reported health benefits of garlic date back thousands of years. Garlic has been used in Greece, Egypt, Rome, China, and Japan for many centuries. In Africa, garlic has even been used to treat typhus and cholera. As knowledge about the benefits of garlic continues to spread from antiquity and folklore to mainstream medicine, recent research conducted around the world has substantiated that garlic may be a significant aid in lowering blood cholesterol levels, thereby lowering the risk of coronary artery disease. One of the chemical compounds into which garlic breaks down, ajolene, may protect the digestive system from turning fat into cholesterol by inhibiting the production of human gastric lipase, an enzyme involved in the metabolism of dietary fats. The best evidence available suggests that ingesting one-half to one clove of garlic per day reduces one's cholesterol level by 9 percent. And, as I just mentioned, garlic provides even more protection against heart disease by preventing the formation of blood clots that can block arteries and lead to heart attack and stroke.

One clove of garlic contains a meager four calories and a variety of vitamins, minerals, and nutrients. For example, garlic contains selenium, a powerful antioxidant. Garlic also contains immune-enhancing properties that help combat many types of bacteria, fungi, and viruses. Allicin and other sulfur components of garlic are capable of killing twenty-three types of bacteria, including salmonella, and at least sixty types of fungi and yeast, including candida. Thus garlic has been touted as a potent immune system stimulant. It is best to take garlic raw and crushed, as much of the allicin is destroyed in overcooking.

By now you probably see the need for garlic in your daily diet, especially if you have a history of coronary artery disease. But how do you deal with the infamous "garlic breath"? Let's face it: Having garlic breath isn't exactly the best way to make friends. The sulfur smell can not only be distributed by the breath, but also can come out of the skin. Where does the odor come from? To receive the benefits of garlic, our bodies activate the internal enzyme allicinase to act on a sulfur-containing amino acid to produce the reactive sulfur compound allicin. It is this sulfur component that causes the smell to be so pungent.

To counteract garlic breath, try chewing on fresh parsley or rosemary. A piece of grapefruit or orange peel may also be helpful, or you can rinse your mouth with a mixture of freshly squeezed lemon juice and water. Some people have found that chewing on fennel and raw carrots can also eliminate the symptoms. If all else fails, try taking a hot, soapy bath to help get the sulfur smell out of your skin.

Raw garlic or commercially produced garlic extract contains significant allicin potential, and can be a tremendous asset in lowering one's cholesterol. Besides the odor, the only problems that may occur with overuse of garlic are stomach upset or an occasional allergic reaction.

Garlic and onions constitute a major portion of my diet, and I frequently use them in many of my sauces and salad dressings. Garlic is great to use with fish, particularly when marinating. It works well with swordfish, bluefish, and flounder. I will frequently marinate a fish with a dressing of chopped garlic, small amounts of white wine, freshly squeezed lemon juice, and freshly chopped basil, with one to two tablespoons of olive oil. Pour this over fish and sprinkle with fresh parsley. Marinate in the refrigerator for several hours or perhaps overnight. This type of marinade works in taking the fishy taste out of bluefish. When used in cooking, garlic can be chopped into fine pieces, julienned, sliced into thin pieces, or used as whole cloves.

COMMON HERBAL CONDIMENTS

As you will see, I recommend garnishing most dishes with parsley. Parsley contains a high concentration of chlorophyll, a chemical found in plants that is similar to the hemoglobin found in red blood cells. In animal studies, chlorophyll has been shown to combat the effects of radiation; this may be why it is considered an anticancer agent. Parsley is an excellent source of protein and, in addition to chlorophyll, contains high quantities of iron as well as vitamins A and C. Fresh parsley not only tastes great, but also gives a beautiful green color to freshly prepared foods, and green is the color associated with good health. I also recommend chlorophyll derivatives in my natural healing approach to arthritis, as well as in my nutritional remedies to support patients undergoing chemotherapy or radiation therapy.

Chlorophyll helps remove heavy metals from the joints. Heavy metals cause accumulation of free radicals and reactive compounds that enhance inflammation, damage joints, and cause arthritis pain. Other common herbs that we use on a daily basis have health-promoting properties. For example, chives contain vitamins A and C; sage is a powerful antioxidant; oregano inhibits the growth of bacteria and fungi; rosemary is also an antioxidant; and paprika has also been used to treat arthritis.

Fourteen

Nutritional Healing for the Year 2001

PHYTONUTRIENTS/PHYTOTHERAPY

My gradual transition toward nutritional/metabolic healing started in the early 1980s with my own personal use of vitamin and mineral supplements. However, it was not until 1984 that I began to prescribe vitamin and mineral support to my patients. Two years later I began to use low doses of coenzyme Q_{10} in my practice. I administered it to patients about to undergo coronary artery bypass surgery and to patients who suffered from heart failure. I also prescribed 10 mg of coenzyme Q_{10} three times daily as a nutritional support for patients going on the "heart/lung" machine during cardiac surgery. Since 1986, I have become increasingly comfortable integrating complementary approaches with traditional Western medicine to facilitate healing.

I now have tremendous confidence recommending coenzyme Q_{10} in doses of 360 to 400 mg to treat my most difficult cases of congestive heart failure. I have noticed that as I have become more comfortable using nutritional support systems, many patients have become more confident as well. Frequently, many of my cardiac patients would request that I treat them for other health problems. As a board-certified cardiologist, I lacked confidence in treating illnesses outside my own area of specialty. But I observed many "accidental cures" occurring over the years. For example, when I was treating arthritic cardiac patients, coincidentally many of them reported their arthritic symptoms improved on my treatment plan—a plan that integrated various diets, herbal remedies, and nutritional support systems.

My patients have always been my best teachers. I learn from them every day. When a phytonutrient relieves symptoms in one patient, I then feel more confident recommending it to others with similar symptom constellations. One thing I am sure about is that natural foods, herbs, vitamins, minerals, and other phytonutrients have the potential to reduce or eliminate symptoms, much like prescription drugs; and they do not have the side effects of pharmacotherapy. Because of my experience in treating thousands of patients, listening to them discussing their symptoms, and witnessing their recoveries, I have grown to feel quite comfortable recommending phytonutrients even for ailments outside the field of cardiology.

In addition to my personal and clinical experience, my knowledge base in nutritional supplemental healing expanded during the research for two books I have authored on the subject. When patients ask me to help them with heart disease, depression, sexual dysfunction, psoriasis, constipation, prostate problems, and even cancer, I feel confident in my recommendations.

In this section of the book, I will offer you some of the insights I have obtained from my experience in treating these patients. With rare exceptions, I only prescribe herbs, vitamins, and minerals that I have taken myself. In fact, over the last twenty-five years I have seldom recommended complementary strategies to patients that I have not experienced myself, including psychotherapy, myofascial therapy, deep tissue massage, cranial/sacral therapy, martial arts, herbal remedies, vitamins, and even chelation therapy. Because of my firsthand experience with these healing modalities, I can offer you insights into many of the more common maladies that affect not only cardiac patients, but also most of us in general. Let's start with depression and fatigue.

DEPRESSION AND FATIGUE

Not a day goes by in my office that I fail to meet someone who is fatigued, tired, listless, or just lacking in energy. I often hear complaints such as "Doc, I just don't have my usual spark." Many of these people are mildly depressed, lacking that "bounce in their step." This is my remedy:

1. B vitamin support including folic acid, B-6, B-1, B-2, B-12, and biotin. Take at least 40 mg of vitamins B-1, B-2, and B-6; 40 mcg of B-12 and 300 mcg of biotin. Take pantothenic acid, 50 to 250 mg daily.
2. Coenzyme Q_{10}, 60 mg after each meal.
3. L-tyrosine, 2 grams one to two times daily. (Do not exceed 4 grams daily.) Tyrosine is an essential amino acid that gets into the brain easily, passing the blood-brain barrier. Once absorbed by the brain, tyrosine is a precursor to the neurotransmitters dopamine and norepinephrine. These two neurotransmitters are directly dependent upon dietary tyrosine. Supplementing tyrosine should increase these active neurogenic transmitters in the body. Please note that tyrosine should not be taken in the presence of antipsychotic medications (usually prescribed by physicians) or in the presence of malignant melanoma, a form of skin cancer.
4. Ginkgo biloba, 40 mg three times daily.
5. Saint-John's-wort, 300 mg three times daily. Saint-John's-wort is an herbal remedy for depression. Hypericin, the active ingredient, causes an inhibition of serotonin re-uptake. It has been nicknamed "herbal Prozac."

NUTRIENTS FOR THE AGING BRAIN—
"I CAN'T REMEMBER . . ."

Although memory loss is not an inevitable consequence of aging, it is a fact that the average brain loses about 10 percent of its mass as we approach our golden years. Many of my older patients tell me, "I can't remember this," or "I can't recall that." However, memory problems affect all of us. Each of us knows the frustration of being unable to retrieve or recall a needed piece of information. Because stress and depression affect memory, it is important to consider the nutritional support suggestions I recommended in the fatigue and depression section of this chapter. In addition to those suggestions, I would recommend the following nutrients for the "aging brain":

1. Eat foods high in DMAE (dimethylaminoethanol) such as sardines and anchovies, or take 100 mg of DMAE daily.
2. Take at least 30 mg of lipoic acid daily. (Lipoic acid, like L-tyrosine and

Pycnogenol, can cross the blood-brain barrier to protect cellular membranes from oxidation. As a polypeptide, lipoic acid is also a chelator of excess iron, copper, and other toxic metals such as cadmium, mercury, and lead. (Because lipoic acid also increases glutathione levels, it has antioxidant potential.)

3. Pycnogenol, 30–60 mg three times a day.

4. Phosphatidylserine, 30 mg one to two times a day. (Phosphatidylserine protects brain cell membranes.)

Most of these nutritionals, including L-tyrosine, B vitamins, and ginkgo, can be purchased in health food stores.

NUTRITIONAL SUPPORT FOR PROSTATE HEALTH

As a cardiologist, I treat many men over the age of fifty. Many of these men have prostate problems as well. While lecturing to the prostate support group at Manchester Memorial Hospital, I was amazed at how many younger men (in their forties) had prostate problems, including cancer. Diet is one of the best ways to protect against prostate cancer. Throughout this book I have been praising the healing capabilities of soybean products. Soybeans contain isoflavones rich in natural phytoestrogens. Extensive research has shown that these compounds have many protective benefits, reducing the incidence of prostate cancer in study populations. There is also experimental evidence that phytoestrogens also protect against colon cancer. Not only do soy products protect the circulatory system, but the phytoestrogen effect of genistin found in soybeans protects against the bone loss that leads to osteoporosis. For men, these phytoestrogens are especially important in reducing the incidence of prostate cancer. It is noteworthy that Japanese men, whose diet is low in fat and high in soy products, have a low incidence of prostate cancer.

Another nutrient associated with the prevention of prostate cancer is lycopene. Lycopene is a protective carotenoid responsible for the red color in tomatoes. Several studies have observed a direct association between increased consumption of tomatoes and a reduction in the risk of prostate cancer. When it comes to prostate health, men should consider the nutritional protection found in tomatoes and tomato sauces, as well as the many soy products I have discussed in previous sections of this book.

However, there are specific herbs and nutritionals that are also useful in prostate healing. In addition to the low saturated fat, lycopene, and a soy-enriched diet, I recommend the following for prostate health:

1. Avoid alcohol and nicotine.
2. Take natural vitamin/mineral preparations including folic acid, vitamin E, zinc, and mixed carotenoids, including beta carotene and lycopene.
3. Take saw palmetto, 160 mg to 320 mg daily, for an enlarged prostate. Saw palmetto is a safe, cost-effective natural alternative for treating BPH (benign prostatic hypertrophy). Clinical studies, such as that described in Michael Murray's *The Healing Power of Herbs*, have determined that it is as effective—if not more effective—than the widely prescribed drug called Proscar. Saw palmetto attacks BPH by reducing levels of DHT (dihydrotestosterone). DHT is the active form of testosterone, the major culprit causing enlargement of the prostate gland. Saw palmetto also blocks the action of 5-alpha reductase, the enzyme that converts testosterone to DHT. Increased 5-alpha reductase activity and high levels of DHT appear to be major contributors to BPH.
4. Pygeum africanum, 50 to 75 mg per day. *Pygeum africanum* is a nontoxic tree native to Africa. Its medicinal properties are derived from the bark of the trunk. It is particularly effective in reducing the size of the prostate gland and in enhancing prostatic secretions.
5. Stinging nettles, 150 mg daily, may help to increase urine flow.
6. GLAs (gamma linolenic acids), 2,000 to 3,000 mg daily (in the form of evening primrose oil, borage oil, or black currant oil).

IMPOTENCE

Whether the result of an enlarged prostate or sexual dysfunction, men of all ages may experience impotence. The following suggestions have helped many of my patients with this problem:

1. Use a multivitamin/mineral formula with zinc, at least 30 mg per day.
2. Take L-tyrosine, 2–3 grams daily.
3. Consume L-arginine 4 grams at bedtime. (Doses greater than 6 grams may increase growth hormone, thus stimulating testosterone production.)
4. Use coenzyme Q_{10}, 60 mg after meals.
5. Take Siberian ginseng, 2 grams per day.
6. Ingest ginkgo biloba, 120 mg daily.

7. Use saw palmetto, 160 to 320 mg daily.

8. Consider Corynanthe yohimbe. (Note that yohimbine, a substance found in the bark of the yohimbe tree, is powerful and can have side effects. Since its primary action is to increase blood flow to erectile tissue, an increase in heart rate and blood pressure may occur. Corynanthe yohimbe should not be used without the supervision of a physician.)

9. Consider Muira puama. (This herb, native to Brazil, has long been used to improve libido and sexual function. Although Muira puama's mechanism of action is unknown, its effectiveness in erectile function may be related to enhancing self-esteem. In one study of 262 patients, 1 to 2 grams of Muira puama extract produced a significant response in at least 50 percent of the subjects. Muira puama is often placed in various male formulas in low dosage. These nutritional support systems can usually be found in health food stores.)

CANCER

As a cardiologist, I am somewhat reluctant to treat my patients for cancer. I often refer patients to the exceptional experienced practitioners available who do treat cancer—either traditionally or nontraditionally—on a regular basis. Some patients may be reluctant or even refuse to engage in traditional cancer treatments such as chemotherapy and radiation. While some cancers do respond to a number of superb conventional treatments available, for those of you who wish to take a more proactive role in combating cancer, consider the following suggestions:

1. Work with a skilled psychotherapist experienced with cancer patients. Employ your emotions as a positive force to channel healing energies in your body. Mental imagery is another way of using the right brain as an integral resource in healing. I have known patients who use mental imagery as an adjunct to traditional cancer treatment. They visualize their cancer cells being destroyed by chemotherapy or radiation.

2. Avoid all animal proteins, including dairy products. Many cancer patients have had tremendous success on a macrobiotic diet.

3. Take advantage of many of the phytochemicals available in fruits and vegetables. Eat as many raw and cooked vegetables as you can on a daily basis.

4. Other important phytonutrients to include in your arsenal are isoflavones from soybeans; thiocyanates from cabbage, broccoli, and kale; quercetin from onions, garlic, and leeks; polyphenols from green tea and grapes; and saponins from beans and legumes.

5. Eat raw almonds and, if you can find them, apricot kernels on a daily basis. These are high in laetrile (vitamin B-17), which has been shown to be an anticancer agent. Some studies, however, have refuted the anticancer potential of laetrile.

6. Take coenzyme Q_{10} in the range of 360 to 400 mg daily. There have been many case reports—even those including metastatic breast cancer—that have responded to high coenzyme Q_{10} supplementation.

7. Take a reputable multivitamin/mineral formula without iron. Not only does excess iron enhance heart disease, but research has also demonstrated that excess iron in the blood can increase the risk of cancer.

8. Take N-acetylcysteine supplements, 500 mg daily.

9. Take high-dose vitamin C in the range of 5 to 10 grams daily. Vitamin C can also be taken intravenously (50 grams every two to three days) and is recommended by some doctors who specifically use alternative treatments in the war against cancer.

10. Take shark cartilage either by mouth or better yet as a rectal suspension on a daily basis.

11. Consume gamma linolenic acids (GLAs) in the form of evening primrose oil, borage oil, or black currant oil, to stimulate the production of prostaglandin E hormones.

12. Take milk thistle, 500 to 1,000 mg per day, to help protect the liver from free-radical stress.

13. Take soy products such as tofu or soy milk every day.

14. Hydrate yourself with at least ten glasses of water a day.

15. Consume two ounces of frozen wheat grass per day.

16. Take chaparral tea or herb in a capsule once a day.

17. Try fasting one day every two weeks (see my twenty-four-hour fasting recipe).

18. Drink essiac herbal tea every day.

19. Follow my suggestions for detoxification in the next section (constipation).

For more information on the exciting research into the clinical applications of phytochemicals, the American Institute for Cancer Research in Washington, D.C., will send you free publications regarding dietary approaches to healing cancer (shipping and handling charges may be applied to orders of more than two publications).

CONSTIPATION

Constipation is an embarrassing but common complaint I hear about every day in my office. The cramping and fatigue can be quite distressing. Constipation is often the result of the drugs that I prescribe for various cardiac conditions. These drugs tend to slow the motility of the gastrointestinal tract. Aging may also predispose individuals to constipation. In most cases, however, constipation actually arises from an insufficient amount of fluids, especially water and fiber, in the diet.

Bowel cleanliness, according to experts in the field such as Bernard Jensen and Victor Irons, is necessary to maintain health and avoid many diseases. Detoxification is often a neglected aspect of healing in the medical profession. Toxic by-products occurring from the metabolic breakdown of foods can accumulate in the bowel, rendering one prone to disease. When the bowel is "boggy" and underactive, these toxic wastes are more likely to be absorbed through the bowel wall and eventually into the bloodstream. Enhancing proper digestion with probiotics, digestive herbs, and other enzymes is extremely important. Listed below are some of the things we can do to protect our bodies from the toxic accumulation of waste products:

1. Increase raw foods in the diet, especially vegetables containing enzymes and other proteins to aid in digestion. The cooking, microwaving, processing, and storage of foods can destroy these important enzyme systems.
2. Take vegetable enzymes and other digestive herbs in supplement form to aid in digestion. Many of these formulas contain plant enzyme blends, that is, amylase, cellulase, protease, lipase, and lactase. Most of these supplements can be purchased in health food stores. There are no recommended dosages because many of these enzymes are blended together.
3. Take prebiotics and probiotics, that is, the friendly bacteria, bifidobacterium and lactobacillus, which will help reestablish and maintain good intestinal health.
4. Drink at least eight to ten glasses of water a day.
5. Have at least three to five servings of fresh fruit per day.
6. Use a multivitamin/mineral formula with folic acid.

7. Consume at least 30 to 35 grams of fiber per day.

8. Use aloe vera juice in the morning and evening. (Aloe vera juice is an ingestible product containing water and at least 50 percent aloe vera gel. It is obtained by cultivating the outer layers of the aloe vera leaf. Aloin, one of the chemical constituents of aloe vera, acts as a tonic and increases colonic secretions and contractions.)

9. Avoid dairy products, processed flour, and white table sugar.

10. Do at least one to two one-day fasts per month (see my "24-Hour Juice and Veggie Fast" recipe) and consider the seven-day bowel cleansing programs recommended by Bernard Jensen, DC, in his book *Tissue Cleaning Through Bowel Management*.

PSORIASIS

Psoriasis, a very common skin disorder, affects some 2 to 4 percent of the population of the United States. It is a condition caused by an accumulation of skin cells (with a characteristic silvery scale appearance) that have replicated too rapidly for the cells to be shed. It is estimated that psoriasis causes skin cells to divide approximately 1,000 times faster than in normal skin. Dietary factors triggering psoriasis include incomplete protein digestion, alcohol consumption, and excessive consumption of animal fats.

Some suggestions for nutritional healing of psoriasis from the inside out are as follows:

1. Drink eight glasses of water per day.

2. Avoid all breads and commercial bread-like products such as bagels, biscuits, cakes, and crackers. Avoid meat and dairy products because of high arachidonic acid content. Add oatmeal, asparagus, or avocado to your daily diet.

3. Take a colonic enema every three to four months.

4. Eat an unlimited amount of apples and take a clear liquid fast one to two days every three to four months.

5. Take vitamin B-5 (pantothenic acid), 100 mg three times a day.

6. Take milk thistle, 500 mg to 1,000 mg per day, as an herbal support for liver regeneration.

7. Take fish, flax, evening primrose, borage, or black currant oil capsules, one to two after each meal.

8. Eat fresh fish one to two times a week.

9. Take coenzyme Q_{10}, 60 mg after meals.

10. Take a multivitamin and mineral formula without iron.

A NUTRITIONAL APPROACH TO LOWERING CHOLESTEROL

I personally use this program with much success and recommend it to my patients. Most of the ingredients in this program can be obtained at your supermarket or local health food store. The plan includes eating high-fiber/healthy-fat foods and consuming vitamins, minerals, and other nutritional supplements.

This simple nutritional strategy for cholesterol lowering contains approximately 30 grams of fiber per day. Most individuals will probably consume an additional 5 to 10 grams of fiber from the rest of their daily diet. This amount of fiber, in combination with psyllium seed and cascara (found in Perfect 7 Psyllium/Herbal Combination supplements), will result in an increased frequency of bowel cleansing. (Some individuals may also experience temporary bloating and excessive gas.)

By following this program, individuals will be getting plenty of bioflavonoids, pectin, and soluble fiber, which will protect the body. The nutritional strategy will also inhibit constipation and bowel irregularity. It also conforms to the National Cancer Institute's recommendation of at least five to nine servings of fresh fruits and vegetables per day. Remember that this program includes no pharmacological drugs; it is perfectly natural. It will not only lower your cholesterol and lipid levels, but also will make you feel considerably healthier.

- Breakfast should include a serving of oatmeal or Fiber-One with fresh fruits such as blueberries, strawberries, raspberries, etc.
- Consume $1/2$ clove of garlic, raw or as a condiment in cooking, or take one Kyolic tablet after each meal.
- Eat $1/2$ grapefruit, including all white pulp (the material between the yellow skin and the fruit).
- Eat one pear or one apple daily.
- Consume one teaspoon of Perfect 7 Psyllium/Herbal Combination three days a week. (Most health food stores carry this mixture as well as Kyolic tablets.)

The following supplements should be taken daily:

1. Take one 1,000 mg flaxseed oil capsule after each meal.

2. Take a reputable multivitamin-multimineral supplement with no iron and less than RDA copper.

3. Take at least 100 to 300 mg of quercetin per day.

4. Take niacin, 250 to 500 mg, one or two times per day, after your largest meals. Niacin (nicotinic acid) is a known lipid-lowering agent and generally the most beneficial of these agents in reducing levels of LDL. Niacin is available in two preparations. One is quick-acting and the other slow-acting. It is the slow-acting group used in large doses that has caused serious liver damage in some individuals, and I would not recommend them because of the possibility of adverse side effects. However, the quick-acting formulation is popular and has been studied extensively over the past three decades. These studies show that niacin not only demonstrates a reduction in cholesterol, but also yields a significant reduction in long-term mortality rates for coronary artery disease.

The unpopularity of niacin has been related to the unpleasant, hot skin sensations that patients may feel in the head and neck area. I remember the first time I took niacin; I thought my entire upper body was on fire. It was a hot day in July, and I took off my shirt because the sensation of heat was so intense. Fortunately, this sensation of heat lasts for only a few minutes, and the reactions can be markedly reduced when taking the vitamin with aspirin or after a large meal. Some people even enjoy the sensation, particularly in cold weather. Nevertheless, it is very important for you to be aware of this minor but unpleasant (for some people) reaction to niacin.

5. If you have high triglycerides in addition to high cholesterol, take 200 mcg of chromium picolinate. Doses of up to 400 mcg of chromium picolinate have been shown to lower triglycerides. There have been studies demonstrating that chromium picolinate has been useful in transforming body fat to lean muscle mass, but I am not yet comfortable with this particular research. More studies are needed. Its role in lowering triglyceride levels, however, is well substantiated.

6. For high cholesterol levels that do not respond readily to other treatments, 2 to 3 grams of L-arginine can be taken daily at bedtime. Because of its membrane-stabilizing properties, this amino acid has been gaining popularity as an antiaging strategy. L-arginine has been known to stimulate the endothelial-cell-releasing factor, which is a nitric oxide derivative

that helps keep blood vessels open. Nitric acid helps to prevent the chain reactions that cause hardening of the blood vessels. In animal studies, L-arginine has been known to reduce cholesterol levels and retard plaque formation in blood vessels. L-arginine has also been reported to increase the immune response, improve wound healing, and retard tumor progression.

7. Consume one green tea beverage after lunch or dinner. Another phytonutrient with not only antioxidant properties, but also anti-platelet-stickiness and cholesterol-reducing activity, green tea is customarily taken after almost every meal in Japan. Some researchers believe that the polyphenol activity in green tea protects you from coronary artery disease by its interaction with cholesterol. Perhaps this is one of the reasons that the Japanese have the lowest incidence of coronary artery disease in the world.

8. Consider taking the phytonutrient guggul—an old yet very new cholesterol-fighting agent. This resin contains a complex mixture of phytonutrients called diterpenes and esters, as well as guggulsterones. Research in the mid-1960s was the first to clearly demonstrate that guggul significantly lowers cholesterol. There have been more than twenty clinical studies since then showing that guggul not only can lower blood cholesterol and triglycerides, but also can lower LDL and raise HDL. Comprehensive pharmacological studies done on animals and humans have shown that this safe and effective agent can lower cholesterol by up to 30 to 40 percent. You can find several brands of guggulipid in health food stores.

In the future, you will certainly see some new, exciting, and creative ways of lowering your cholesterol. All that is needed is an open mind.

NATURAL BLOOD-PRESSURE-LOWERING PROGRAM

Potassium, calcium, and magnesium deficiencies have all been incriminated in blood pressure elevation. In my natural approach to blood pressure control, adequate supplementation of these minerals is crucial. The following nonpharmacological approach to lowering blood pressure includes increasing calcium, potassium, and magnesium intake, decreasing sodium, and adding coenzyme Q_{10} to your daily regimen.

1. Reduce all salt intake and be careful of processed foods. Read labels! Be aware of food additives and food enhancers, particularly monosodium glutamate. Avoid canned vegetables, canned soups, diet soft drinks, preservatives, meat tenderizers, soy sauce, etc. If you are overweight, watch the amount of fats and calories that you consume. Try to lose weight.

2. Consume a high-fiber diet. Eat at least five to nine servings of fresh fruits and vegetables per day. Drink eight glasses of clean, filtered, or bottled water per day.

3. Avoid high-salt meats, including processed meats (as well as bacon, sausage, ham, and hot dogs).

4. Do not take nonsteroidal pain relievers such as Motrin, Advil, Nuprin, etc.

5. Maintain a regular exercise program.

6. Avoid Nutrasweet, aspartame, and antihistamines.

7. Take a 200 to 500 mg magnesium supplement each day.

8. Take a daily multivitamin and mineral formula that contains antioxidants but no iron, copper, oils, preservatives, fillers, or animal products.

9. Take 60 mg of coenzyme Q_{10} after each meal.

10. Consume as much parsley and garlic as possible. Increase your intake of calcium- and potassium-containing foods such as kale, white beans, raisins, figs, and lima beans.

11. Eat fresh fish one to two times per week or take fish- or flaxseed-oil supplements.

12. Be aware of your internalized anger.

A NUTRITIONAL APPROACH TO HEALING ARTHRITIS

As a cardiologist, I have used a natural, nutritional approach in treating heart disease for many years. To my surprise, many of my cardiac patients found that this nutritional therapy also helped reduce the pain and swelling of their arthritic hands, knees, and other joints. This led me to review carefully the medical literature on nutrition and its impact on arthritis. Eventually I developed a program of eating guidelines and nutritional supplements designed specifically to ease the pain and inflammation of arthritic joints. (As a bonus, many of these tips will help promote a healthy heart as well.)

If you follow these guidelines, over time (usually within eight weeks) you should see a significant reduction in pain and stiffness. Begin this program with the twenty-four-hour juice and veggie fast (see chapter fifteen); after the initial twenty-four-hour fast, follow this program:

1. Consume an alkalizing diet including one glass of carrot juice or wheat grass juice daily. Consume only fresh fruits and vegetables but avoid those from the nightshade family such as peppers, eggplant, tomatoes, or potatoes. Do not drink sodas or caffeine; avoid chocolate. Increase the amount of yams in the diet and consume a cup of miso soup daily. Increase your consumption of high-fiber, healthy-fat foods. Decrease the use of citrus fruits, dairy products, and animal proteins (meat and fish).

2. Use one small Certo package or one tablespoon of Certo in cranberry juice daily. Certo is used to thicken jams and jellies and can be found in supermarkets and some health food stores.

3. Drink one cup of ginger tea daily.

4. Take supplements of chlorella, green barley, or wheat grass daily.

5. Consume omega-3 oils, found primarily in flaxseed oil and fish oil. Omega-3 oils inhibit production of leukotrienes, eicosanoids that stimulate inflammation. I recommend taking one 1,000 mg flaxseed capsule after each meal; these can be found in any health food store. Another way to boost your omega-3 intake is to eat at least one to two helpings of fresh fish per day.

6. Eat cayenne and garlic. Both herbs have an anti-inflammatory effect, helping to reduce swelling and pain. I urge my patients to take a cayenne capsule with 40,000 heat units after one meal. If this upsets your stomach, eat bread or crackers with it. If stomach upset is severe, stop taking cayenne. Remember, if you can't tolerate hot chili, you will not tolerate cayenne.

7. Take multivitamin and mineral supplements. (Be sure to select iron-free supplements, since too much iron has been linked to an elevated risk of heart disease.) The supplement you select should also contain no more than 1 mg of copper, half the RDA. It should contain folic acid, vitamin B-6, vitamin D, zinc, and calcium, as deficiency in any of these nutrients may cause arthritic symptoms. The supplement should also contain the antioxidants selenium and vitamin E.

8. Take coenzyme Q_{10} and quercetin. I recommend 30 mg of coenzyme Q_{10} after each meal and at least 100 mg of quercetin a day. Coenzyme Q_{10} works to stabilize membranes, thus preventing cellular breakdown in

the joints. Quercetin blocks the release of histamines (inflammation-producing chemicals) into the bloodstream.

9. Take GLAs (evening primrose oil, borage oil, or black currant oil), 1,000 mg a day.

10. Take glucosamine sulfate, 500 to 1,000 mg a day.

I have also had much success in some patients using shark cartilage, boswellin, and cat's claw. These nutrients can be purchased in health food stores and can be considered on an individual basis.

NUTRITIONAL HEALING FOR INDIVIDUALS ON CHEMOTHERAPY OR RADIATION THERAPY

Begin this program with a twenty-four-hour juice and veggie fast (see chapter fifteen). After the initial twenty-four-hour fast, follow this program:

1. Consume a vegan diet (a vegetarian diet that excludes all dairy or animal protein).

2. Drink ginseng tea daily.

3. Consume one cup of miso soup with parsley and shiitake mushrooms daily.

4. Consume frozen wheat grass, green barley, or green magna extract as a daily supplement.

5. The following supplements should be taken: N-acetylcysteine, 500 mg; glutathione, 100 mg; a multivitamin and mineral supplement, copper-free and iron-free; quercetin, 100 mg to 300 mg; and coenzyme Q_{10}, 60 mg after each meal.

Fifteen

Recipes for
Preventive Medicine

The following recipes are ones I use in my daily life. Although I eat pasta and rice, I consume small portions; I try to use pastas made from Jerusalem artichoke, spelt, and rye whenever possible, and I always eat brown rice. For protein, I consume fish at least two or three times a week, frequently eat chicken or turkey, and eat red meat on occasion. I also use soy milk on a regular basis and have tofu once or twice a week.

I usually accompany my meals with a simple salad of lettuce and tomatoes or vegetables marinated in olive oil. I am, however, not perfect. I do indulge now and then and eat less healthy foods when they are prepared for me by someone else (by a friend, or at a restaurant or party). I enjoy them, too. My point here is that I have discovered ways to eat healthy foods more often and unhealthy foods less often without feeling deprived.

In the following recipes, note the frequent use of olive oil. Although it is best to use as little oil as possible, I wholeheartedly endorse the use of olive oil for salads and cooking. Since many of the recipes require two tablespoons of olive oil and most of the recipes will serve four or five, the grams of fat per person is still quite reasonable. For example, two tablespoons of olive oil have 28 grams of fat; divided by four people, this comes out to only seven grams of fat per serving. This will not affect your insulin levels. Other ingredients are also low in fat, yielding recipes that are healthy-fat and, in most instances, high-fiber.

Whenever possible, use fresh ingredients when preparing food, particularly lemons, basil, parsley, watercress, and lots of garlic and onions, all of which are heart-healing. Try to steam as many items as you can. When cooking with oil, use low heat and short cooking times to prevent overcooking and oxidation of the oil. Always try to minimize the use of salt. Some of the following menu suggestions, especially the rice and pasta selections, are moderate glycemic. I suggest you use additional protein in the form of some three to four ounces of seafood and/or meat with these recipes. Consider doing the following twenty-four-hour fast once a month for bowel cleansing, reduction of free-radical stress, and longevity, as it increases melatonin levels.

24-HOUR JUICE AND VEGGIE FAST

Begin the fast by squeezing half a fresh lemon into a glass of pure water and adding one-half teaspoon of maple syrup. Drink the mixture.

Breakfast: One glass of cranberry juice
Lunch: One glass of carrot juice with either frozen wheat grass, green barley, or chlorella added; one cup of ginger tea
Dinner: One glass of grapefruit juice and two bowls of miso broth (recipe on page 217)
Bedtime: One cup of either chamomile, ginger, or echinacea tea

In addition to the above, drink eight glasses of water per day. You will find the majority of the products listed above at your local health food store.

MISO BROTH

Ingredients

2 quarts water
4 or 5 carrots
2 potatoes with skins
1 onion
4 shiitake mushrooms
3 celery stalks
2 garlic cloves
$^1/_2$ bunch parsley
$^1/_2$ cabbage or $^1/_2$ cup Brussels sprouts
$^1/_2$ bunch broccoli
$^1/_2$-inch piece ginger root
2 tablespoons miso

Directions

Cut up vegetables and simmer ingredients except miso for 30 minutes, then discard all solids. Add miso. Stir and simmer at low heat for at least $^1/_2$ hour.

MISO-VEGETABLE SOUP

Ingredients

3 quarts water
2 onions, chopped
3 carrots, sliced
1 clove garlic, crushed
10 to 15 mushrooms, cut into quarters
1 tablespoon toasted-sesame-seed oil
4 teaspoons miso
Freshly ground pepper and sea salt
1 bay leaf
Olive oil

½ cup cooked short-grain brown rice, barley, lentils, peas, millet, wheat berries, or adzuki beans (optional)

Fresh parsley, watercress, or scallions, chopped

Directions

Bring water to a boil and add onion, carrots, and garlic; cover and simmer until vegetables are tender. Sauté mushrooms in sesame-seed oil; add to soup. Add miso and simmer for approximately 5 to 10 minutes. Do not boil. Add pepper and sea salt to taste, one bay leaf, and a dash of sesame or olive oil. Add ½ cup of cooked rice or other grains or beans if using them. Cook for 10 more minutes. Garnish with freshly chopped parsley, scallions, or watercress.

Variation

Add chopped kale, cut-up string beans, or chopped spinach before adding rice or other grains.

SEA VEGETABLE SOUP—NATURE'S WONDER

This recipe, with slight modifications, was taken from *Fighting Radiation with Foods, Herbs, and Vitamins: Documented Natural Remedies That Boost Your Immunity and Detoxify*, by Steven R. Schechter, ND (Vitality, 1990).

Ingredients

1 cup mixed sea vegetables (dulse, kelp, wakame, kombu, etc.)

3 quarts water

1 large onion, chopped

1 carrot, chopped

1½ cups broccoli, chopped

2 cloves garlic, minced

3 tablespoons toasted–sesame-seed oil

1 teaspoon thyme

1 teaspoon marjoram

Dash of cayenne pepper, freshly ground pepper, or finely chopped fresh ginger

2 tablespoons miso

Fresh parsley, chopped
Optional ingredients: mushrooms, brown rice

Directions

Soak sea vegetables for thirty minutes and discard water (this takes out the excess sodium). Now place in 3 quarts water and simmer. Sauté onion, carrot, broccoli, and garlic in oil for five minutes, or until onion is partially translucent. Add vegetables to water with remaining ingredients except miso and parsley. Simmer for thirty minutes. Turn off heat. Remove $1/2$ cup of liquid and dissolve miso in it. Return to soup and heat for three minutes; do not boil. Adjust seasonings to taste. Garnish with parsley.

ANTIGUAN BLACK BEAN SOUP

Ingredients

2 tablespoons olive oil
$1/2$ green pepper, chopped
1 onion, chopped
$1/2$ clove garlic, minced
$1/2$ pound dried black beans, cooked according to package directions, or substitute 2 one-pound cans of black beans and drain
2 quarts water
Freshly ground pepper
2 tablespoons red wine vinegar
1 bay leaf
1 cup short-grain brown rice, cooked
Fresh parsley, chopped

Directions

In a large saucepan, combine olive oil, green pepper, onion (reserve some raw onion as a topping), and garlic. Sauté until tender. Add precooked or canned black beans, pepper, vinegar, and bay leaf. Add water and then simmer for 30 to 40 minutes. Remove bay leaf before serving. Top with raw onion and brown rice. Garnish with parsley.

BEET SALAD WITH LEMON AND HONEY

Ingredients

1 tablespoon olive oil
1 tablespoon red wine vinegar
$^1/_2$ cup lemon juice
1 tablespoon honey
1 teaspoon tamari
3 medium beets, peeled and finely chopped
Fresh chopped parsley

Directions

Make the dressing by combining the olive oil and red wine vinegar. Add the lemon juice, honey, and tamari and stir briskly. Pour over beets and toss. Sprinkle with parsley.

BOSTON LETTUCE AND WATERCRESS SALAD

Ingredients

1 head Boston lettuce
1 bunch watercress
1 teaspoon prepared mustard
Sea salt and freshly ground pepper
2 teaspoons finely minced garlic
1 tablespoon red wine vinegar
$^1/_2$ tablespoon balsamic vinegar
2 tablespoons extra-virgin olive oil
Fresh parsley, chopped

Directions

Remove the core of the lettuce and pull the leaves apart. Cut off the tough ends of the watercress. Rinse greens well and pat dry.

Put the mustard in a salad bowl with sea salt and pepper to taste. Add the garlic and vinegars and beat with a wire whisk. Gradually add the oil, beating briskly with the wire whisk until well blended. Pour dressing over the lettuce and watercress. Toss well and serve. Garnish with parsley if desired.

DAD'S ITALIAN-STYLE TOMATOES

Ingredients

4 medium to large tomatoes
1 tablespoon olive oil
1 clove garlic, finely chopped
1 tablespoon balsamic vinegar
Sea salt and freshly ground pepper to taste
Fresh basil or oregano to taste (do not use both)

Directions

Wash and dry tomatoes and place in the refrigerator to chill. Cut tomatoes into $1/4$-inch slices and place on a plate. Sprinkle tomatoes with olive oil, garlic, vinegar, sea salt, pepper, and basil or oregano.

EASY ITALIAN-STYLE TOMATO SAUCE

Ingredients

2 tablespoons olive oil
3 cloves garlic, finely chopped
2 medium onions, chopped
2 cans Italian-style plum tomatoes or 2 pounds fresh plum or cherry tomatoes, chopped
1 ounce red or white wine
1 tablespoon fresh basil, chopped
1 teaspoon fresh oregano, crushed
Sea salt and freshly ground pepper to taste
Hot cooked spaghetti or linguini
Fresh parsley, chopped

Directions

Place the olive oil in a pan and sauté garlic and onions for approximately 30 seconds to 1 minute. Add tomatoes and wine and cook for 3 to 4 minutes. Add basil, oregano, sea salt, and pepper. Serve over hot cooked spaghetti or linguini and sprinkle with parsley. Spelt, Jerusalem artichoke, or protein-enriched pastas have a better glycemic index than traditional white pastas and are preferred for this and subsequent pasta dishes.

MEDITERRANEAN SEAFOOD SAUCE WITH JERUSALEM ARTICHOKE PASTA

Ingredients

2 to 3 tablespoons olive oil
2 small onions, chopped
8 cloves garlic, minced
1 ounce fresh parsley, chopped
1 bunch fresh basil, chopped
$1/2$ teaspoon fresh oregano, chopped
1 teaspoon anchovy paste
1 dozen fresh clams, chopped
4 ounces fresh tuna, chopped
White wine or vegetable broth or bottled clam juice
Hot cooked Jerusalem artichoke pasta
Freshly ground pepper
Grated Asiago or Parmesan cheese

Directions

Into a frying pan over very low heat, place 2 to 3 tablespoons of olive oil, onions, and garlic. Sauté for a few minutes. Add chopped fresh parsley and basil (reserve a small amount of the basil), oregano, and anchovy paste. Then add clams and tuna. You may add your choice of 1 ounce of white wine, 3 ounces of vegetable broth, or 2 ounces of bottled clam juice. Cook for a few minutes. Toss with hot cooked Jerusalem artichoke pasta. Add freshly ground pepper to taste and/or Asiago or Parmesan cheese. Top with the remaining chopped basil.

PASTA À LA SINATRA

Ingredients

    2 tablespoons olive oil
    4 garlic cloves, minced
    3 small onions, chopped
    1 8-ounce jar sun-dried tomatoes in olive oil, pureed in food
        processor to desired consistency
    2 medium summer squash, finely chopped
    Fresh chopped basil and freshly ground pepper to taste
    Hot cooked fettucine
    Grated Parmesan cheese
    Chopped parsley

Directions

Place olive oil in a saucepan. Add garlic and onions and sauté for a few minutes. Add tomatoes and sauté for a few minutes more. Add squash and sauté a few minutes. Add fresh basil and pepper. Pour sauce over hot cooked fettucine. Add grated cheese and garnish with chopped parsley.

PASTA WITH GARLIC, MUSHROOMS, AND PARSLEY

Ingredients

    2 tablespoons olive oil
    6 cloves garlic, minced
    1 12-ounce carton mushrooms, finely chopped
    1 large bunch parsley, finely chopped
    1 ounce white wine
    Freshly ground pepper
    Hot cooked linguini or fettucine
    Freshly grated Parmesan cheese

Directions

Into a pan place the olive oil and garlic. Gently sauté for a couple of minutes. Add mushrooms and parsley (reserve a small amount of fresh

---

parsley). Simmer 5 to 7 minutes. Add white wine and pepper. Serve over hot cooked linguini or fettucine. Sprinkle with remaining fresh parsley and add grated Parmesan cheese.

JERUSALEM ARTICHOKE PASTA WITH FRESH TOMATO SAUCE

Ingredients

6 medium tomatoes, skinned and sliced thinly
2 tablespoons olive oil
1 clove garlic, minced
2 medium onions, chopped
Fresh basil, one small bunch, cut into thin strips
Hot cooked Jerusalem artichoke pasta
Freshly grated Parmesan cheese
Freshly ground pepper

Directions

To skin tomatoes, dip in boiling water for 30 seconds. Remove and let cool. Skins should slip off easily.

Place olive oil, garlic, and onions in a pan and gently sauté. Add tomatoes and sauté for a few minutes. Add basil. Pour sauce over hot cooked pasta. Sprinkle with grated cheese and pepper to taste. (This is a "dry" pasta dish, yielding little extra sauce.)

RYE PASTA WITH SPINACH

Ingredients

2 tablespoons olive oil
3 cloves garlic, minced
12 mushrooms, finely sliced
2 bags spinach, stems removed and leaves washed well and spun dry
Freshly ground pepper to taste

Hot cooked spelt-rye pasta
2 tablespoons grated Parmesan cheese

Directions

Into a large pan put olive oil, garlic, and mushrooms. Sauté over medium heat for a couple of minutes. Add spinach. Cover pan and steam for 2 minutes. Add pepper. Mix sauce and pour over pasta. Sprinkle with grated Parmesan cheese.

PASTA WITH FENNEL AND TUNA

Ingredients

1 pound fresh fennel
1 pound fresh tuna, cut into 1-inch pieces
1 large onion, chopped
2 tablespoons olive oil
$^1/_2$ cup tomato sauce
$^1/_2$ tablespoon pine nuts
3 tablespoons dried black currants
Sea salt and freshly ground pepper to taste
6 threads saffron
Hot cooked pasta
Fresh parsley, chopped

Directions

Boil the fennel until tender; drain and chop. Sauté the tuna and onion in olive oil. Add tomato sauce and simmer. Add fennel, pine nuts, currants, salt, and pepper. Cook over low heat for approximately 20 minutes.

Dissolve saffron in two tablespoons of warm water. Add saffron to drained pasta and mix thoroughly. Spoon tuna mixture over pasta and garnish with freshly chopped parsley as desired.

Rice with Steamed Vegetables

Ingredients

3 ounces water
2 or 3 medium carrots, sliced
2 medium zucchini, chopped
1 small bunch broccoli, chopped
2 medium summer squash, chopped
12 mushrooms, chopped
1/4 head cauliflower, chopped
3 cloves garlic, minced
2 teaspoons dried basil
2 tablespoons olive oil
2 tablespoons grated Parmesan cheese
Fresh parsley, chopped
1 1/2 cups hot cooked short-grain brown rice

Directions

Place water in a wok or frypan. (Use a steaming rack if available.) Place the prepared vegetables into the wok or frypan. Sprinkle garlic, basil, and olive oil on top. Cover and steam for several minutes, until the vegetables are tender. Stir frequently if not using a rack. When tender, sprinkle Parmesan cheese and parsley over the steamed vegetables and serve with brown rice.

Fried Rice

Ingredients

1 tablespoon dark sesame oil
1 medium onion, sliced
12 mushrooms, sliced
1/2 package frozen peas (usually a 10-ounce package)
1 tablespoon shredded daikon
4 cups cooked short-grain brown rice

¹/₂ tablespoon tamari

Chopped scallions or fresh chopped parsley

Directions

Brush skillet with sesame oil. Heat for a minute or less but do not let oil start to smoke. Add onion, mushrooms, peas, and daikon; place rice on top. If rice is dry, moisten with a few drops of water. Cover skillet and cook over low heat for 10 to 15 minutes. Add tamari and cook for another 5 minutes. Stir to mix before serving.

Garnish with chopped scallions or parsley.

BUCKWHEAT PANCAKES WITH BLUEBERRIES

This is my version of a recipe taken from *Fighting Radiation with Foods, Herbs, and Vitamins: Documented Natural Remedies That Boost Your Immunity and Detoxify,* by Steven R. Schechter, ND (Vitality, 1990).

Ingredients

1 cup buckwheat flour

1 cup other whole-grain flour

2 cups soy milk or water

2 eggs

1 tablespoon grapeseed oil

1 tablespoon honey

¹/₂ cup fresh unsweetened blueberries

Directions

Stir dry ingredients together. Add soy milk, eggs, oil, and honey and mix briefly. Add blueberries and stir gently. Cook on hot lightly oiled griddle.

Blueberry or Apple-Cinnamon Bran Muffins

Ingredients

2 cups bran cereal
1 cup skim milk
2 tablespoons grapeseed oil
2 egg whites
1 tablespoon honey
$^1/_3$ cup molasses
$1^1/_2$ cups whole-wheat flour or Soy Quik flour
$^1/_2$ tablespoon sea salt
1 cup blueberries or 1 apple, grated, and 1 teaspoon cinnamon

Directions

Mix bran cereal and milk and let stand 5 minutes. Add oil, egg whites, honey, and molasses. Add flour and salt. Add blueberries or apple-cinnamon mixture. Stir until just mixed. Bake in a muffin tin at 400 degrees for 15 minutes.

Chicken with Pea Pods and Zucchini

Ingredients

8 ounces boneless breast of chicken
2 tablespoons peanut or olive oil
12 mushrooms, sliced
1 teaspoon dried basil
2 cloves garlic, crushed
1 tablespoon onion, chopped
1 medium zucchini, chopped
1 cup pea pods
1 ounce white wine (optional)
Cooked brown rice
Fresh parsley, chopped

Directions

Slice boneless breast of chicken into strips 2 inches by $^1/_2$ inch. Heat oil in wok or frypan. Add chicken, mushrooms, basil, garlic, onion, zucchini, and pea pods. Sauté until chicken is done. Add wine. Simmer gently until zucchini and pea pods are tender. Serve with brown rice. Garnish with parsley.

CHICKEN WITH ARTICHOKES

Ingredients

8 ounces boneless breast of chicken
2 tablespoons peanut or olive oil
1 teaspoon dried basil
2 cloves garlic, minced
12 mushrooms, thinly sliced
1 ounce white wine (optional)
1 large (12-ounce) or two small (6-ounce) jar(s) marinated artichoke hearts, drained
$^1/_2$ lemon
Fresh parsley, chopped

Directions

Slice chicken into strips 2 inches by $^1/_2$ inch. Heat oil in wok or frypan. Add chicken, basil, and garlic. Sauté for 2 minutes. Add mushrooms, wine, and artichoke hearts. Simmer on low heat for 10 minutes. Squeeze lemon on top and mix. Garnish with parsley and serve.

Variations

Additional ingredients: bread crumbs and freshly ground pepper. Slice chicken into larger pieces, 4 inches by 2 inches. Sprinkle chicken with olive oil, parsley, garlic, bread crumbs, and pepper. Broil $1^1/_2$ minutes or until chicken is cooked and bread crumbs are brown. Place chicken in bowl and squeeze lemon juice over it; add artichokes and chopped basil, and serve.

Santiago's Chicken

Ingredients

4 boneless half breasts of chicken
4 cloves garlic, minced
$^1/_2$ cup dry sherry or white wine
1 lime
1 teaspoon paprika
$^1/_2$ teaspoon ground coriander
$^1/_2$ teaspoon cumin
$^1/_2$ teaspoon grated ginger root
Sea salt and freshly ground pepper to taste
Fresh parsley, chopped

Directions

Place chicken in a dish and add remaining ingredients, excluding parsley, to form a marinade. Place in refrigerator for at least 1 to 2 hours. Turn the chicken every so often to coat evenly with marinade.

Broil chicken until tender, continuing to baste with marinade while cooking. Garnish with freshly chopped parsley.

Spinach Salad with Grilled Chicken, Mango, and Raspberries

Here's a great recipe from Sandy Szwarc of Albuquerque, New Mexico. I found it in the July 1996 issue of *Gourmet,* modified it slightly, and would like to share it with you.

Ingredients

For dressing:

2 tablespoons raspberry vinegar
1 tablespoon balsamic vinegar
1 tablespoon soy sauce
$^1/_4$ teaspoon Dijon mustard
2 teaspoons minced, peeled fresh ginger root

3 garlic cloves, minced and mashed into a paste with salt to taste

$1/4$ teaspoon freshly ground black pepper, or to taste

$1/2$ cup extra-virgin olive oil

For salad:

1 whole skinless, boneless chicken breast (about $3/4$ pound), halved

3 bunches spinach (about 2 pounds), coarse stems discarded and leaves washed well and spun dry

2 firm, ripe mangoes, cut into $1/4$-inch-thick slices

1 cup raspberries, picked over

4 scallions, chopped finely

$1/2$ cup walnuts, toasted and chopped coarsely

Directions

In a bowl, whisk together all dressing ingredients except oil. Add oil in a stream, whisking, and whisk until emulsified. Dressing may be made 2 days ahead and chilled, covered.

In a shallow dish or resealable plastic bag, coat chicken with 3 tablespoons dressing. Marinate chicken, covered and chilled, 2 hours.

Heat an oiled, well-seasoned, ridged grill pan over moderately high heat until hot but not smoking. Drain chicken and grill until cooked through, about 7 minutes on each side. Transfer chicken to a platter and cool. Chicken may be made up to this point 1 day ahead and then chilled, covered.

Cut chicken into $1/4$-inch-thick slices, and in a large bowl combine with remaining salad ingredients. Drizzle remaining dressing over salad and toss gently to combine well.

GRILLED HALIBUT MEDITERRANEAN STYLE WITH LEMON-BASIL VINAIGRETTE

Ingredients

1 lemon

2 tablespoons olive oil (preferably extra-virgin)

3 garlic cloves, crushed

$^1/_2$ teaspoon grated lemon peel

3 tablespoons thinly sliced fresh basil or 3 teaspoons dried

2 teaspoons drained capers

Salt and freshly ground pepper

4 (5- to 6-ounce) halibut steaks, about $^3/_4$ inch thick

Directions

Squeeze lemon. Whisk lemon juice, olive oil, garlic, and lemon peel in a small bowl to blend. Stir in 2 tablespoons fresh basil and the capers. Season vinaigrette to taste with salt and pepper. (Can be prepared 1 hour ahead. Let stand at room temperature.)

Preheat broiler (medium-high heat). Season halibut steaks with salt and pepper. Brush fish with 1 tablespoon vinaigrette. Grill or broil halibut steaks until just cooked through, about 4 minutes per side. Transfer fish to plates. Rewhisk remaining vinaigrette; pour over fish. Garnish fish with remaining basil and serve.

BREADED SOLE, FLOUNDER, OR FLUKE

Ingredients

2 tablespoons olive oil

1 ounce white wine

1 juiced lemon

$^1/_2$ teaspoon dried basil

Fresh parsley, chopped

Sea salt and freshly ground pepper to taste

1 pound sole, flounder, or fluke fillets

1 cup Italian-style bread crumbs

Lemon slices

Watercress, chopped, if desired

Directions

Mix olive oil, wine, lemon juice, basil, and parsley; add salt and pepper. Dip fish in this marinade and then gently roll it in bread crumbs. Broil for a minute or two on each side. Serve with lemon slices and garnish with chopped parsley and/or watercress.

GRILLED TUNA OR SWORDFISH WITH SPINACH

Ingredients

1 tablespoon olive oil
1 bunch spinach
1 fresh lemon
1 pound fresh tuna or swordfish
Sea salt and freshly ground pepper to taste
1 teaspoon dried basil
Fresh parsley, chopped

Directions

Into a saucepan put olive oil. Rinse the spinach well, discarding the stems, and place it wet into the pan. Cover and cook for a few minutes, but do not overcook. Squeeze lemon over fish and sprinkle with sea salt, pepper, and basil. Grill fish for 2 to 3 minutes per side. Tuna should be slightly red in the middle; rare tuna, like rare meat, tastes very good. If you use swordfish, cook longer, until it is cooked through. After the fish is cooked, take the spinach out of the pan and place on a platter. Place the fish on top of the spinach. Squeeze some fresh lemon juice over it. Sprinkle with fresh parsley and serve.

MARINATED BLUEFISH

Ingredients

2 medium-sized bluefish steaks
$1/2$ lemon
2 tablespoons olive oil
1 ounce white wine
$1/2$ teaspoon dried basil
3 cloves garlic, minced
Sea salt and freshly ground pepper to taste
Fresh parsley, chopped

Directions

Place bluefish steaks on a platter and squeeze lemon over them. Mix olive oil, white wine, basil, garlic, sea salt, and pepper and pour over fish. Marinate for several hours, or overnight if desired. Sauté fish in a lightly oiled pan, or grill. Sprinkle with fresh parsley and serve. This dish is nice over rice and accompanied by a watercress salad.

ROAST EYE OF ROUND WITH ROSEMARY AND POTATOES

Ingredients

2 pounds eye of round
1 teaspoon rosemary, crushed in a small bowl
Sea salt and freshly ground pepper to taste
8 small red potatoes, cut in half
2 onions, sliced
2 tomatoes, sliced
Fresh parsley, chopped

Directions

Preheat oven to 350 degrees. Trim off excess fat from the roast and sprinkle with crushed rosemary, salt, and pepper. Place the roast on a rack in a roasting pan and add 1 ounce of water to bottom of pan. Place potatoes on rack around roast and sprinkle with rosemary. Roast until tender, approximately $1^1/_2$ hours. Slice thin and serve with raw sliced onions and tomatoes sprinkled with parsley.

LOW-FAT EXCEPTIONAL HAMBURGERS

This is an excellent recipe for those who desire red meat. Each quarter-pound burger has only four to five grams of fat per serving.

Ingredients

>   2 pounds top round steak or London broil, all fat trimmed and meat
>   ground
>   Few drops extra-virgin olive oil
>   Sea salt and freshly ground pepper to taste
>   Fresh parsley, chopped

Directions

Form meat into quarter-pound hamburgers.

Into a glass or steel frypan, add a few drops of extra-virgin olive oil and place the hamburgers over high heat. Sprinkle with salt and pepper. When cooked, serve with freshly chopped parsley.

TOFU WITH SESAME SEEDS

Ingredients

>   1 block firm tofu
>   2 tablespoons sesame seeds
>   1 clove garlic, minced
>   8 scallions, chopped
>   4 tablespoons salt-free or reduced-sodium soy sauce
>   2 ounces rice wine

Directions

Chop tofu into 1-inch cubes. Sprinkle sesame seeds into tofu. Add garlic, scallions, soy sauce, and rice wine to the tofu cubes and mix well.

Salad Dressings

Sour Cream and Chive Dressing

Ingredients

$^1/_2$ cup light sour cream
1 clove garlic, crushed
1 tablespoon apple cider vinegar
1 teaspoon Dijon mustard
2 teaspoons fresh chopped chives or finely chopped fresh parsley

Lemon-Honey Dressing

Ingredients

Juice of one large lemon
2 tablespoons honey
2 tablespoons olive oil
$^1/_2$ teaspoon dried basil

Olive Oil–Balsamic Dressing

Ingredients

2 tablespoons olive oil
1 tablespoon balsamic vinegar
Pinch of finely chopped fresh parsley
Pinch of garlic powder
Pinch of freshly ground black pepper

Directions

Shake or beat all ingredients in a glass jar.

VEGETABLE RECIPES

Asparagus

Directions

Steam asparagus until almost tender, approximately 5 minutes. Place on plate; add 1 teaspoon olive oil. Sprinkle with fresh lemon and garlic powder to taste.

Steamed Spinach

Directions

Use wok or covered pan. Sauté 1 or 2 cloves minced garlic in 1 teaspoon olive oil; add spinach with 2 ounces water and cook until tender. Sprinkle with lemon juice and garlic powder to taste.

FOODS TO AVOID

Lard, margarines, coconut oil, palm oil, salt pork, meat drippings, gravies, cream sauces, ketchup, mayonnaise, butter, whole milk, cream, nondairy coffee creamer, whipped topping, and high-fat cheeses.

Red fatty meats, spareribs, ham, corned beef, regular ground meat, cold cuts, hot dogs, sausages, bacon, meats canned or frozen in sauces or gravies, frozen packaged dinners, fried fish, fried meats, poultry skin, fish roe, and organ meats.

White flour and its commercial products, including biscuits, muffins, sweet rolls, doughnuts, waffles, and bagels.

French fries, white potatoes, potato chips, junk foods, popcorn with salt or butter.

Olives, creamed or fried vegetables.

Cream soups, dehydrated soups, and commercial bouillon.

All beverages with added sweeteners, alcohol, or caffeine. (Limit coffee to one cup per day.)

Pies, cakes, cookies, chocolate, coconut, candies, jams, jellies, granulated sugar, molasses, gourmet ice cream.

Avoid the mortal sins:

1. Margarine
2. High-fat gourmet ice cream
3. Lard
4. White table sugar
5. Peanut butter
6. Palm oil
7. Corn oil
8. Safflower oil

FOODS TO SUBSTITUTE

Cold-pressed extra-virgin olive oil; almond, flax-, and grapeseed oils; meat juices.

One-percent or skim milk, low-fat cottage cheese, skim-milk cheese, ricotta cheese, soy milk.

Fresh fish one to two times per week, lean beef one to two times per week, eggs, lean Canadian bacon, lean veal and lamb, lobster, scallops, crab in small amounts, chicken, turkey, wild goose, canned tuna (water packed), dried beans, lentils, barley, buckwheat, seaweeds, tofu.

Whole-grain baked goods containing no whole milk or sugar, unsweetened nonprocessed cereals, unsalted and unbuttered popcorn, oatmeal.

Celery, cauliflower, zucchini, daikon (white radish), green beans, broccoli, squash, kale, onions, garlic, cabbage, parsley, watercress, spinach.

Chicken soup (no fat), clear broth, fat-free vegetable soup, miso soup.

Fresh-squeezed juice, mineral water, herbal teas.

Angel food cake, puddings made with skim milk, cooked apples, fresh fruit, unsweetened frozen or canned fruit (drained), rice pudding, chestnuts, almonds, walnuts, macadamia nuts.

CHAPTER
Sixteen

The Agony and Ecstasy of Change

T his chapter deals with the many repercussions, both positive and negative, of weight loss, and will support you in handling the multitude of new challenges you will now face, including keeping the weight off.

Since any change often elicits deep feelings and emotions, losing a great deal of weight may create some unforeseen problems. As these feelings and situations arise, it will be tempting for you to regress to your previous maladaptive, yet familiar, ways of handling them. Remember, we often use food as a substitute when we are really hungry for something else. We eat when we are alone, sad, depressed, frustrated, or even happy. Unconsciously, we often turn to food to console us; however, the toxic effects of repressed anger can also drive us to eat voraciously.

Since unconscious drives are what really motivate us and, at times, control us, it is important to get feedback and support in our attempt to learn more about ourselves. Overweight people have many experiences in common. In emotional support groups, we can experience the sharing and caring of others who have experienced the same pain and conscious struggles over obesity. While we may not be aware of our own unconscious issues, group support can sometimes evoke them. As we relate and react to the issues of others, we may realize that these issues are ours as well; others can serve as mirrors for ourselves. Mood swings, for example, are common after losing a considerable amount of weight. You may feel elated, proud of yourself, excited about your future, and sexy; yet you may also feel sad, scared, defensive, and lost. These feelings often subside with time, but in the meantime it helps to have someone who understands what you are going through and who can encourage and support you.

Not only will you view yourself differently after your weight loss, but people you have known for years will often view you and treat you differently. Their responses to you will range from total support and pride to jealousy. They may judge you, reject you, or even come on to you sexually. Be prepared! If you are oversensitive to others' opinions of you, their reactions may be counterproductive to all your hard work. No one is able to be consistent all of the time. We all have our ups and downs. You might have a friend who constantly validates you. If you begin to rely on him or her for a sense of yourself, what happens when this person is having a terrible day, week, or even year? Or feeling particularly insecure or angry? In these instances this individual may fail to provide you with the validation to which you have become so accustomed. Consequently you may begin to feel negated or worthless.

When you stop basing your sense of self-esteem on the presence or absence of a particular physical (material or intellectual) attribute, you will feel one hundred percent better about yourself. *Self-worth is not about anything you do; it is about who you are.* It is wonderful to heal, grow, and change for the better, but it is not as if you will be more worthy when you achieve these goals. In our society, unfortunately, we are programmed to have relentless expectations of what we *have* to change or what we *have* to own in order to be loved, lovable, happy, worthy, or successful. *Only you can change yourself*—your beliefs and perceptions. Unfortunately, it will take longer for society to change its erroneous and stereotypical beliefs.

Developing a stronger sense of self, of who you are and what's great about you—without undue reliance on external validation—is an important task for us all, fat and thin. While support groups may help you along the way, ultimately you must do the hard work by yourself. It is particularly crucial for you to be self-motivated if you are going to keep the weight off, since old friends and foes alike may tempt you to return to the way you were, the person they knew or loved, that is, someone with whom they felt safe and unchallenged. But you can't stay stuck for anyone. People may begin to view you as a threat, but this may be a gift to others. You might elicit feelings that cause them to reflect on their behavior, just as you have reflected on your own. You may have a close friend who is still overweight express delight to you verbally, but you may feel the opposite energy coming toward you from "underneath." He or she may not mean to act in a rejecting or cruel manner, but when a person gets frightened or jealous, deep emotions are triggered, and that person can act out on you in one way or another.

Any strong negative reaction is an indication that *the other person* wants very much to change for the better too but feels stuck, believes they can't, or is terrified to do so. Don't fall into the trap of feeling guilty about your own good fortune. You've worked hard for this new body—and attitude. You deserve it. Stop feeling that it is your job to protect people from their pain. They have the same potential for change, growth, and healing that you do. Let others grow.

WEIGHT LOSS IS GREAT—CHANGE IS DIFFICULT

There are going to be many other changes that accompany your weight loss. You might find yourself asking some of the following questions:

Should I go out and buy a new wardrobe?
Do I have enough money to buy the clothes I need?
What if I gain the weight back after I buy all these clothes?
Should I change my image? My hairstyle?
Does my new body look too sexy?

Such questions will arise, and you will need to make many decisions. My advice here is to *take your time*. The changes will come automatically. The new you will become more integrated, and you will develop a deeper sense of your own identity. Trust your instincts to guide you. Although you may change your look two or three times before you find the one that feels right, don't think of this as a struggle; enjoy the process.

You may begin to feel more sexual energy. With weight loss, your body may look more appealing to yourself and to others. This may cause you to feel more alive and happy, or perhaps even guilty and frightened. But sexuality is a healthy part of life, and once viewed as such can bring much pleasure and satisfaction. If you feel a new sexual energy being directed at you, use it as a tool. Flirt, play, have fun. Do not try to suppress these feelings for fear that something uncontrollable will happen to you. Your body is awakening and moving toward its natural urges. Accept it and allow it to happen. If, on the other hand, your newly discovered sense of sexuality frightens you, you may want to explore it with a professional counselor.

Realize also that a husband, wife, or partner may express fear of losing you because you now look so terrific. Do your best to express your love and commitment to them. Accentuate the positive effects your transformation has on them as well as you. Go out dancing. Create more romance. This could be an opportunity to ignite a delightful fire in your marriage. If, on the other hand, you are in an unfulfilling relationship, this may be the time to explore it. While I don't recommend taking on too many emotional issues at one time, neither do I suggest remaining stuck in a bad relationship. It is often difficult to let go of relationships, even destructive ones. It takes a certain conviction to heal your life, to want to surround yourself with people who are there for you most of the time and are not trying to manipulate you, control you, or use you to satisfy their own needs at your expense. People hold on to destructive relationships for various reasons, sometimes out of fear of being alone. If you have connections that no longer work for you or that hurt you, then you owe it to yourself to explore letting them go or to work on them by restructuring the dynamics of the connection.

Be aware that in any recovery process you need to take more responsibility for your actions and examine the negative patterns that you would like to change in your relationships as well as in yourself. If you have a tendency to manipulate loved ones with your weight, the old pattern can show up in times of domestic stress. For example, if your spouse wanted you to lose weight and is now thrilled that you did, be careful not to reach for food if he or she upsets you. Remind yourself that you are the one who ultimately pays the price for this action. Continue to find and utilize healthier ways to handle any intense emotions. If you are feeling angry and your old pattern was to eat, take more note of the anger. Once you are in charge of it, instead of it being in charge of you, you can channel it in a different, more positive, direction. You can go out and take a walk, go into the woods and scream, turn on some music and dance, walk the dog, go to a movie, or call a friend and share your feelings. Remember, patterns change with the repetition of new behavior. The more you act differently, the more you acknowledge your commitment to yourself. When you care enough to change, the new behavior will become reinforced and become easier.

Let's say you go home to visit your family. At dinner your mother tries to serve you foods that you know are harmful. If you say, "No, thank you," you may hear, "But I made this especially for you"; you will then know that you need to change your usual way of interacting with her. You may feel enraged. You may feel guilty and compelled to eat what you don't want to eat. But perhaps it is better to disappoint your mother than to betray yourself. If your mother expresses love through food, and if your refusal indicates in her mind that you don't love her, you might try expressing that you appreciate the time she took to cook for you and that you love her; however, also let her know that you have worked hard to change your eating habits and that you must honor your commitments.

BE YOUR OWN BEST FRIEND

This brings to mind the case of Sally, a schoolteacher who was in the weight loss program I supervised. Sally weighed about 225 pounds when she started the program. At five feet three inches, she was round, to say the least. Over the course of the program, she lost seventy pounds and really felt great about herself. In the two years after the program ended, Sally kept off at least fifty pounds of the original weight, always fluctuating within a ten- to thirteen-pound range. I spoke with her recently, and she is still determined to lose more weight. Her twin sister, on the other hand, was also in the program, and while she lost weight in the program, she has regained it all. Now the relationship between the two sisters is strained. Sally sometimes feels responsible for the tension, for having succeeded where her sister did not, yet she knows she must honor herself and not go back to her old way of punishing herself. After she lost the weight, Sally wrote me the following letter. You might be able to relate to it.

"Smile tho' your heart is aching," a corny song I suppose, and the rest of it just gets worse. What happens if you actually lived that line all your life?

There have been a multitude of lines ingrained into my being over the past thirty-eight years, lines such as "keep busy, don't make waves," "a quitter never wins," "SMILE, it will be okay," "what you give you gather," "do for others even if it means sacrifice," "do your best," "make believe you are happy and you will be," "show everyone you can cope as well as deal with everything for everyone else," "never say no or I'm too busy right now," "always ask how you can help." Do things you really don't want to do, Sally, just to please others so they will give you praise, a pat on the shoulder, a hug and/or a compliment. But hugs, compliments, smiles, and words of encouragement aren't quite enough right now. I've got to do more.

Smile. Smile. Smile. Try to help others. Feel sorry for them instead. Be a candle, burn yourself out lighting the way for everyone else, and then sit home in the dark and smile and EAT, EAT, EAT. That was my cure. Who needs help? Keep busy. It will cover up the loneliness, emptiness, lack of self-worth, self-doubt, insecurity, the side of me I won't accept as part of me right now. Stop wondering who will help me when I need it. Forget it. Tuck the thought away. I'll never need help. What a joke! I do need help.

I was taught how to love everyone. It helps build self-confidence and self-esteem in others, but what about me? These characteristics are now growing within me with the weight loss. I now have more energy to do more for others—WRONG! That's the energy I need to turn inward toward myself. That's part of becoming the WHOLE me, not just the me who's becoming thinner. I have to do this for me, the person who needs to learn to relax and do things just for me. If I take the time to love and nurture myself, people will love me and I will love me, even though I have faults. People won't love me because I'm the person who can do it all.

I need to take little steps instead of diving into this concept. I am starting to chip away at my smiling facade and peek inside, discovering that there really is a beautiful person underneath who is slowly learning to become satisfied.

What am I doing for ten weeks this summer? No more two-aspirin or Band-Aid cures! I wouldn't think of doing that to others or, God forbid, to the children I teach. I want to dig into who I really am and find those roots to help ground me. What's wrong with not smiling for a while? Not a thing because I AM growing with patience, love, caring, intelligence, dedication, time, sharing, God's help, and all the energy that I take pleasure in giving to others every day of my life. I'm not only going to have strong roots and growth, I'm going to BLOOM!

Love, as we can see, has incredible healing powers. Filling yourself up with food or even someone else's love will not fill the emptiness within you. But loving yourself will. And if you become upset with yourself or suffer a setback and go through some turmoil that results in overeating, be careful not to turn your self-love into self-hatred. If this does occur, catch it as soon as possible and apologize for turning against yourself. This may sound silly, but it works. Self-hatred, or anger turned inward, will only cause you to feel even more turmoil and possibly prolong or create another binge. If you slip up, remember to forgive yourself. Understand that it takes time to change these old patterns completely, and don't become greedy. If you have lost twenty-five pounds or have toned your stomach but your legs still need work, look in the mirror with approval. Don't knock those legs. Love them as they are. In all the therapy I've done with women, their biggest issue seems to be the size and shape of their legs. Perhaps this is because women feel that men place too much emphasis on legs. However, in the men's self-awareness group that I run, I've learned this is not the case.

FRIENDS OR FOOD POLICE?

Weight reduction means recovery and self-healing. Perfection is not the key to happiness. Be patient, but keep the momentum going. Take a few moments occasionally to praise yourself and express gratitude. Look in the mirror and thank yourself for your achievement out loud. While you may feel self-conscious, your mind needs this type of reinforcement, and speaking to yourself while looking into your own eyes is a powerful exercise. As previously mentioned, while others may support you or even unconsciously try to undermine you, you are the one who is ultimately responsible for your own feelings, growth, behavior, happiness, and body.

As a result of your weight loss, you may experience an emotional loss as well. If you have been overweight for many years, or you have lost sixty to a hundred pounds, it may feel as though you have lost a friend. Or if you have been using your weight to hide, you may feel a sense of fear about how you will survive. This is when it is especially beneficial to look yourself in the eye in the mirror and find comfort where you once may have seen rejection. In time, you will adjust and develop healthy ways to feel safe.

Friends may think they are being encouraging by being "food police," suggesting what you should or shouldn't eat. You can choose to respond to each situation accordingly. If they do indeed care, you can thank them for their suggestions. On the other hand, a friend may think that something you are eating is bad for you, while you know that in your program of awareness, you can balance the food with other, less caloric items. If you are doing something that is not in your best interest, you will know it, and a gentle reminder may be all that you need to put you back on track. You are writing your own program and can create it according to your own taste and preferences. While support from friends is fine, intrusion is not. Stay firmly within your own boundaries.

Again, taking quiet time to acknowledge that you love yourself is one such way to do this. Rejoicing in your weight loss is another. You may reward yourself by buying clothes in the regular-size department instead of the plus-size department. If you have been leading a reclusive life and begin to feel more alive and want to go out more often, do so. Or, like Roger, about whom I wrote earlier, if you had trouble fitting into cars before, you may now physically and metaphorically love the pleasure of riding comfortably. As you participate in more activities that satisfy you and occupy your thoughts, you will be relieved of your preoccupation with your body. Allow yourself to enjoy your meals; put love into your food, especially when you prepare it for yourself and others. Food made with love tastes better. I know. My father taught me this, and his meals were always outstanding. While I appreciate food and the love that goes into it, I know it is only a symbol of the love of the people behind it.

As you adopt a new lifestyle that supports you in making changes, losing weight, and keeping it off, you will have helped everyone around you. You will have more energy available to give to others because you first gave to yourself; and you will give authentically only what and when you choose. You may be an inspiration to those who are close to you and even exude a positive energy that says, "I've changed for the better. You can too." Our society desperately needs role models who offer hope. We can look back on that old self in the mirror and see our growth reflected in the symbol of our new image—an image of integration and self-love.

Seventeen

The Search for the Fountain of Youth

G reek mythology discussed the myth of aging in one of the most famous and ancient riddles of the Sphinx. The question was, "What is it that has one voice and yet becomes four-footed, two-footed, and three-footed?"

Oedipus provided the obvious answer: a human being. A human being crawls on all fours in infancy, walks on two legs as an adult, and then leans on a cane as old age approaches. The assumption in the riddle of the Sphinx is that as we grow older we become stiff and debilitated.

As we age, a gradual degenerative process occurs. Aging has become synonymous with degeneration. Science has shown that many of our hormone systems decline with age.

But do we really have to age? Can we interrupt the gradual deterioration of the body? Many people in every generation age yet continue to function without developing degenerative diseases. Geriatric analysis shows that humans age in very different ways. Perhaps some age successfully while others don't. The question we need to ask ourselves is: "What is it that makes one person age more quickly than another?"

AGING GRACEFULLY

Certainly, people are different. I have often asked myself why some of my very old patients look much younger than their actual age, and some of my younger patients look older than their age. Recently, a Russian gerontologist tried to answer this question. He examined 15,000 individuals age eighty and above in the Soviet Union, and found four common denominators for longevity:

1. Long-lived people worked outside with lots of physical activity.
2. They ate a diet of grains, fresh fruits, and vegetables. Many sometimes lacked for food, which obviously caused calorie restrictions.
3. They enjoyed good relationships, with love, intimacy, and support in their lives.
4. Many of these individuals continued to have an active sex life, even in their eighties and nineties.

Thus, the common factors for longevity appear to include a high-fiber diet, exercise, and supportive, loving relationships. In addition, these people had optimistic outlooks on life. There is nothing like intimacy, support, and an emotional connection to keep life feeling worthwhile.

On the other hand, a pessimistic outlook on life with negative emotions, hostility, anger, and resentment depresses not only one's personality, but also one's immune response. Therefore when considering longevity, one should consider mind and body interactions.

Before we discuss aging, we need to be clear about the symptoms of aging. The most obvious symptom of aging is disease. Diseases related to aging include coronary artery disease, arthritis, osteoporosis, low back pain, Alzheimer's, and cancer. We need to ask ourselves whether modern medicine is really useful in curing these illnesses. As a physician, I have to say that the answer is no.

Other symptoms of aging can be very subtle, such as diminished sexual activity, poor sleep habits, constipation, joint stiffness, or poor skin tone. More obvious symptoms include memory loss, diminished immunity, and a susceptibility to infections, allergies, or disease.

Many of my patients really don't understand that we gain weight as we get older because our metabolic rate falls. Ask any man in his forties and he will tell you that his waist size is increasing. I know it is happening to me! Many of us also get little exercise after the age of forty. And then there is the most obvious symptom of aging that I see: the patient who comes into my office taking multiple drugs for various symptoms and illnesses. Although many of my patients don't specifically ask me to prescribe antiaging therapies, many would like to see an increase in sexual libido, would prefer a better memory, and would like to sleep better.

WE CAN BE FRIENDS WITH AGE

Age does not have to be an enemy. The only enemies that I see are illnesses such as cancer, severe depression, resignation, and despair. So what can we do to give us a better quality of life, full of vitality, energy, and enthusiasm for living?

There are many ways to attack the aging process. There are nutritional and food therapies involving vitamins, minerals, herbs, and enzymes; exercise therapies; and other recommendations such as good personal hygiene and minimizing exposure to sunlight, microwaves, and X rays. Maintaining a normal or even less than normal body weight will also retard aging.

More advanced antiaging therapies include the use of hormones, amino acids, and powerful antioxidants. Later in this chapter, I will give you my prescription for health, healing, and longevity which combines all of these therapies.

Previously in this book, I discussed important health maintainers. I also spoke about cholesterol levels, preferably with low LDL and high HDL as positive markers. I also discussed iron overload and the harmful effects of homocysteine. But there are also two other exciting markers of health. They include serum albumin in your body and the hormone called DHEA (dehydroepiandrosterone).

Think of the Ice Man found in the European Alps. Although he had some arthritis and possibly even some vascular disease, he was a very healthy individual. They found a grain pouch among his belongings. This man probably ate seeds, grains, plants, and roots. Biochemically, the Ice Man was in good shape. He had high levels of DHEA and low levels of insulin. This is modern man in reverse. We have low DHEA and high insulin levels, making us prone to the degenerative diseases I have mentioned.

What causes degenerative diseases and aging? The answer is free-radical oxidative stress, causing cellular deterioration. What can we do to protect ourselves from unnecessary free-radical damage and optimize our health? Read on.

As I've mentioned, dehydroepiandrosterone is the mother steroid, precursor of some eighteen hormones in the body. As we age, our DHEA levels fall. Remember when you were eighteen? How much energy did you have? We find the highest levels of DHEA at this time.

If our DHEA levels decline too rapidly with age, we get sick more often. For example, a recent article indicated that lower levels of DHEA were found in patients with premature coronary artery disease. Declining levels have also been noted in cancer patients and individuals with HIV. And when DHEA falls to very low levels, HIV turns into full-blown AIDS.

In animal studies, supplementation with DHEA leads to an increased life span, reduced risk of degenerative diseases, and reduced body fat. DHEA is also known to be a factor in weight reduction. Other uses of DHEA include enhancing immunity by increasing the antibody effect. It also reduces undesirable blood clotting. DHEA increases levels of sex hormones in men and women, which may help to activate sexual libido.

Wild yam (*Dioscorea villosa*) extract is a natural form of DHEA. Wild yam actually contains very low doses of DHEA. However, remember that before taking any of these agents, whether DHEA, wild yam extract, or pregnenolone (a precursor of DHEA) you should consult a physician, as these therapies may cause some side effects. Men who take DHEA should be evaluated periodically for prostate size and gland activity. For women, excessive DHEA may increase facial hair. Discussing these concerns with your physician should eliminate any problems when you undertake these treatments.

STRESS AND HEALTH

It's also interesting to note that DHEA levels have an inverse relationship to emotional stress. That is, the more stress we are under, the more serum cortisol (the body's natural hormonal response to stress, coming from the adrenal glands) is released into the body. As cortisol increases, DHEA levels decrease. It isn't any wonder that when we're under stress, our immunity decreases.

Frequently one may get a cold, an infection, or even a heart attack in situations of severe emotional stress. Sometimes, when we are under stress, our memory fails. Research seems to indicate that higher serum cortisol levels can be associated with structural changes in brain cells, causing cell death. As a result, our memory fails. Since the effects of stress can be cumulative over time, our memory, as well as our brain, is affected. Severe and unrelenting stress may be a risk factor for Alzheimer's disease and premature death. There is a lot of merit to the expression "Don't worry, be happy." Simple meditation can be used in reducing stress. Meditation can be a way to lower serum cortisol levels, thereby improving memory. Meditation not only enhances mental and physical health, it supports memory. In Alzheimer's disease, as memory decreases, DHEA levels fall and albumin (the body's master protein) levels deteriorate.

YOU AND YOUR ALBUMIN

Multiple studies have indicated that lower levels of serum albumin are also a predictor of health and disease; for example, the lower serum albumin, the more severe the dementia. Albumin is the most abundant serum protein found in the cerebrospinal fluid as well as other tissues. Albumin is our most versatile antioxidant. It stabilizes and strengthens our immunity and transports vitamins A, D, and C, along with the minerals zinc, copper, and magnesium throughout the body. It is important to keep your albumin as high as possible. If the body contains at least 48 grams per liter, this demonstrates excellent health.

Although increasing nutritional defenses by eating a healthy diet and taking vitamins, minerals, and herbs will help maintain our albumin, increasing our levels of personal hygiene is one of the best ways of keeping our albumin levels elevated. Antibodies claim a large percentage of the body's plasma proteins. In response to immune system challenges such as bacteria and allergies, the percentage of antibodies rises while the albumin drops. It works something like this: Plasma proteins are maintained at approximately 75 grams per liter in the body. Albumin makes up 60 percent of the protein, antibodies 20 percent, and carrier proteins another 20 percent. If we are under stress or have an acute infection or allergy, our antibodies rise to meet the offending invaders. As antibody levels grow higher, albumin must get lower.

If albumin gets lower, this creates an overall weakened condition. So why is it vital during situations of infection and higher allergy states to increase our levels of personal hygiene? Cleaning our fingernails, eyes, nose, skin, and nasal cavity helps to eliminate sources of bacterial contamination. This reduces stress on the immune system and allows albumin to be maintained at a healthy level.

Albumin and DHEA are certainly terrific partners in maintaining health and delaying aging. But I still have not defined the biochemistry of aging. In other words, I have not gone into detail as to why aging occurs in the first place.

HOW AGING OCCURS

I believe that aging is really a disease. Although there are many theories to explain why we age, including hormonal, neuroendocrine, and immunologic theories, perhaps the best and most reasonable theory is the free-radical theory. Aging, in simple terms, is related to accumulated damage to membranes and cells as a consequence of oxidative stress.

Remember that oxidative stress occurs when there is a high amount of free radicals present in the body, overwhelming the body's natural antioxidant defenses. Excessive amounts of free radicals tend to impair cellular membranes. The destruction of cellular membranes is, therefore, the sine qua non of the aging process. If cellular membranes are kept intact, cellular function remains intact. However, if cellular membranes suffer permanent damage due to free-radical attacks, our health deteriorates and we fall prey to degenerative diseases. Earlier I gave you a simple explanation of the free-radical theory. For a more comprehensive evaluation of aging, however, I will discuss the free-radical theory in deeper detail.

Although oxygen is necessary for life, the metabolism of oxygen has an ominous consequence: the formation of free radicals. A free radical is a molecule with an odd number of electrons (negatively charged particles). Stable compounds such as gaseous oxygen contain paired electrons. In contrast, highly unstable and reactive compounds (free radicals) contain unpaired electrons.

The normal metabolism of oxygen by cells in the body proceeds via a pathway known as reduction. During this process, oxygen is "reduced" to water by the addition of four electrons by a sequential transfer. The oxygen molecule acquires electrons one at a time, thereby forming at each stage molecular fragments (free radicals) with unpaired electrons having a very high chemical reactivity. As unpaired electrons are transferred to a nonradical, another free radical is created, setting up a chain of reactions of electron transfer. Such chain reactions may occur thousands of times before the reaction is terminated.

Under normal conditions, 95 to 98 percent of the molecular oxygen consumed by cells is reduced to water. The remaining 2 to 5 percent, however, gives rise to reactive free radicals, even under the best of circumstances. Free-radical generation reaches much higher levels during situations such as infection, inflammation, radiation exposure, and the high oxygen–tension states that occur during vigorous exercise. It also occurs in situations in which one has a heart attack.

Although research shows that free radicals may play a fundamental role in supporting some basic life processes, such as hormone synthesis, these unstable and deleterious highly charged particles cause extensive damage to cell membranes, cell contents (called organelles), and even the DNA itself. The paradox of free-radical chemistry has generated considerable interest among health care professionals, especially those interested in preventative medicine.

I have already told you that free radicals, over time, cause biological changes that may lead to acceleration of aging and the development of a variety of chronic diseases such as heart disease, cancer, and cataracts. Fortunately, the body has its own complex antioxidant defense systems against free radicals. If not for these antioxidant defense systems, the thousands of chain reactions of free radicals generated within seconds could quickly cripple and destroy cellular functions. Most of the body's natural antioxidants deactivate free radicals by using them to generate safer chemical reactions. However, these antioxidant systems can be overwhelmed during extraordinary oxidative stress such as an acute heart attack or the period after the ingestion of a heavy, fat-laden meal.

Another key factor in free-radical damage is one's intrinsic metabolic rate, that rate at which energy is consumed to maintain basic bodily functions. The higher the metabolic rate, the greater the number of free radicals released by oxygen reduction. Over time, the oxidative damage combines with age-related DNA mutations to leave us more susceptible to cancer and other degenerative diseases. By contrast the metabolic rate and free-radical damage that follows can be slowed by caloric or protein restriction. This has been demonstrated both in the animal studies and among survivors of World War II. Individuals who were starved or were survivors of concentration camp conditions had a significantly lower incidence of coronary artery disease later in life. This was a by-product of sharply restricted caloric intake.

The most potent free-radical invader in these oxidative processes is the hydroxyl radical (OH). The hydroxyl radical is a key factor in the oxidation of polyunsaturated fatty acids. When oxidized, polyunsaturated fatty acids are extremely toxic and damaging to the cardiovascular system. They also play a role in the aging of the eye, causing lens opacity and cataract formation. They are also related to nerve degeneration.

Polyunsaturated fatty acids, like free radicals, represent a paradox. Although they are essential building blocks for the body, providing cellular elasticity and pliability, they are easily broken down by free radicals. Since polyunsaturated fatty acids play a major role in the development of atherosclerosis and cancer, I recommend avoiding polyunsaturated fats, such as margarines, and polyunsaturated oils in the diet. Again, the safest oil that you can consume from the cardiological point of view is olive oil, a monounsaturated fat.

OTHER ANTIAGING STRATEGIES

L-Arginine

A newer antiaging agent on the horizon is L-arginine. Briefly introduced in my chapter on cholesterol and women, L-arginine has received favorable press for preventing both heart disease and cancer.

To refresh your memory, recall that animal studies have shown that the amino acid L-arginine reduces cholesterol blockages in the aorta. It works like nitric oxide, which is a substance that keeps blood vessels open. Physicians call this vasodilation. L-arginine may be used in people with high cholesterol levels that cannot be lowered by other means. I take 1 to 2 grams of L-arginine prior to my exercise sessions, as it stimulates the secretion of growth hormone.

Recent research also advocates high dosages of L-arginine for stimulating immune function. In one review, 30 grams of L-arginine per day, in combination with the traditional therapies, was said to increase immune function in patients with breast cancer. If you are considering L-arginine in this dose I strongly recommend that you discuss it with your physician beforehand.

Melatonin

Melatonin is a hormone excreted from the pineal gland, deep in the brain, almost exclusively during periods of darkness. Research has suggested that raising melatonin levels may be one method to slow aging. In some experimental animal studies melatonin definitely produced an increase in longevity. In some populations of rats and mice, melatonin has been shown to stimulate immunity by increasing antibodies while promoting enhanced lymphocyte function at the same time.

Many physicians and researchers whom I know take melatonin for promoting sleep. I can personally attest to the benefits of taking low-dose melatonin for the relief of jet lag. However, I do not recommend melatonin to everyone. Certainly, children, pregnant women, and nursing mothers should not take it. I would also not give it to patients who are suffering from depression. Although melatonin has been used with some success in Europe in treating breast cancer and prostate cancer, melatonin should not be given in any case of cancer involving the immune system, such as leukemia. In some patients with severe allergies or in others with an autoimmune illness, such as lupus or rheumatoid arthritis, melatonin may make the condition worse.

Melatonin does, however, have a definite upside. Melatonin is also a powerful free-radical scavenger. It helps to eliminate the hydroxyl radical, one of the most devastating free radicals in the body. Like DHEA and albumin, the natural production of melatonin decreases with age, particularly for those over the age of forty. Fasting and dieting increase the natural body stores of melatonin. This in itself is a bonus when we lose weight. If you do consider taking melatonin for sleep, I would start not at milligram doses, which are commonly found in health food stores, but at microgram doses which can be found in some commercial products, especially those mixed with valerian root, hops, passionflower, and other tranquilizing herbs. I strongly recommend that you consult with your physician before supplementing with melatonin.

DMAE

Another interesting compound to consider is DMAE (dimethylaminoethanol). This substance is found in anchovies and sardines, among other foods. A precursor of choline, DMAE increases levels of acetylcholine in the brain. Acetylcholine is needed for learning and memory. DMAE can be taken as a supplement of as little as 100 mg daily and has been found to improve mood, memory, learning, sleep, and energy. I strongly recommend that before taking DMAE, you consult your physician.

L-Deprenyl

Lately I have been writing more and more prescriptions for the agent L-deprenyl, marketed as Eldepryl in this country. L-deprenyl has tremendous merits.

As we age we produce a substance called monoamine oxidase (MAO). In patients with Alzheimer's disease, monoamine oxidase levels are extremely high. To lower the body's amount of monoamine oxidase, we must inhibit its development. This is where L-deprenyl comes in. It is actually a monoamine oxidase inhibitor, lowering the levels of MAO while increasing the body's levels of dopamine. By stimulating the body's natural level of dopamine, L-deprenyl has been said to enhance mental alertness and memory. It has also been touted to increase libido by raising the amount of certain neurotransmitters in the brain. Thus L-deprenyl not only may heighten one's overall energy and mental alertness, but also may affect one's libido.

Dopamine is one of the most important hormonal transmitters of our brains. Without dopamine, people become stiff, immobile, and unable to function on a musculoskeletal level. In Parkinson's disease, dopamine levels often drop very low as the disease progresses. This lack of dopamine is why patients with Parkinson's have a fixed stare, resting tremors, rigidity of limbs, and often a shuffling walk they cannot stop.

The production of dopamine in our brain decreases with advancing age, usually after the age of forty-five. Therefore, L-deprenyl may serve an antiaging function. Unfortunately, L-deprenyl is not popular in the United States. Nevertheless, European physicians who have much more experience with L-deprenyl prescribe it frequently.

Proanthocyanidins

I am very comfortable with taking proanthocyanidins, remarkable plant-derived substances originating from standardized extracts of grapeseed and pine bark. Arguably they are the most powerful natural antioxidants available. The proanthocyanidins go by popular names such as Pycnogenol and OPC (oligomeric proanthocyanidin) which are trademarks. While Pycnogenol was patented by a French researcher in 1987, for centuries Native Americans have used as a remedy a tea made from the bark and needles of certain evergreen trees. Currently, Pycnogenol is often made from the *Pinus maritima* tree.

Proanthocyanidins such as Pycnogenol contain many bioflavonoids such as catechins and epicatechins, as well as organic acids. They are very powerful antioxidants, enhancing memory, stimulating the immunity, and improving circulation. They have also been used to treat diabetic retinopathy.

Pycnogenol also improves skin smoothness and elasticity, reduces phlebitis, and assuages the inflammation from allergic disorders. Furthermore, Pycnogenol serves an important function for the brain. Since it is one of the few dietary antioxidants that can readily cross the blood-brain barrier, Pycnogenol is able to protect brain cells, resulting in stimulated memory and retarded aging. Because of this ability, I believe Pycnogenol has considerable potential as an antiaging agent.

Human Growth Hormone (HGH)

Like melatonin and DHEA, HGH declines with age. It declines significantly after age thirty, and in some older people, production may actually cease. Low levels of HGH, which is secreted by the pituitary gland, are associated with age-related changes such as weight gain, sagging skin, and a fall in libido. Further, a deficiency can result in diminished immune capacity, lower energy levels, sleep difficulties, short-term memory loss, and even a predisposition to cardiovascular disease.

At the December 1996 Anti-Aging Conference in Las Vegas, Nevada, I heard Dr. Bengt-Ake Bengtsson, one of the leading human growth hormone researchers in the world, discuss his landmark study of 333 patients with low levels of HGH. Dr. Bengtsson discovered that these patients were twice as likely to die from heart disease as the age-matched control group. Among patients treated with HGH replacement therapy, there was a uniform decrease in cardiovascular risk, as well as weight loss and a favorable increase in HDL and lower LDL blood fractions.

Another promising aspect of HGH is its ability to improve congestive heart failure. In the March 28, 1996 issue of the *New England Journal of Medicine,* Italian investigators reported that seven cardiomyopathy patients who received HGH by injection all increased the percentage of blood pumped from the left ventricle with each heartbeat, an improvement that translated into enhanced feelings of well-being and quality of life.

HGH therapy of this nature, however, needs to be given under the administration of a physician. The therapy costs approximately 100 to 250 dollars a week and usually lasts for six months. However, you can increase your HGH naturally by either fasting, exercising, or taking niacin in combination with amino acids. As little as 200 mg of niacin has been known to increase HGH secretion. Amino acids such as L–arginine, L–glutamine, and L–ornithine have also been shown to have a dramatic effect. These amino acids can be taken on an empty stomach, one hour prior to exercise, or before sleep. You can find these nutrients in almost any health food store, and there are no side effects at the recommended doses of 1 to 2 grams each. For an excellent book on HGH, I would suggest *Grow Young with HGH* by Dr. Ronald Klatz.

A STRATEGY OF PREVENTION

The search for the fountain of youth has been going on for centuries. Today, people are especially concerned with delaying the process of aging. In my mind, the best method for halting disease and delaying aging is prevention. A good prescription for disease prevention and antiaging tactics includes a healthy diet: targeted nutritional supplementation with vitamins, minerals, and herbs; chlorophyll–containing foods; and mild to moderate exercise regimens. Those seeking a more aggressive approach may consider the leading hormonal and protein therapies.

When fighting age and disease, we must not forget the environment. I am genuinely concerned about the deterioration of the water supply in this country. In my office and home, we use bottled water and central water filters to filter out chlorine, heavy metals, and harmful bacteria. I also advocate air filters, which extract carbon monoxide, pollens, and other impurities from the air.

Lighting is another area of interest for me. Full-spectrum lighting is much more natural and safe than the usual incandescent and fluorescent light bulbs. It also helps to nurture the body, particularly the eye and the pineal gland, which stimulates the body's production of melatonin. Recently I placed full-spectrum lighting in my home and office.

In summary, I believe that futuristic medicine will engage the antiaging process, because if you can delay aging, you can delay disease. For instance, take the problem of cataracts. If cataracts could be delayed by a mere ten years, this country could perhaps save billions of dollars in reduced health care costs.

Searching for the fountain of youth can be very exciting when done in a way that supports one's continuing vitality and promotes living a stable, satisfying, and enthusiastic life. Getting old is not bad; it's inevitable. Premature aging with its accompanying degenerative diseases is an unnecessary hardship. This pathological aging process certainly can be a tragedy. But we have the opportunity to delay and even prevent it. Think about it.

MY RECOMMENDATIONS FOR HEALTH, HEALING, AND LONGEVITY

1. Nutritional and Food Therapy

1. Consume a high-fiber (greater than 30 grams per day), healthy-fat diet.
2. Increase consumption of fresh fruits and vegetables (organic preferred) to five to nine servings per day.
3. Consume fewer simple carbohydrates such as pastas made from white flour, white rice, potatoes, breads, etc.
4. Consume less red meat, fewer dairy products, and more fish, turkey, and lamb.
5. Omit table sugar, margarine, high-fat ice cream, and peanut butter.
6. Use more monounsaturated fats such as olive oil or almond oil.
7. Avoid polyunsaturated fatty acids such as corn oil, safflower oil, and canola oil.
8. Use more omega-3 oils.
9. Use miso preparations one to two times per week.
10. Increase garlic and onion in the diet; consider using sea vegetables.
11. Substitute green tea in place of coffee.
12. Maintain an adequate calcium intake greater than 1,000 mg per day.
13. Use less alcohol and caffeine. Drink six to eight glasses of pure water daily.

14. Limit sodium intake to less than 3 grams per day.
15. Take targeted nutritional supplements daily.

2. Vitamin, Mineral, Enzyme, and Nutritional Supplementation

Multivitamin and mineral combinations should be ingested on a daily basis. The supplement you choose should contain the following fifteen essential ingredients:

Beta carotene	12.5 to 25,000 IU
Vitamin C	300 to 600 mg
Vitamin E	200 to 400 IU
Selenium	100 to 200 mcg
Folic acid	400 to 800 mcg
Vitamin B-6	20 to 40 mg
Pantothenic acid	25 to 50 mg
Vitamin B-12	20 to 40 mcg
Magnesium	200 to 400 mg
Chromium picolinate	50 to 100 mcg
Coenzyme Q_{10}	30 to 60 mg
Quercetin	10 to 40 mg
Vanadium	200 to 400 mcg
Bromelain	50 to 100 mg
N-acetyl cysteine	50 to 100 mg

3. Herbal Therapy (optional)

Ginger—enhances immunity, controls nausea

Garlic—lowers cholesterol, acts as an anti-inflammatory and antithrombotic agent

Ginseng—enhances immunity and energy

Gotu kola—enhances memory and combats depression

Ginkgo—enhances memory, controls dizziness, benefits central nervous system

Cayenne—enhances energy, helps lower cholesterol, reduces symptoms of arthritis

Echinacea—enhances immunity and T cells

Goldenseal—enhances immunity and T cells

Hawthorn berry—improves health of heart and lowers blood pressure

Saint-John's-wort (hyperium)—combats depression

4. Green Chlorophyll Therapy (optional)

Chlorella, wheat grass, green barley, or magna extract; one dose per day.

5. Other Recommendations

1. Maintain normal or less than normal body weight.
2. Consider a juice-cleansing fast once a month (see chapter fifteen).
3. Avoid heavy metals, pollutants, toxins, and smoking.
4. Exercise regularly.
5. Avoid prolonged exposure to sunlight, microwaves, televisions, and computers (electromagnetic contamination). Avoid unnecessary X rays.
6. Use good personal hygiene for eyes, nose, fingers, and fingernails, especially during infection or allergy season.
7. Consider installing water filters, air filters, and full-spectrum lighting.

General Markers of Health

1. DHEA levels greater than 800 mg/dl
2. Serum albumin levels greater than 48 g/l
3. Cholesterol levels less than 180, with HDL greater than 45 and LDL less than 130
4. Serum ferritin levels less than 100 (index of iron stores)
5. Serum homocysteine levels less than 14

Eighteen

Optimum Health

This book may be the first step in a process that enables you to take charge of your own health, nutrition, and well-being. Although attitudes and belief systems are deeply ingrained and resistant to change, understand that each one of us is up to the challenge. Being able to change our prejudices, our negative habits, and our lifelong self-defeating patterns opens us up to growth. It is growth that makes life truly rewarding and worth living.

The goal of this book is to help you integrate your body, mind, and spirit as you seek true aliveness and satisfaction in your life. We are each responsible for our own health and happiness. While life may strike us unexpected blows, we can do much to reframe negative experiences; furthermore, we can try to prevent them. Healthy eating, exercise, and emotional release can be regarded as preventive medicine. These are good habits that will be with us the rest of our lives once we begin to participate in them fully. They do not require much self-sacrifice, merely awareness.

A healthy-fat, high-fiber diet with appropriate portions of protein and complex carbohydrates is the first step to optimal health. Throughout the book I have stressed that we cannot deprive ourselves of good-tasting meals and foods that we like. I included several of my own recipes that were created with a healthy heart and a trim, fit body in mind. I recommend eliminating very few products from the diet; rather, I recommend simply using less of certain foods and substituting healthy-fat versions of old comfort foods for the ones that no longer fit a healthy lifestyle.

Enough said. You now know my favorite foods and my personal and professional recommendations for a healthy diet. Much, if not everything, that I have written about in this book I have incorporated into my own life. For me, life has been a continuous journey of self-discovery. I hope that you share the road with me.

On this same path is a new breed of progressive doctors who are being educated in complementary healing techniques and alternative medicine. They are learning that the allopathic model of medicine does not adequately treat the mind, body, and spirit of their patients. They are learning that our lives are governed and influenced by thoughts, beliefs, and lifestyle patterns that can be as damaging to the mind and spirit as to the body. My waiting room is full of patients who have both chronic and acute illnesses. With their all-American diets, maladaptive habits, and tendencies toward obesity, some have waited too long. They have come to my office wanting and expecting to be cured, yet they rarely take responsibility for their own condition or attempt to change it. My patients want me to give them relief, but I am not a magician, nor do I have any powers that can induce healing. I can't make a new body with pharmaceutical agents. I can't replace a heart that is ravaged with disease with a new healthy one. Good health has to come from lifestyle patterns and decisions—the way you live in the world now. Granted, many older people who now have heart disease were not taught how to take care of themselves. While it is hard to believe, *preventive medicine in this country is not a major component of mainstream medical training, instruction, or energy.* Much of my generation, for example, grew up on junk foods. But as a medical student, I was never taught about the negative effects of junk food. Fortunately, attitudes are slowly changing.

FROM MY HEART TO YOURS

This book explains in simple terms how to follow a lifestyle awareness program that utilizes nutritional and dietary approaches to healing the whole person.

Inevitably, the physicians of the future will be involved in environmental matters as they impact on the health of us all. Hazardous chemicals ravaging the air, earth, and water supply are slowly and insidiously infiltrating our bodies as well. Constantly contaminated by oil spills, radiation leakage, the receding ozone layer, and man-made toxic wastes, the planet, as well as its inhabitants, is engaged in a bitter struggle for survival. It is true that our planet is on the verge of a biological Armageddon.

And then there is AIDS. Life-threatening, malignant diseases and conditions abound and are subjects that every human being needs to be concerned about. Although I ponder these things, I have greater dread about what my children's children will have to face.

However, I do have some hope for the future. As I said, there is a new generation of doctors who believe in taking responsibility for themselves, the environment, and the planet. As a physician and healer, I feel a responsibility to communicate my knowledge, experience, and dreams to as many people as possible, so that they may begin to transform themselves and adopt new ways of living.

THE CORE OF OUR BEING

As a clinical cardiologist, I know that the heart is the place where everything comes together. After all, the heart is the core of our being. *Unfortunately, the hearts of many of us have been broken.* We all have experienced heartbreak on some level or another. Many of us are lonesome and need to be fed on many different levels. Some of us need to be touched. Some need to give. Others need to receive. We are all searching for solutions, happiness, and joy. We all want cures.

But the best kind of healing, in my opinion, comes from within. It comes from deep in our core. It comes from intuition, awareness, insight, and a genuine feeling of knowing.

Are you hungry? Are you hungry for a healthier, happier, and more productive life? The possibilities for self-healing are endless. Like you, I have fantasies. My search continues, and my path has taken me to a higher emotional and spiritual level. It is my hope that this book will stimulate you to utilize your highest power to obtain growth and satisfaction in your own life.

Believe it or not, heart disease or any catastrophic illness can indeed be a gift in disguise. It can help you re-examine your priorities, refocus your life, and get in touch with your spiritual needs. I have seen many patients transform themselves as a result of a life-threatening disease, and they tell me, from the bottom of their hearts, that their illness was one of the best things that ever happened to them. For many patients, heart disease was a motivating force that made them look deeper into their own emotional and spiritual selves.

Spirituality is a journey that each of us can embark upon. All that is necessary is an open heart and a willingness to contemplate the mysteries of life. But actually, what is spirituality? Is it religion—going to church every Sunday? Is it searching for a guru? Or is it getting in touch with nature? While spirituality can embrace any one or all of these, drawing on the power of the divine can have tremendous implications in healing. Think of spirituality as your beliefs about the life force or God that is both within and outside yourself. It is about having faith in that power and turning to it for courage, strength, and healing.

You may be wondering why a cardiologist is advocating spirituality. Aren't medicine and spirituality at opposite ends of the spectrum? Isn't one grounded in fact, the other in faith? Actually, I believe that medicine and religion are indeed the twin traditions of healing. More and more, physicians and health care providers are discovering spirituality as an untapped resource and tool in healing. In a recent conference at Harvard Medical School, for example, research was cited showing that people who attended church frequently or prayed regularly had lower rates of heart disease, hypertension, and even suicide. In addition, those who prayed even lived longer than those who did not.

I have spent many precious moments with patients taking their last breaths and literally going over to the "other side." My patients have taught me that life is so precious and ever so short. I have learned so much from them. Health is not just a physical condition, but also a condition of the mind and the divine spirit. This is the basis and essence of optimum health.

Are you ready to choose optimum health and make a commitment to your life? Are you emotionally and spiritually connected? Is this the body in which you really wish to live? You need to continually ask yourself these questions because *if you wear out this body, where are you going to live?*

Following is a healthy eating regimen that I have prepared for optimum health as well as weight loss. This is a balanced program of eating with awareness. Since it is not a "diet," it may be repeated over and over or mixed with other foods recommended in this book. The asterisks mark those recipes that I include in the "Recipes for Preventive Medicine" chapter. Here are a few suggestions, and remember to include fats, proteins, and carbohydrates at every meal.

Breakfasts

1 glass fruit juice
fresh fruit
1/2 grapefruit
1 bran muffin★
2 whole-grain pancakes with
  pure maple syrup or fresh
  blueberries

1 ounce Nova Scotia smoked
  salmon
1–2 organic eggs
1 bowl oatmeal
1 cup low-fat yogurt
1 cup soy milk
Lean Canadian bacon (nitrate
  free)

Lunches

Leaf lettuce and tomato salad
Low-fat goat or cottage cheese
Salad of greens, turkey, feta
  cheese, and raw veggies
Bowl of pasta and vegetables,
  served hot or cold

Salad of greens and cold
  veggies
Bean salad
Tuna packed in water
Veggie soy burger with
  cucumbers and sprouts
1 cup soup

Lunches

$^1/_2$ sandwich (tuna, hummus, turkey)
Miso broth★
2 eight-ounce glasses water
1 cup low-fat yogurt with fresh fruit

Spinach, raw or sautéed
Tomatoes with olive oil and lemon
Tofu with sesame seeds★

Dinners

Fish
Steamed broccoli
Steamed asparagus
Santiago's chicken★
Green salad
Stir-fried vegetables
Lentils and chickpeas
Miso broth★
Spinach salad
Peaches
Pasta with clam sauce or chicken
Dad's Italian-style tomatoes★

Green beans
Sautéed spinach
Yellow and green summer squash
Spelt pasta sprinkled with Parmesan cheese
Barley soup
Low-fat exceptional hamburgers★
Tossed salad
Watermelon

FINDING YOUR IDEAL WEIGHT

The following charts may be used to determine your ideal weight. First find your height in the left-hand column. Then move across the page to the body frame that best describes you. For the purpose of this table, your body frame is small if you can wrap your left thumb and middle finger around your right wrist and have these two digits overlap. If the thumb and finger barely touch, then you have a medium body frame. If they don't touch at all, you have a large build.

HEIGHT/WEIGHT TABLE

Men

Height in Inches	Small Frame	Medium Frame	Large Frame
62	128–134	131–141	138–150
63	130–136	133–143	140–153

APPENDIX

Height in Inches	Small Frame	Medium Frame	Large Frame
64	132–138	135–145	142–156
65	134–140	137–148	144–160
66	136–142	139–151	146–164
67	138–145	142–154	149–168
68	140–148	145–157	152–172
69	142–151	148–160	155–176
70	144–154	151–163	158–180
71	146–157	154–166	161–184
72	149–160	157–170	164–188
73	152–164	160–174	168–192
74	155–168	164–178	172–197
75	158–172	167–182	176–202
76	162–176	171–187	181–207

Women

Height in Inches	Small Frame	Medium Frame	Large Frame
58	102–111	109–121	118–131
59	103–113	111–123	120–134
60	104–115	113–126	122–137
61	106–118	115–129	125–140
62	108–121	118–132	128–143
63	111–124	121–135	131–147
64	114–127	124–138	134–151
65	117–130	127–141	137–155
66	120–133	130–144	140–159
67	123–136	133–147	143–163
68	126–139	136–150	146–167
69	129–142	139–153	149–170
70	132–145	142–156	152–173
71	135–148	145–159	155–176
72	138–151	148–162	158–179

Courtesy of Metropolitan Life Insurance Company.

269

BEVERAGES

Food	Serving Size	Calories	Sodium (mg)
Club soda	12 oz.	0	75
Cola, regular	12 oz.	150	14
Gatorade	12 oz.	39	123
Ginger ale	12 oz.	125	25
Root beer	12 oz.	150	49
Beer, regular	12 oz.	145	19
Beer, light	12 oz.	100	10
Wine, dessert	3.5 oz.	70	10
Wine, red	3.5 oz.	75	6
Wine, white	3.5 oz.	70	5
Apple juice	4.0 oz.	58	3.5
Apricot nectar	4.0 oz.	70.5	4.5
Carrot juice	4.0 oz.	55	36
Cranberry juice	4.0 oz.	75	5
Pineapple juice	4.0 oz.	70	1
Prune juice	4.0 oz.	90	5.5
Tomato juice	4.0 oz.	21	438
V–8	4.0 oz.	25	378
Grapefruit juice	4.0 oz.	50	1
Grape juice	4.0 oz.	80	3.5
Orange juice	4.0 oz.	55	1

BEANS/NUTS/SEEDS

Food	Serving Size	Cal.	Fat (g)	Cal. from fat (%)	Chol. (mg)	Fiber (g)
Soybeans, cooked	1 cup	234	10	38	0	
Soybean curd (tofu)	4 oz.	86	5	52	0	1
Peanuts, roasted	1/4 cup	210	18	77	0	
Peanut butter	2 tbsp.	188	16	76	0	
Almonds, roasted	1/4 cup	246	23	84	0	
Walnuts, black (shelled and chopped)	1/4 cup	196	18	82	0	
Chickpeas	1/2 cup	135	2.2	15	0	6.2
Kidney beans	1/2 cup	110	Trace .5	4	0	5.8
Lentils	1/2 cup	115	Trace .4	3	0	2.0
Pinto beans	1/2 cup	115	Trace .5	4	0	5.3
Split peas	1/2 cup	115	Trace .8	6	0	5.1
Pork and beans in tomato sauce	1 cup	311	6.6	19	6	
Lima beans (frozen or cooked)	1 cup	168	0.2	1	0	10
Lima beans (canned)	1 cup	163	0.5	2	0	
Green beans (fresh or frozen)	1 cup	34	0.1	2	0	1.1
Green beans (canned)	1 cup	32	0.3	8	0	0.7
White beans, cooked	1 cup	212	1.1	4	0	8
Wax beans (frozen)	1 cup	28	0.3	9	0	
Wax beans (canned)	1 cup	32	0.4	11	0	2
Sunflower seeds (hulled)	1 tbsp.	51	4.3	75	0	0.5
Water chestnuts	4 nuts	20	0.1	4	0	0.5
Macadamia nuts	1 oz.	196	20.3	93	0	1
Pecans (chopped or pieces)	1 tbsp.	51	5.2	91	0	0.5

CEREALS

Food	Serving Size	Cal.	Fat (g)	Cal. from Fat (%)	Chol. (mg)	Fiber (g)
All-Bran	1/3 cup	70	1	13	0	8.6
Bran (unprocessed)	1/4 cup	29	0.6	17	0	6
Bran Buds	1 cup	216	1.8	11	0	30
Cheerios	1 1/4 cups	110	2	16	0	1.6
Cornflakes	1 cup	110	0.1	.01	0	1
Corn grits	1 cup	125	0.5	4	0	0
Cream of Wheat	3/4 cup	105	0.5	.05	0	0.6
40% Bran Flakes	3/4 cup	95	1	.9	0	6.0
Froot Loops	1 cup	110	1	.9	0	0.3
Frosted Flakes	1 cup	147	0	0	0	0.2
Granola	1/3 cup	125	5	36	0	3
Grape-Nuts	1/4 cup	100	0.2	.02	0	2.2
Oatmeal	3/4 cup	108	2	17	0	2.8
Product 19	1 cup	110	0.2	.02	0	1.2
Puffed rice	1 cup	55	0		0	0
Raisin bran	3/4 cup	90	1	1	0	3.6
Rice Krispies	1 cup	110	0.2	.02	0	0
Shredded Wheat	2/3 cup	100	0.3	.03	0	3.3
Special K	1 cup	110	0.1	.001	0	0.1
Total	1 cup	100	1	.9	0	2.5
Wheat Chex	1/3 cup	110	1	.8	0	2
Wheat germ	1 tbsp.	23	0.7	27	0	1
Wheaties	1 cup	100	1	.9	0	2.6

CURED MEATS

Food	Serving Size	Cal.	Fat (g)	Cal. from Fat (%)	Chol. (mg)
Bacon	3 slices	110	9	73	16
Bologna	1 oz.	90	8	80	16
Corned beef brisket	3 oz.	215	16	66	83
Frankfurter	1	145	13	80	23
Ham	3 oz.	205	14	61	52
Ham (lean only)	3 oz.	135	5	33	47
Liverwurst	1 oz.	65	7.8	97	45
Pork sausage	1 link	50	4	72	11
Salami, cooked	1 oz.	116	10	78	30
Salami, hard	1 oz.	126	10	71	16

DAIRY PRODUCTS

Food	Serving Size	Cal.	Fat (g)	Cal. from Fat (%)	Chol. (mg)
Cheeses					
Parmesan, grated	1 tbsp.	25	2	72	3
Ricotta, part skim milk	1/2 cup	170	10	53	38
Ricotta, whole milk	1/2 cup	215	16	67	62
Swiss	1 oz.	105	8	68	26
American	1 oz.	105	9	77	27
American (spread)	1 tbsp.	47	3	57	9
Brie	1 oz.	95	8	76	28
Cheddar	1 oz.	115	9	70	30
Cottage cheese (creamed)	1/2 cup	110	5	41	16
Cream cheese	1 oz.	100	10	90	31
Mozzarella, part skim milk	1 oz.	80	5	56	15
Mozzarella, whole milk	1 oz.	80	6	68	22
Blue cheese	1 oz.	100	8.2	74	21
Feta	1 oz.	75	6.0	72	25
Romano	1 oz.	110	7.6	62	29
Velveeta	1 oz.	82	3.8	42	16
Milk, Creams, and Milk Products					
Milk, nonfat (dry)	1/4 cup	81	0.2	0	0
Milk, skim	1 cup	85	Trace	0	4

273

Food	Serving Size	Cal.	Fat (g)	Cal. from Fat (%)	Chol. (mg)
Milk, 1%	1 cup	102	2.6	23	10
Milk, 2%	1 cup	120	5	37	18
Milk, whole	1 cup	150	8	48	33
Milk, evaporated (whole)	1 cup	338	19.1	51	74
Milk, evaporated (skim)	1 cup	200	0.6	2.7	10
Buttermilk	1 cup	100	2	18	9
Chocolate milk	1 cup	210	8	34	30
Cocoa mix with water	1 cup	100	1	.9	1
Condensed milk (sweetened)	1 cup	980	27	25	104
Cream, light	1 tbsp.	29	2.9	90	10
Cream, whipping (light)	1 cup	699	73.9	95	265
Cream, whipping (heavy)	1 cup	821	88.1	96	326
Cream, heavy	1 tbsp.	50	6	90	21
Creamer, nondairy	1 tbsp.	33	2.1	57	0
Half and half	1 tbsp.	20	2	90	6
Sour cream	1 tbsp.	25	3	95	5
Dessert topping	1 tbsp.	33	2.1	69	0
Yogurt, low-fat (plain)	8 oz.	145	4	25	14
Yogurt, low-fat (with fruit)	8 oz.	230	2	7.8	10
Yogurt (whole milk)	8 oz.	139	7.4	48	29
Yogurt, frozen	8 oz.	244	3.0	11	10
Milk shake, vanilla	10 oz.	315	9	26	33
Ice cream, premium	1 cup	349	23.7	61	88
Ice cream, regular	1 cup	269	14.3	48	59
Eskimo Pie	1	270	19.1	64	35
Ice cream sandwich (3 oz.)	1	238	8.5	32	34
Ice milk, soft-serve	1 cup	223	4.6	19	13
Ice milk, hard	1 cup	131	5.6	38	18
Pudding mix, regular (with whole milk)	1 cup	322	7.8	22	36
Pudding mix, instant (with whole milk)	1 cup	325	6.5	18	36
Pudding mix, low-cal (dry)	4 oz.	100			

Eggs

Food	Serving Size	Cal.	Fat (g)	Cal. from Fat (%)	Chol. (mg)
Egg, boiled	1 large	80	6	68	274
Egg, fried	1 large	95	7	66	278

Food	Serving Size	Cal.	Fat (g)	Cal. from Fat (%)	Chol. (mg)
Egg, scrambled	1 large	110	8	65	282
Egg white	1 large	15	Trace	0	0
Egg yolk	1 large	65	6	83	272

DESSERTS

Food	Serving Size	Cal.	Fat (g)	Cal. from Fat (%)	Chol. (mg)
Cookies					
Brownie with nuts and frosting	1 small	100	4	36	14
Chocolate chip cookie	1 medium	45	2	40	1
Fig bars	1 bar	55	1	16	7
Gingersnap	3 small	50	1	16	0
Marshmallow cookie with chocolate coating	1 cookie	55	2	38	0
Oatmeal raisin	1 medium	60	2	30	0–1
Sandwich cookie	1 medium	50	2	36	0
Sugar cookie	1 medium	60	3	45	7
Ice Creams (See Dairy)					
Pies (9″ Pie)					
Apple	1/6 pie	405	18	40	0
Banana custard	1/6 pie	335	14	38	45
Blueberry	1/6 pie	380	17	40	0
Cherry	1/6 pie	410	18	39	0
Lemon meringue	1/6 pie	355	14	35	143
Mincemeat	1/6 pie	430	18	38	0
Pecan	1/6 pie	575	32	50	95
Pumpkin	1/6 pie	320	17	48	109
Puddings					
Butterscotch	1/2 cup	170	4	21	17
Chocolate	1/2 cup	150	4	24	15
Custard	1/2 cup	150	8	48	139
Rice	1/2 cup	155	4	23	15
Tapioca	1/2 cup	145	4	25	15

Cakes

Food	Serving Size	Cal.	Fat (g)	Cal. from Fat (%)	Chol. (mg)
Angelfood	1/12 cake	125	Trace	0	0
Carrot with cream cheese icing	1/16 cake	385	21	49	74
Cheesecake, plain	1/12 cake	280	18	58	170
Chocolate with icing	1/16 cake	235	8	31	37
Danish, plain	1 medium	220	12	49	49
Doughnut, yeast	1 medium	235	13	50	21
Pound cake	1/8 loaf	246	10	39	33
Spice with icing	1/16 cake	270	8	26	NA

FATS/VEGETABLE OILS

Food	Serving Size	Cal.	Fat (g)	Cal. from Fat (%)	Chol. (mg)
Butter	1 tbsp.	108	12.2	100	33
Lard (animal shortening)	1 tbsp.	115	13	100	12
Chicken fat	1 tbsp.	126	14	100	9
Margarine, imitation or diet	1 tbsp.	50	5	90	0
Margarine, regular, soft	1 tbsp.	100	11	100	0
Coconut oil	1 tbsp.	120	14	100	0
Corn oil	1 tbsp.	125	14	100	0
Cottonseed oil	1 tbsp.	120	14	100	0
Olive oil	1 tbsp.	120	14	100	0
Palm kernel oil	1 tbsp.	120	13.6	100	0
Peanut oil	1 tbsp.	125	14	100	0
Soybean oil	1 tbsp.	120	14	100	0
Sunflower oil	1 tbsp.	125	14	100	0
Vegetable shortening	1 tbsp.	115	13	100	0

FISH/SHELLFISH

Food	Serving Size	Cal.	Fat (g)	Cal. from Fat (%)	Chol. (mg)
Bluefish	3 oz.	135	4	26	59
Clams, raw	2 clams	25	1	36	59

Food	Serving Size	Cal.	Fat (g)	Cal. from Fat (%)	Chol. (mg)
Cod	3 oz.	100	3	27	50
Crab, soft-shell, fried	1 medium	215	13	54	87
Crab, steamed	3 oz.	80	2	22	79
Crabmeat, canned	3 oz.	85	2	21	84
Flounder	3 oz.	100	6	54	50
Herring, pickled	3 oz.	190	13	61	85
Lobster tail, steamed	1 medium	100	1	9	88
Mackerel	3 oz.	215	15	62	94
Mussels, steamed	3 oz.	80	2	22	42
Oysters, raw	3 oz.	55	1	16	42
Salmon, canned	3 oz.	120	5	37	34
Salmon	3 oz.	150	7	42	36
Sardines, canned in oil	3 oz.	175	9	46	85
Scallops, steamed	3 oz.	95	1	9	45
Shrimp	7 medium	200	10	45	168
Swordfish	3 oz.	150	7	42	56
Trout	3 oz.	215	14	58	55
Tuna, chunk light in oil, drained	3 oz.	169	7	37	16
Anchovies, canned in olive oil	5 fillets	42	2	43	20
Herring, Pacific	3 oz.	166	12	65	65
Catfish	1 oz.	29	1	31	0
Halibut, broiled	1 oz.	28	0.3	9	14
Sole	1 oz.	26	0.3	10	0

FRUITS

Food	Serving Size	Cal.	Fat (g)	Cal. from Fat (%)	Chol. (mg)	Fiber (g)
Apple	1 medium	90	Trace	0	0	2.8
Applesauce	1/2 cup	95	Trace	0	0	2
Apricots	3	50	Trace	0	0	2.2
Avocado	1 medium	325	31	86	0	4.5
Banana	1 medium	105	1	0	0	2.1
Blueberries	1/2 cup	40	Trace	0	0	2.5
Cantaloupe	1/2 medium	95	1	0	0	2.7

Food	Serving Size	Cal.	Fat (g)	Cal. from Fat (%)	Chol. (mg)	Fiber (g)
Cherries, canned	½ cup	105	Trace	0	0	1.7
Coconut, packaged	1 cup	277	28	91	0	11.1
Cranberry sauce (canned)	¼ cup	105	.1	0	0	1
Dates	10	219	0.4	0	0	0.2
Figs, dried	1	50	Trace	0	0	3.7
Fruit cocktail (canned in water)	1 cup	91	0.2	0	0	0.2
Grapefruit	½ medium	40	Trace	0	0	1.7
Grapes, seedless	10	35	Trace	0	0	0.4
Honeydew cubes	1 cup	60	Trace	0	0	1.2
Lemons	1 medium	15	.2	0	0	1
Mangoes	1 medium	135	.6	0	0	4
Nectarines	1 medium	65	1	14	0	1.9
Oranges	1 medium	60	.2	0	0	4
Peaches	1 medium	35	.1	0	0	1
Pears	1 medium	100	1	9	0	5
Pineapple	½ cup	40	.3	0	0	1.2
Plums	1 medium	35	.6	0	0	3
Prunes, dried	5 large	115	.2	0	0	7.9
Raisins	½ cup	220	.4	0	0	4.9
Raspberries, raw	1 cup	70	.6	0	0	6
Rhubarb, frozen (sweetened)	1 cup	381	.3	0	0	6
Strawberries	1 cup	55	.7	0	0	3
Tangerines	1 large	46	.2	0	0	4
Watermelon (diced pieces)	1 cup	42	.3	0	0	1

GRAIN PRODUCTS: BREADS/PASTA/RICE

Food	Serving Size	Cal.	Fat (g)	Cal. from Fat (%)	Chol. (mg)	Fiber (g)
Bagel	1 bagel	200	2	9	0	2
Cornbread	1 piece	200	7	31	0	1.7

Food	Serving Size	Cal.	Fat (g)	Cal. from Fat (%)	Chol. (mg)	Fiber (g)
Frank or burger bun	1	115	2	15	Trace	1
French bread	1 slice	100	1	9	0	1.3
French toast	1 slice	155	7	40	112	0
Hard roll	1	155	2	11	1	1 less than
Pancake, plain	1	60	2	30	16	1
Rye bread	1 slice	65	1	13	0	0.9
Taco shell	1	50	2	36	0	1
Tortilla, corn	1 cake	65	1	13	0	1
White bread	1 slice	65	1	13	0	0.5
Whole-wheat bread	1 slice	70	1	12	0	1.4
Graham crackers	2	60	1	15	0	2.1
Melba toast	1 piece	20	Trace	0	0	0
Saltine crackers	4	50	1	18	5	0.5
Blueberry muffin from mix	1	135	5	33	19	0
Bran muffin, homemade	1	125	6	43	24	2
Corn muffin	1	145	5	31	23	1
English muffin	1	140	1	6	0	1
Egg noodles, cooked	1 cup	200	2	9	50	1.7
Macaroni, cooked	1 cup	190	1	4	0	1.2
Spaghetti, cooked	1 cup	190	1	4	0	1.6
Rice, brown, cooked	1/2 cup	115	1	7	0	2.4
Rice, white, cooked	1/2 cup	110	Trace	0	0	0.1

MISCELLANEOUS

Food	Serving Size	Cal.	Fat (g)	Cal. from Fat (%)	Chol. (mg)
Beef and vegetable stew	1 cup	220	11	45	71
Chili with beans	1 cup	340	16	42	28
Corned beef hash	1 cup	290	10	31	NA
Macaroni and cheese	1 cup	340	22	46	44
Spaghetti, canned	1 cup	260	9	31	8

Food	Serving Size	Cal.	Fat (g)	Cal. from Fat (%)	Chol. (mg)
Biscuit with sausage and egg	1	555	37	60	259
Cheeseburger patty	4 oz.	525	31	53	104
Chicken nuggets	6	265	16	54	60
Chicken sandwich	1	615	34	49	68
Enchilada	1	235	16	61	19
Fish sandwich with cheese	1	420	23	49	56
Frankfurter	1	280	16	51	45
French fries	15 pieces	230	12	46	0
Ham and cheese sandwich	1	400	22	49	60
Hamburger patty	4 oz.	445	21	42	71
Onion rings	1 serving	260	15	51	NA
Pizza with cheese	1/4 of 12" slice	290	9	27	18
Roast beef sandwich	1	345	13	33	55
Taco	1	195	11	50	21
Bacon bits	1 tsp.	14	0.6	38	0
M&M's	1/4 cup	230	9.7	37	3
Potato chips	10 chips	114	7	63	
Olives, green	10	33	4	99	
Beef tongue	1 slice	49	3.3	60	18
Beef liver	1 oz.	40	1.1	24	86
Beef tallow, suet	1 tbsp.	120	13.2	99	11
Deviled ham	1/4 cup	198	18.2	82	5
Sausage, Vienna (canned)	1	56	5.2	3	10

POULTRY

Food	Serving Size	Cal.	Fat (g)	Cal. from Fat (%)	Chol. (mg)
Chicken, dark meat (with skin)	4 oz.	286	17	54	103
Chicken, dark meat (no skin)	4 oz.	233	11	41	105
Chicken, white meat (with skin)	4 oz.	253	12	42	96

Food	Serving Size	Cal.	Fat (g)	Cal. from Fat (%)	Chol. (mg)
Chicken, white meat (no skin)	4 oz.	193	5	24	96
Chicken breast (no skin)	1/2 breast	140	3	19	73
Chicken breast (no skin, fried)	1/2 breast	160	4	22	78
Chicken drumstick (with skin)	1	110	6	49	48
Chicken drumstick (no skin)	1	75	2	24	41
Duck (with skin)	4 oz.	380	32	75	101
Duck (no skin)	4 oz.	227	13	52	95
Turkey, dark meat (with skin)	4 oz.	253	13	47	101
Turkey, dark meat (no skin)	4 oz.	213	8	33	96
Turkey, white meat (with skin)	4 oz.	220	9	38	86
Turkey, white meat (no skin)	4 oz.	180	4	20	79
Chicken gizzards	4 oz.	108	2.4	20	142

RED MEAT

Food	Serving Size	Cal.	Fat (g)	Cal. from Fat (%)	Chol. (mg)
Beef chuck roast	4 oz.	413	32	69	117
Beef flank steak	4 oz.	306	17	57	80
Beef rib roast	4 oz.	433	36	74	96
Beef top round★	4 oz.	210	5	21	70
Beef short ribs	4 oz.	533	48	81	107
Beef sirloin★	4 oz.	233	9	36	101
Beef T-bone★	4 oz.	240	12	45	91
Beef tenderloin	4 oz.	233	10	41	96
Hamburger (lean)	4 oz.	326	21	58	112
Porterhouse steak★	4 oz.	246	12	43	90

Food	Serving Size	Cal.	Fat (g)	Cal. from Fat (%)	Chol. (mg)
Lamb leg	4 oz.	213	8	33	80
Lamb loin chop★	1 large	250	14	50	60
Lamb rib chop★	1 large	290	22.5	70	75
Pork loin chop★	1 medium	275	19	62	84
Pork tenderloin	4 oz.	186	5	25	87
Spareribs	4 oz.	453	37	68	137
Veal cutlet	4 oz.	207	5.3	23	112
Veal loin chop	4 oz.	246	13	34	116
Veal rib roast	4 oz.	344	24	63	119

★All visible fat removed before cooking.

SOUP: CANNED/CONDENSED

Food	Serving Size	Cal.	Fat (g)	Cal. from Fat (%)	Chol. (mg)
Bean with bacon	1 cup	170	6	31	3
Beef consommé	1 cup	15	1	60	Trace
Chicken broth	1 cup	40	1	22	1
Chicken noodle	1 cup	75	2	24	7
Chicken rice	1 cup	60	2	30	7
Clam chowder (red)	1 cup	80	2	22	2
Clam chowder (white)	1 cup	165	7	38	22
Minestrone	1 cup	85	3	31	2
Mushroom with milk	1 cup	205	14	61	20
Split pea with ham	1 cup	190	4	18	8
Tomato	1 cup	85	2	21	0
Vegetable (vegetarian)	1 cup	70	2	25	0
Vegetable (with beef)	1 cup	80	2	22	5
Cream of celery with water	1 cup	86	5.5	57	7
Cream of chicken with water	1 cup	94	5.8	55	8
Canned onion with water	1 cup	65	2.4	33	6
Dehydrated onion	1 pack	150	4.6	27	0

VEGETABLES

Food	Serving Size	Cal.	Fat (g)*	Cal. from Fat (%)	Chol. (mg)	Fiber (g)
Artichoke, bud or globe (frozen)	1 whole	52	0.2	3	0	
Asparagus	½ cup	20	.3	14	0	2.2
Beets	½ cup	25	.3	11	0	2.2
Broccoli	½ cup	46	.4	8	0	4.5
Brussels sprouts	1 cup	51	0.3	5	0	
Cabbage, cooked	½ cup	15	.2	12	0	2
Cabbage, raw (shredded)	½ cup	10	.1	9	0	0.7
Carrot, raw	1 medium	30	.2	6	0	2.4
Carrot, sliced (cooked)	½ cup	35	.1	3	0	2.3
Cauliflower	½ cup	15	.1	6	0	1.6
Celery, raw	1 stalk	5	.1	18	0	0.7
Corn, kernels	½ cup	90	1	1	0	3.9
Corn, creamed canned	½ cup	93	.4	4	0	
Cucumber, raw	½ cup	5	.1	18	0	0.5
Eggplant, cubes	1 cup	25	.2	7	0	4
Greens, collard	1 cup	51	0.7	12	0	
Lettuce, iceberg	1 cup	5	0	0	0	0.5
Lettuce, leaf	1 cup	10	.2	18	0	1.2
Mushrooms, raw (sliced)	½ cup	10	.2	18	0	0.9
Okra, frozen (cooked)	1 cup	70	0.2	2	0	
Onion, raw (chopped)	½ cup	25	.2	7	0	2.6
Pea pods, Chinese	½ cup	35	0	0	0	1.3
Peas, green	½ cup	65	.2	3	0	4.1
Pepper, green (raw)	1 medium	20	.3	14	0	0.8
Pepper, jalapeño (raw)	1	7	0		0	
Pepper, jalapeño (canned)	½ cup	17	.4	21	0	
Pickles, dill	1 large	15	0.3	18	0	
Pickles, sweet	2 slices	11	0	0	0	

Food	Serving Size	Cal.	Fat (g)*	Cal. from Fat (%)	Chol. (mg)	Fiber (g)
Potatoes, baked (no skin)	1 medium	145	.1	1	0	3.7
Potatoes, boiled	1 medium	115	.1	1	0	2.7
Radishes	4 medium	5	.1	18	0	0.5
Sauerkraut, canned	1/2 cup	20	.2	9	0	2.4
Spinach, frozen	1/2 cup	30	.2	6	0	2.1
Squash, summer	1 cup	25	0.2	7	0	
Squash, winter	1/2 cup	40	1	22	0	3.6
Sweet potato (mashed)	1/2 cup	170	.5	3	0	3.8
Tomato, raw	1 medium	25	.3	11	0	1
Tomato juice	1/2 cup	20	.1	5	0	0
Tomato puree	1/2 cup	50	.2	4	0	3
Yam, cubes	1/2 cup	80	.1	1	0	2.6
Vegetable juice cocktail	1/2 cup	20	.1	5	0	0
Zucchini, sliced (cooked)	1/2 cup	15	.1	6	0	2.7

* 0 represents the equivalent of less than 1 gram of fat per serving.

VITAMINS

VITAMIN A (Beta carotene)—Beta carotene is a powerful antioxidant involved with enhancing the immunity of the body. It is particularly important in the growth and maintenance of healthy skin, hair, and eyes. Multiple clinical studies have shown its positive impact on heart disease, stroke, and cancer.

VITAMIN D—Vitamin D is crucial in building strong bones and teeth. It is extremely important in calcium metabolism. Children and pregnant or nursing women will need additional vitamin D.

VITAMIN E—Like vitamin A, vitamin E is a potent antioxidant. It is particularly important in the prevention of atherosclerosis. Vitamin E aids in the healing of wounds and protects the respiratory system from pollution. When combined with selenium, it is known to be a potent immune stimulant.

VITAMIN C—Vitamin C must be taken in the diet, as we cannot synthesize it in our bodies. It is extremely effective in enhancing immunity and building resistance to infections and fatigue. It helps protect blood vessels and improves healing after surgery. It favorably affects cholesterol in the blood and is extremely important in delaying cataract formation. Multiple clinical studies also show its unique effectiveness in combating heart disease and cancer.

VITAMIN B-1—Vitamin B-1 helps strengthen the nervous system and is necessary in the treatment of beriberi and alcoholism. It is extremely important in the metabolism of sugar. It also can be effective in improving one's memory.

VITAMIN B-2 (Riboflavin)—Riboflavin is important in healing and in digesting fat, protein, and carbohydrates. It aids in growth and reproduction.

VITAMIN B-3 (Niacin)—Niacin is important in the healthy functioning of the nervous system. It is essential in the production of male and female sex hormones. It improves circulation and lowers cholesterol.

VITAMIN B-6—Vitamin B-6 is crucial in the proper chemical balance of the body. It helps convert fats and proteins into energy. Combined with vitamin B-1, it may be helpful in seasickness. It is particularly important in relieving premenstrual swelling. It has been touted as enhancing the immune system and alleviating depression.

VITAMIN B-12—Vitamin B-12 is extremely important as a supplement for strict vegetarians. It helps to prevent anemia and to improve digestion and memory. It supports the immune system and the nervous system.

BIOTIN—Biotin is necessary in the support of protein, fat, and carbohydrates. It helps prevent skin disorders, especially eczema, and builds resistance in allergic situations.

PANTOTHENIC ACID—Pantothenic acid is frequently referred to as a "stress" vitamin. It is necessary in the proper functioning of the adrenal glands. It also helps stimulate the immune system.

FOLIC ACID—Folic acid is crucial in supporting the immune system. It has particular utility in the nervous system and has been used in the treatment of senility. Folic acid helps prevent anemia and has recently been reported to help in the prevention of cervical cancer as well as coronary artery disease. It prevents malformation of the nervous system in fetuses.

MINERALS

CALCIUM AND PHOSPHORUS—Calcium and phosphorus are extremely important in the proper functioning and healthy maintenance of bones and teeth. Calcium is also particularly useful in the regulation of the irritability of nerves and muscles. Calcium supplements are useful in helping prevent osteoporosis.

MAGNESIUM—Magnesium is involved in over three hundred enzymatic reactions in the body. It has particular utility in the prevention of cardiovascular disorders. It is useful in PMS, especially when combined with vitamins B-6 and E. It is also useful in chronic fatigue syndrome because it enhances energy.

MANGANESE—Manganese is a powerful antioxidant that helps in the prevention of atherosclerosis. It helps reduce fatigue and improve memory. It also helps in regulating blood sugar.

IODINE—Iodine is crucial in the proper synthesis of thyroxine in the thyroid gland. It aids in maintaining mental alertness. It is important in the overall functioning of the immune system.

SELENIUM—Selenium is a powerful antioxidant that has been touted in the prevention of heart disease and cancer. It is particularly important as an immune system stimulant. It is helpful in combating harmful metals in the environment.

ZINC—Zinc is crucial in wound healing as well as the immune system. It plays a role in the healthy sexual functioning of the male, as it supports the prostate gland.

CHROMIUM PICOLINATE—Chromium plays a vital role in the body's utilization of sugar. It has been reported to lower cholesterol. Chromium may also reduce triglycerides. Clinical studies have also demonstrated the utility of chromium as a "fat buster," especially when used in combination with L-carnitine. Some researchers indicate that chromium is useful in increasing longevity. Up to 90 percent of us may be deficient in chromium. Chromium picolinate is the most easily absorbable form of chromium.

POTASSIUM—Potassium is particularly crucial in the overall functioning of nerves and muscles, especially the heart. It helps counteract the blood-pressure-raising effects of sodium. It is useful in treating allergies and in maintaining proper heart rhythms.

BORON—Boron has particular usefulness in the musculoskeletal functioning of the body. Some investigators indicate that it is especially helpful in combination with calcium in preventing osteoporosis.

VANADIUM—Vanadium has been touted as an antiaging mineral. A deficiency in vanadium has been associated with heart disease. It has been shown to have cholesterol-lowering ability.

LIPOTROPIC FACTORS—NUTRITIONALS THAT SUPPORT THE METABOLISM OF FAT

CHOLINE—Choline is particularly important in cholesterol metabolism and in protecting the liver against toxic chemicals. Choline supplements have also been said to improve memory.

INOSITOL—Like choline, inositol helps protect the liver and nervous system. It regulates cholesterol levels and aids in the treatment of atherosclerosis. It has been known to counteract the negative effects of caffeine.

METHIONINE—Methionine, like choline, inositol, and betaine, is a lipotropic factor that helps prevent excessive fat in the liver. It also helps prevent cholesterol buildup. It is an antioxidant and free-radical scavenger. It is an important amino acid, particularly for those who consume high levels of alcohol and sugar.

BETAINE HCL—Betaine HCL is important in stimulating the production of hydrochloric acid in the gut. This is useful in the digestion of proteins.

L-CARNITINE—L-carnitine is particularly helpful in fat metabolism. Although L-carnitine can be manufactured by the body, adequate quantities of the amino acids lysine and methionine are required for L-carnitine synthesis. A deficiency of L-carnitine may result in a fatty liver, a weakened immune system, muscle wasting, and perhaps even heart failure.

ENZYMES

PAPAIN AND BROMELAIN—Papain is an extract of papaya, and bromelain is an extract of pineapple. They not only aid in digestion, but also have been reported to reduce soreness and speed healing of bruises and swelling after minor trauma. Bromelain also acts to help with the absorption of quercetin.

ALOE VERA—Aloe vera is a healing remedy that has been used in the healing of mucous membranes and skin. It is especially helpful in healing ulcers and has been effective in helping burns to heal.

ACIDOPHILUS—Acidophilus is a friendly bacterium in our bowel. It protects the colon from cancer and aids digestion of food. Acidophilus

can be destroyed by caffeine, antibiotics, and birth control pills. It also
reduces putrefaction in the bowel.

NUTRITIONALS

COENZYME Q_{10}—Coenzyme Q_{10} is helpful in enhancing energy. It does
this by stimulating energy production in the mitochondria, the
"powerhouses" of cells. It has particular utility in heart efficiency and
exercise tolerance. It is used as a treatment for heart failure and angina
and is believed to enhance immunity and to prevent cancer. Coenzyme Q_{10} is now being utilized in AIDS patients.

L-GLUTATHIONE—L-glutathione is a powerful antioxidant. As a free-
radical scavenger, it has been known to bolster immunity. It is now
receiving considerable scrutiny as an effective agent in reducing HIV
activity. It also has been reported to be useful in converting oxidized
vitamin C back to a form that can serve again as an antioxidant.
Glutathione also combines with selenium to form glutathione peroxidase, a potent free-radical scavenger.

QUERCETIN—Quercetin is a polyphenol found in high concentrations in
red grapes and onions that inhibits the oxidation of LDL. It is the
major nutrient responsible for the "French Paradox."

SELECTED REFERENCES

BOOKS

Achterberg, J., and G. E. Lawlis. 1978 *Imagery and Disease*. Champaign, IL: Institute for Personality and Ability Testing.

Achterberg, J., B. Dossey, et al. 1994 *Rituals of Healing: Using Imagery for Health and Wellness*. New York: Bantam.

American College of Sports Medicine. 1986 *Guidelines for Exercise Testing and Prescription*. Philadelphia: Lea and Febiger.

Bailey, C. 1978 *Fit or Fat?* Boston: Houghton Mifflin.

Balch, J. F., and P. A. Balch. 1990 *Prescription for Nutritional Healing*. Garden City Park, NY: Avery.

Bass, E., and C. Davis. 1988 *The Courage to Heal*. New York: Harper and Row.

Bland, J. 1983 *Medical Applications of Clinical Nutrition*. New Canaan, CT: Keats.

Bliznakof, E. G., and G. L. Hunt. 1986 *The Miracle Nutrient Coenzyme Q$_{10}$*. New York: Bantam.

Bruch, E. 1973 *Eating Disorders*. New York: Basic Books.

Carper, J. 1988 *The Food Pharmacy: Dramatic New Evidence That Food Is Your Best Medicine*. New York: Bantam.

Cortis, B. 1995 *Heart and Soul*. New York: Villard.

Cowmeadow, O. 1987 *An Introduction to Macrobiotics: The Natural Way to Health and Happiness*. Wellingborough, UK: Thorsons.

Eades, M. R., and M. D. Eades. 1996 *Protein Power*. New York: Bantam.

Eastwood, M. A., W. G. Brydon, and K. Talese. 1980 "Effects of fiber on colon continence." In G. A. Spiller and R. McP. Kay, eds., *Medical Aspects of Dietary Fiber*. New York: Plenum.

Eddy, M. B. 1934 *Science and Health with Key to the Scriptures*. Boston: Publishers Agent.

Eliot, R. S. 1994 *From Stress to Strength: How to Lighten Your Load and Save Your Life*. New York: Bantam.

Eliot, R. S., and D. L. Breo. 1986 *Is It Worth Dying For?* New York: Bantam.

Fletcher, A. M. 1989 *Eat Fish, Live Better*. New York: Harper and Row.

Folkers, K., ed. 1981 *Biomedical and Clinical Aspects of Coenzyme Q_{10}*, vol. 3. Amsterdam: Elsevier.

Gillespie, C. 1994 *Hormones, Hot Flashes, and Mood Swings: The Menopausal Survival Guide*. New York: Harper Perennial.

Goodwin, J., et al. 1989 *Sexual Abuse*. Chicago: Yearbook.

Hirschmann, J. R., and C. H. Munter. 1988 *Overcoming Overeating*. New York: Fawcett Columbine.

Hirschmann, J. R., and L. Zaphiropoulos. 1985 *Are You Hungry?* New York: Random House.

Hubert, E., and A. Soben. 1970 "Properties and fatty acid composition of fats and oils." In *Handbook of Biochemistry*, pp. E20–21. Cleveland: CRC.

Jarvis, D. C. 1958 *Folk Medicine*. New York: Fawcett Crest.

Jensen, B. 1981 *Tissue Cleaning Through Bowel Management*. Escondido, CA: Bernard Jensen.

1983 *Food Healing for Man*. Escondido, CA: Bernard Jensen.

Johnston, J. M., J. R. Johnston, R. S. Passwater, and E. Mindell. 1990 *Flaxseed (Linseed) Oil and the Power of Omega-3: How to Make Nature's Cholesterol Fighters Work for You*. New Canaan, CT: Keats.

Keul, J., E. Doll, and D. Koppler. 1972 *Energy Metabolism of Human Muscle*. Basel: S. Karger.

Kushi, M., with A. Jack. 1985 *Diet for a Strong Heart*. New York: St. Martin's.

Lark, S. M. 1984 *PMS: Premenstrual Syndrome Self-Help Book*. Berkeley: Celestial Arts.

Lesser, M. 1980 *Nutrition and Vitamin Therapy*. New York: Grove.

Lowen, A. 1976 *Bioenergetics*. New York: Pelican.

1977 *The Way to Vibrant Health*. New York: Harper and Row.

1980 *Fear of Life*. New York: Macmillan.

1980 *Stress and Illness: A Bioenergetic View*. New York: Lowen.

1988 *Love, Sex, and Your Heart*. New York: Macmillan.

Masquelier, J. 1959 "The bactericidal action of certain phenolics of grapes and wine." In *The Pharmacology of Plant Phenolics*. New York: Academic.

Meiselman, K. 1986 *Incest*. San Francisco: Jossey-Bass.

Miller, A. 1981 *Prisoners of Childhood*. New York: Basic Books.

1983 *For Your Own Good*. New York: Farrar, Straus, and Giroux.

Miquel, J. 1986 "Theoretical and experimental support for an 'oxygen radical-mitochondrial injury' hypothesis of cell aging." In J. E. Johnson, R. Walford, D. Harmon, and J. Miquel, eds., *Free Radicals, Aging, and Degenerative Diseases*. New York: Alan R. Liss.

1995 *The Healing Power of Herbs*. Rocklin, CA: Prima Publishing.

National Academy of Sciences. 1989 *Diet and Health: Implications for Reducing Chronic Disease Risk*. Washington, D.C.: National Academy Press.

Niazi, S. K. 1987 *The Omega Connection: The Facts About Fish Oils and Human Health*. Chicago: Esquire Books.

Ornish, D. 1990 *Dr. Dean Ornish's Program for Reversing Heart Disease*. New York: Random House.

Ornstein, R., and C. Swencionis. 1990 *The Healing Brain: A Scientific Reader*. New York: Guilford.

Page, Linda. 1994 *Healthy Healing: An Alternative Healing Reference*. Sonora, CA: Healthy Healing.

Passwater, R. A., and C. Kanddaswami. 1994 *Pycnogenol: The Super "Protector" Nutrient*. New Canaan, CT: Keats.

Pearson, D., and S. Shaw. 1982 *Life Extension: A Practical Scientific Approach*. New York: Warner.

Pennington, J.A.T. 1989 *Food Values of Portions Commonly Used*. New York: Harper and Row.

Pfeiffer, C. C., et al. 1975 *Mental and Elemental Nutrients: A Physician's Guide to Nutrition and Health Care*. New Canaan, CT: Keats.

Porter, N. A. 1980 "Prostaglandin endoperoxides." *Free Radicals in Biology*, vol. 4. New York: Academic Press.

Poston, C., and K. Lison. 1989 *Reclaiming Our Lives*. New York: Little, Brown.

Pritikin, N., with P. M. McGrady Jr. 1979 *The Pritikin Program for Diet and Exercise*. New York: Bantam.

Reich, W. 1945 *Character Analysis*. New York: Farrar, Straus, and Giroux.

1973 *The Function of the Orgasm*. New York: Simon and Schuster.

Remington, D., G. Fisher, and E. Parent. 1983 *How to Lower Your Fat Thermostat: The No-Diet Reprogramming Plan for Lifelong Weight Control*. Provo: Vitality House International.

Ross, R. 1992 "The pathogenesis of atherosclerosis." In E. Braunwald, ed., *Heart Disease: A Textbook of Cardiovascular Medicine*. 4th ed. Philadelphia: W. B. Saunders.

Rush, R. 1980 *The Best-Kept Secret*. New York: McGraw-Hill.

Sattilaro, A. J., with T. Monte. 1984 *Living Well Naturally*. Boston: Houghton Mifflin.

Schechter, S. R., with T. Monte. 1988 *Fighting Radiation with Foods, Herbs, and Vitamins*. Brookline, MA: East-West Health Books.

Sears, B., with B. Lawren. 1995 *The Zone: A Dietary Road Map*. New York: Regan.

Seibin, and T. Arasaki. 1983 *Vegetables from the Sea*. Tokyo: Japan Publications.

Siegel, B. S. 1989 *Peace, Love, and Healing.* New York: Harper and Row.

Sinatra, S. T. 1987 "Stress management and cardiovascular rehabilitation." In R. Cantu, ed., *The Exercising Adult.* New York: Macmillan.

Somer, E. 1993 *Nutrition for Women: The Complete Guide.* New York: Henry Holt.

Story, J. A. 1980 "Dietary fiber and lipid metabolism: an update." In G. A. Spiller and R. McP. Kay, eds., *Medical Aspects of Dietary Fiber.* New York: Plenum.

Tarnower, H., and S. S. Baker. 1978 *The Complete Scarsdale Medical Diet Plus Dr. Tarnower's Lifetime Keep-Slim Program.* New York: Bantam.

Walters, R. Avery. 1992 *Options: The Alternative Cancer Therapy Book.* Garden City Park, NY.

PERIODICALS

Alession, H. M., A. H. Goldfarb, and R. C. Cutler. 1988 "MDA content increases in fast- and slow-twitch skeletal muscle with intensity of exercise in a rat." *Am J Physiol* C874–77.

Alession, H. M., and A. H. Goldfarb. 1988 "Lipid peroxidation and scavenger enzymes during exercise: adaptive response to training." *J Appl Physiol* 64:1333–36.

Ames, B., M. Shigenaga, and T. Hagent. 1993 "Oxidants, antioxidants, and the degenerative diseases of aging." *Proc Nat Acad Sci* 90:7915–22.

Anderson, J. W., et al. 1986 "Dietary fiber: hyperlipidemia, hypertension, and coronary heart disease." *Am J Gastroenterology* 81(10):907–17.

Anderson, J. W., and N. J. Gustafson. 1987 "High-carbohydrate, high-fiber diet: is it practical and effective in treating hyperlipidemia?" *Postgraduate Medicine* 82(4):40.

Anderson, J. W., N. J. Gustafson, C. A. Bryant, and J. Tietyen-Clark. 1987 "Dietary fiber and diabetes: a comprehensive review and practical application." *J Am Diet Assoc* 87:1189–97.

Anderson, K. M., et al. 1991 "An updated coronary risk profile: a statement for health professionals." *Circulation* 83:356–62.

Aro, A., et al. 1995 "Adipose tissue isometric trans-fatty acids and risk of myocardial infarction in nine countries: the EURAMIC study." *The Lancet* 345:273–78.

Ascherio, A., E. B. Rimm, et al. 1995 "Dietary intake of marine n-3 fatty acids, fish intake, and the risk of coronary disease among men." *NEJM* 332:977–82.

Augusti, K. T., et al. 1975 "Partial identification of the fibrinolytic activators in onion." *Atherosclerosis* 21:409–16.

Babior, M. B. 1978 "Oxygen-dependent microbial killing of phagocytes." *New England Journal of Medicine* 298:659.

Beaglehole, R., R. Jackson, J. Watkinson, R. Scragg, R. L. Yee. 1990 "Decreased blood selenium and risk of myocardial infarction." *Int J Epidemiol* 19(4):918–22.

Becker, A. B., et al. 1984 "The bronchodilator effects and pharmacokinetics of caffeine in asthma." *New England Journal of Medicine* 310:743–46.

Bell, L. P., K. Hectome, H. Reynolds, et al. 1989 "Cholesterol-lowering effects of psyllium hydrophilic mucilloid: adjunct therapy to a prudent diet for patients with mild to moderate hypercholesterolemia." *Journal of the American Medical Association* 261:3419–23.

Benfante, R., and D. Reed. 1990 "Is elevated serum cholesterol a risk factor for coronary heart disease in the elderly?" *Journal of the American Medical Association* 263:393–96.

Benson, J. A., Jr., et al. 1975 "Simple chronic constipation." *Postgraduate Medicine* 57:55.

Bhaskaram, C., and V. Reddy. 1975 "Cell-mediated immunity in iron- and vitamin-deficient children." *BMJ* 3(5982):522.

Blair, S. N., H. W. Kohn, R. S. Paffenbarger, et al. 1989 "Physical fitness and all-cause mortality." *Journal of the American Medical Association* 262:2395–401.

Blake, D. R., et al. 1989 Letter. "Hypoxic-reperfusion injury in inflamed human joints." *The Lancet* 289–93. May 6; 1(8645):1023.

Blankenhorn, D. H., and D. M. Kramsch. 1989 "Reversal of atherosis and sclerosis: the two components of atherosclerosis." *Circulation* 79:1–15.

Block, G. 1991 "Vitamin C and cancer prevention: the epidemiologic evidence." *Am J Clin Nutr* 53:270S–282S.

Boadella, A. 1986 "Personal observations." Paper presented at the International Bioenergetic Conference, Belgium.

Bohigian, M. D. 1988 "Dietary fiber and health." Information report of the Council on Scientific Affairs, American Medical Association, April: 1–14.

Bordia, A. K. 1981 "Effect of garlic on blood lipids in patients with coronary heart disease." *Am J Clin Nutr* 34:2100.

Bordia, A. K., et al. 1977 "Effect of essential oil of garlic on fibrinolytic activity in patients with coronary artery disease." *Atherosclerosis* 28(2):155–59.

Borish, E. T., and W. A. Prior. 1987 "Cigarette smoking, free radicals, and free radical DNA damage." *Ann Int Med* 107:526–45.

Boxer, L. A., A. M. Watanabe, et al. 1976 "Correction of leukocyte function in Chediak-Higashi syndrome by ascorbate." *New England Journal of Medicine* 295:1041–45.

Bray, G. A. 1982 "The energetics of obesity." Paper presented at the annual meeting of the AC Sports Medicine, May.

Brownlee, S. A. 1991 "Alzheimer's: Is there hope?" *U.S. News and World Report,* August 12:40–49.

Bulrum, R. R., C. K. Clifford, and E. Lanza. 1988 "NCI dietary guidelines: rationale." *Am J Clin Nutr* 48:888–95.

Burkitt, D. P. 1973 "Some diseases characteristic of modern Western civilization." *BMJ* (1)848:274–78.

Burkitt, D. P., A.R.P. Walker, and N. S. Painter. 1974 "Dietary fiber and disease." *Journal of the American Medical Association* 229(8):1068–74.

Burton, G. W., and K. U. Ingold. 1984 "Beta carotene: an unusual type of lipid antioxidant." *Science* 224:569–73.

Camaione, D. N., and S. T. Sinatra. 1981 "Beneficial effects of exercise and current concepts in adult fitness." *CT Med* 45(10):620–25.

Cardiology World News. 1991 "Pectin may reduce cholesterol, colon cancer incidence." September: 8.

Castell, W. P. 1988 "Cardiovascular disease in women." *Am J Obstet Gynecol* 158:1153–60.

Chan, J. K., V. M. Bruce, and B. E. McDonald. 1995 "Dietary alpha-linolenic acid is as effective as oleic acid and linoleic acid in lowering blood cholesterol in normolipidemic men." *Am J Clin Nutr* 55(1):140–41.

Chandra, R. J., et al. 1993 "Vitamins for the elderly." *The Lancet* 340:1124–27.

Chen, T.-Y., Y.-T. Lin, and S.-C. Wu. 1994 "Effectiveness of coenzyme Q_{10} on myocardial preservation during hypothermic cardioplegic arrest." *J Thorac Cardiovasc Surg* 107:242–47.

Chihara, G., et al. 1970 "Fractionation and purification of the polysaccharides with marked antitumor activity, especially lentinan, from *Lentinus edodes* (Berk.) Sing. (an edible mushroom)." *Cancer Res* 30:2776–81.

Choices in Cardiology. 1991 "Twelve weeks to a healthier diet." *Choices in Cardiology* 5(4):167–68.

Clark, R., L. Daly, K. Robinson, et al. 1991 "Hyperhomocysteinemia: an independent risk factor for vascular disease." *New England Journal of Medicine* 17:1149–55.

Cleary-Merker, L. 1991 "Childhood sexual abuse as an antecedent to obesity." *The Bariatrician: American Journal of Bariatric Medicine,* spring: 17–22.

Colditz, G. A., S. E. Hankinson, et al. 1995 "The use of estrogen and progestins and the risk of breast cancer in postmenopausal women." *New England Journal of Medicine* 332:1589–93.

Connett, J. R., I. H. Kuller, M. O. Kjelberg, et al. 1989 "Relationship between carotenoid and cancer: the MRFIT study." *Cancer* 64:126–34.

Conrad, C. C. 1981 "The president's council on physical fitness and sports." *Am J Sports Med* 9:199–202.

Cooper, K. H. 1988–89 "Coronary combat." *Modern Maturity,* December: 78–84.

Cosgrove, D. M. 1994 "Coronary artery surgery in women." *CVR&R,* September: 54–59.

Costill, D. L., et al. 1978 "Effects of caffeine ingestion on metabolism and exercise performance." *Medicine and Science in Sports* 10(3):155–58.

Cox, I. M. 1991 "Magnesium therapy improves symptoms of chronic fatigue syndrome." *The Lancet* 337:757–60.

Crawford, M. A. 1993 "The role of essential fatty acids in neural development: implications for perinatal nutrition." *Am J Clin Nutr* 57(5 Suppl):703S–709S; discussion 709S–710S.

Cross, C. E., et al. 1987 "Oxygen radicals and human disease." *Ann of Int Med* 107(4):526–45.

Cummings, J. H., et al. 1978 "Colonic response to dietary fiber from carrot, cabbage, apple, bran." *The Lancet,* January 7: 5–8. Vol. 1(8054):5–9.

Cunnane, S. C., S. Ganguli, C. Menard, A. C. Liede, M. J. Hamadeh, Z.-Y. Chen, T. M. Wolever, and D. J. Jenkins. 1993 "High alpha-linolenic acid flaxseed *(Linum usitatissimum):* some nutritional properties in humans." *Br J Nutr* 69(2):443–53.

D'Agostino, R. B., A. J. Belanger, and W. B. Kannel. 1991 "Relations of low diastolic blood pressure to coronary heart disease death in presence of myocardial infarction: the Framingham study." *BMJ* Aug 17; 303(6799):385–89.

Davis, K.J.A., et al. 1982 "Free radical and tissue damage produced by exercise." *Biochem Biophys Res Comm* 107:1178–205.

DeLorgeril, M., et al. 1994 "Mediterranean alpha-linolenic acid-rich diet in secondary prevention of coronary heart disease." *The Lancet* 343:1454–59.

Delver, E., and B. Pence. 1993 "Effects of dietary selenium levels on UV-induced skin cancer and epidermal antioxidant status." *FASEB J* 7:A290.

Donoghue, S. 1977 "The correlation between physical fitness, absenteeism, and work performance." *Can J Pub Health* 69:201–3.

Dyckner, T., and P. O. Wester. 1987 "Potassium/magnesium depletion in patients with cardiovascular disease." *Am J of Med* 62:11–17.

Enstrom, J. E., L. E. Kanim, and M. E. Klein. 1992 "Vitamin C intake and mortality among a sample of the United States population." *Epidemiology* 3:194–202.

Esterbauer, H., et al. 1991 "Role of vitamin E in preventing the oxidation of low-density lipoprotein." *Am J Clin Nutr* 53:314S–21S.

Esterbauer, H., M. Rotheneder, G. Striegel, et al. 1989 "Vitamin E and other lipophilic antioxidants protect LDL against oxidation." *Fat Sci Technol* 91:316–24.

Facchinetti, F., P. Borella, G. Sances, et al. 1991 "Oral magnesium successfully relieves premenstrual mood changes." *Obstetrics and Gynecology* 78(2):177–81.

Fardy, P. S., et al. 1976 "An assessment of the influence of habitual physical activity, prior sports participation, smoking habits, and aging upon indices of cardiovascular fitness: preliminary report of a cross-sectional and retrospective study." *J Sports Med Phys Fit* 16:77–90.

Felson, D. T., Y. Zhang, et al. 1993 "The effect of postmenopausal estrogen therapy on bone density in elderly women." *New England Journal of Medicine* 329:1141–46.

Ferrier, L. K., et al. 1995 "Alpha-linolenic acid– and docosahexaenoic acid– enriched eggs from hens fed flaxseed: influence on blood lipids and platelet phospholipid fatty acids in humans." *Am J Clin Nutr* 62:81–86.

Folkers, K., P. Langsjoen, et al. 1990 "Lovastatin decreases coenzyme Q_{10} levels in humans." *Proc Nat Acad Sci* 87:8931–34.

Folkins, D. H., et al. 1972 "Psychological fitness as a function of physical fitness." *Arch Phys Med Rehabil* 53:503–8.

Foster, W. R., and B. T. Burton. 1985 "Health implications of obesity." *Ann Int Med* 103:1024–30.

Frambach, D. A., and E. B. Rick. 1991 Letter to the editor. *Journal of the American Medical Association* 265:879.

Frankel, E. N., J. Kanner, J. B. German, et al. 1993 "Inhibition of oxidation of human low-density lipoprotein by phenolic substances in red wine." *The Lancet* 341:454–56.

Freese, R., M. Mutanen, L. M. Valsta, and I. Salminen. 1994 "Comparison of the effects of two diets rich in monounsaturated fatty acids differing in their linoleic/alpha-linolenic acid ratio on platelet aggregation." *Thromb Haemost* 71:73–77.

Gaziano, J. M., J. E. Manson, et al. 1990 "Beta carotene therapy for chronic stable angina." *Circulation* 82:111–201.

Gaziano, J. M., L. G. Brach, J. E. Manson, et al. 1995 "Prospect study of beta-carotene in fruits and vegetables and decreased cardiovascular mortality in an elderly cohort." *Ann Epidemiol* 5:255–60.

Gey, K. F., and P. Puska. 1989 "Plasma vitamins E and A inversely correlated to mortality from ischemic heart disease in cross-cultural epidemiology." *Ann NY Acad Sci* 570:268–82.

Gey, K. F., et al. 1991 "Inverse correlation between plasma, vitamin E, and mortality from ischemic heart disease in cross-cultural epidemiology." *Am J Clin Nutr* 53:326S–44S.

Giles, T. D. 1990 "Magnesium deficiency: an important cardiovascular risk factor." *Advances in Cardiology* 1 (5).

Gloth, F. M., III, et al. 1991 "Can vitamin D deficiency produce an unusual pain syndrome?" *Arch Intern Med* 151:1662–64.

Goldman, I. S., and N. E. Canturwitz. 1982 "Cardiomyopathy associated with selenium deficiency." *New England Journal of Medicine* 305:701.

Goldschmidt, M. G. 1994 "Dyslipidemia and ischemic heart disease mortality among men and women with diabetes." *Circulation* 89:991–97.

Goldsmith, M. 1988 "Will exercise keep women away from oncologists or obstetricians?" *Journal of the American Medical Association* 259:1769–70.

Gorsky, R. D., J. P. Koplan, et al. 1994 "Relative risks and benefits of long-term estrogen replacement therapy: a decision analysis." *Obstet Gynecol* 83:161–66.

Gotto, A. M., Jr. 1992 "Hypertriglyceridemia: risks and perspectives." *Am J Cardiol* 70(19):19H–25H.

Greenberg, S. M., and W. H. Frishman. 1988 "Coenzyme Q_{10}: a new drug for myocardial ischemia?" *The Medical Clinics of North America* 72(1):243–58.

1990 "Coenzyme Q_{10}: a new drug for cardiovascular disease." *Journal of Clinical Pharmacology* 30:596–608.

Greiser, E. M., U. Maschewski-Schneider, G. Tempel, and U. Helmert. 1991 "Smoking, medication found to increase cholesterol levels." *Cardiology World News,* September: 26–27.

Grundy, S. M. 1986 "Comparison of monounsaturated fatty acids and carbohydrates for lowering plasma cholesterol." *New England Journal of Medicine* 314:745–48.

1989 "High serum cholesterol: treatment by diet." *Cardiology Board Review* 6(3):32–38.

1990 "Cholesterol and coronary heart disease: future directions." *Journal of the American Medical Association* 264:3053–59.

Haber, J. B., K. W. Heaton, D. Murphy, and L. F. Burroughs. 1977 "Depletion and disruption of dietary fiber: effect on satiety, plasma, glucose, and serum insulin." *The Lancet* 2:679–82.

Halevy, O., and D. Sklan. 1987 "Inhibition of arachidonic acid oxidation by beta-carotene, retinol, and alpha-tocopherol." *Biochem Biophys Acta* 918:304–7.

Hankinson, S. E., and M. J. Stampfer. 1994 "All that glitters is not beta-carotene." *Journal of the American Medical Association* 272:1455–56.

Hardy, S. C., and R. E. Kleinman. 1994 "Fat and cholesterol in the diet of infants and young children: implications for growth, development, and long-term health." *J Pediatr* 17:119–46.

Harman, D. 1994 "Aging: prospects for further increases in the functional life span." *Age* 17:119–46.

Hartman, I. S. 1995 "Alpha-linolenic acid: a preventive in secondary coronary events?" *Nutr Rev* 53:194–97.

Harvey, R. F., E. W. Pomare, K. W. Heaton. 1973 "Effects of increased dietary fibre on intestinal transit." *The Lancet* 1(815):1278–80.

Heaton, K. W., E. W. Pomare. 1974 "Effect of bran on blood lipids and calcium." *The Lancet* 1(846):49–50.

Henderson, B. E., R. K. Ross, et al. 1986 "Estrogen use and cardiovascular disease." *Am J Obstet Gynecol* 154:1181–86.

Hennekens, C. H., et al. 1989 "Final report on the aspirin component of the ongoing physicians' health study." *New England Journal of Medicine* 321:129–35.

Hennekens, C. H., and J. M. Gaziano. 1993 "Antioxidants and heart disease: epidemiology and clinical evidence." *Clin Card* 1(16): Apr; 16 (4 Suppl.) I10–3. discussion I13–5.

Herbert, J. 1995 "The age of dehydroepiandrosterone." *The Lancet* 345:1193–94.

Herbert, V. 1993 "Does mega-C do more good than harm, or more harm than good?" *Nutr Today* 28:28–32.

Herold, K. C., and B. C. Herold. 1983 Letter to the editor. *Journal of the American Medical Association* 249:21.

Hertog, M. G., et al. 1993 "Dietary antioxidant flavonoids and risk of coronary heart disease: the Zutphen Elderly Study." *The Lancet* 342(8878):1007–11.

Hodis, H. N., et al. 1995 "Serial coronary angiographic evidence that antioxidant vitamin intake reduces progression of coronary artery atherosclerosis." *Journal of the American Medical Association* 273:1849–54.

Horrobin, D. F. 1993 "The effects of gamma-linolenic acid on breast pain and diabetic neuropathy: possible non-eicosanoid mechanisms." *Prostaglandins Leukot Essent Fatty Acids* 48(1):101–4.

Huag, A. 1964 "*Composition and Properties of Alginates.*" Report no. 30. Trondheim: Norwegian Seaweed Research Institute.

Hunter, D. J., J. E. Manson, G. A. Colditz, et al. 1993 "A prospective study of the intake of vitamins C, E, A and the risk of breast cancer." *New England Journal of Medicine* 329:234–40.

Internal Medicine News. 1991 "Nutritional trends." *Internal Medicine News,* July 15–31: 30.

Jackson, R., R. Scragg, and R. Beaglehole. 1991 "Alcohol consumption and risk of coronary heart disease." *BMJ* July 27; 303(6796):211–6.

    1992 "Does recent alcohol consumption reduce the risk of acute myocardial infarction and coronary death in regular drinkers?" *Am J Epidemiol* 136(7):819–24.

Jacques, P. F., and L. T. Chylack Jr. 1991 "Epidemiological evidence of a role for the antioxidant vitamins and carotenoids in cataract prevention." *Am J Clin Nutr* 53:3525–55.

Jacques, P. F., L. T. Chylack Jr., R. B. McGandy Jr., et al. 1988 "Antioxidant status in persons with and without senile cataract." *Arch Ophth* 106:337–40.

Jain, R. C., et al. 1969 "Onion and blood fibrinolytic activity." *BMJ* 258:514.

Jain, R. C., C. R. Vyas, and O. P. Mahatma. 1973 "Letter. Hypoglycaemic action of onion and garlic." *The Lancet* 2(844):1491.

Jain, R. C. 1971 "Effect of onion on serum cholesterol, lipoproteins and fibrinolytic activity of blood in alimentary lipaemia."*J Assoc Physicians India* 19(4):305–10.

Jancin, B. 1994 "Exercise study may point to hormones as the breast cancer culprit." *Family Practice News,* November: 5.

Jialal, I. 1992 "Can vitamins slow the atherosclerotic process?" Paper presented at the American Heart Association, Science Writer's Forum, Texas, January. Apr; 16(4 Suppl) I6–9.

Jialal, I., and C. J. Fuller. 1993 "Oxidized LDL and antioxidants." *Clin Card* 1(16):9.

Jialal, I., C. Fuller, B. Huet, et al. 1995 "The effect of alpha-tocopherol supplementation on LDL oxidation: a dose response study." *Artérioscler Thromb Vasc Biol* 15:190–98.

Jialal, I., and S. M. Grundy. 1992 "Vitamin E inhibits LDL oxidation, may help prevent atherosclerosis." *J Lipid Res* 33:899–906.

Jialal, I., E. P. Norkus, L. Cristol, and S. M. Grundy. 1991 "Beta carotene inhibits the oxidative modification of low-density lipoprotein." *Biochem Biophys Acta* 1086:134–38.

Jialal, I., G. L. Vega, and S. M. Grundy. 1990 "Physiologic levels of ascorbate inhibit the oxidative modification of low-density lipoprotein." *Atherosclerosis* 82:185–91.

Johnson, C., C. Meyer, and J. Srilakshmi. 1993 "Vitamin C elevates red blood cell glutathione in healthy adults." *Am J Clin Nutr* 58:103–5.

1982 "Multiple risk factor intervention trial." *Journal of the American Medical Association* 248:1465–77.

Joosten, E. 1993 "Metabolic evidence that deficiencies of vitamin B-12 (cobalamin), folate and vitamin B-6 occur commonly in elderly people." *Amer J Clin Nutr* 58:468–76.

Kamikawa, T., A. Kobayashi, T. Yamashita, et al. 1985 "Effects of coenzyme Q_{10} on exercise tolerance in chronic stable angina pectoris." *Am J Card* 56(4):247–51.

Kannel, W. B., and P. Wilson. 1995 "Risk factors that attenuate the female coronary disease advantage." *Arch Intern Med* 155:57–61.

Kanter, M. M., L. A. Nolte, et al. 1993 "Effects of an antioxidant vitamin mixture on lipid peroxidation at rest and postexercise." *J Appl Physiol* 74(2):965–69.

Kaplan, J. R., S. B. Manuck, T. B. Clarkson, et al. 1982 "Social status, environment, and atherosclerosis in cynomolgus monkeys." *Arteriosclerosis* 2(5):359–68.

Kardinaal, A. F., F. J. Kok, et al. 1991 "Antioxidants in adipose tissue and risk of myocardial infarction." *The Lancet* 337:1–5.

Keen, H., J. Payan, J. Allawi, J. Walker, G. A. Jamal, A. I. Weir, L. M. Henderson, E. A. Bissessar, P. J. Watkins, M. Sampson, et al. 1993 "Treatment of diabetic neuropathy with gamma-linolenic acid: the gamma-linolenic acid multicenter trial group." *Diabetes Care* 16(1):8–15.

Keys, A., et al. 1986 "The diet and fifteen-year death rate in the seven countries study." *Am J Epid* 124(6):903–15.

Kirby, R. W., et al. 1981 "Oat bran intake selectivity lowers serum low-density lipoprotein cholesterol concentrations of hypercholesterolemic men." *Am J Clin Nutr* 34:824–29.

Koplan, J. P., K. E. Powell, R. K. Silkes, et al. 1982 "An epidemiological study of the benefits and risks of running." *Journal of the American Medical Association* 248:3118–21.

Korthuis, R. J., and D. N. Granger. 1993 "Reactive oxygen metabolites, neutrophils, and the pathogenesis of ischemic-tissue/reperfusion." *Clin Card* Apr; 16 (4 Supp. 1): I119–26.

Langsjoen, P. H., and K. Folkers. 1993 "Isolated diastolic dysfunction of the myocardium and its response to CoQ_{10} treatment." *Clin Invest* 71:S140–S144.

Lanza, E., Y. Jones, G. Block, and L. Kessler. 1987 "Dietary fiber intake in the US population." *Am J Clin Nutr* 46:790–97.

Lau, B.H.S., et al. 1983 "*Allium sativum* (garlic) and atherosclerosis: a review." *Nutr Res* 3:119–28.

Lauer, M. S., K. M. Anderson, W. B. Kannel, et al. 1991 "The impact of obesity on left ventricular mass and geometry: the Framingham heart study." *Journal of the American Medical Association* 266:231–36.

Leaf, A., and P. C. Weber. 1988 "Cardiovascular effects of n-3 fatty acids: an update." *New England Journal of Medicine* 318:549–57.

Leibovitz, B., M.-L. Hu, and A. L. Tappel. 1990 "Dietary supplements of vitamin E, beta-carotene, coenzyme Q_{10}, and selenium protect tissues against lipid peroxidation in rat tissue slices." *J Nutr* 120:97–104.

Levine, M., et al. 1996 "Vitamin C pharmacokinetics in healthy volunteers: evidence for a recommended daily allowance." *Proc Nat Acad Sci* 93(8):3704–9.

Lobstein, D. D., et al. 1983 "Depression as a powerful discriminator between physically active and sedentary middle-aged men." *J Psychosom Res* 217:69–76.

Lockwood, K., S. Moesgaard, et al. 1994 "Partial and complete regression of breast cancer in patients in relation to dosage of coenzyme Q_{10}." *Biochem and Biophys Res Comm* 199:1504–8.

Lowe, T. W. 1995 "Cardiovascular disease and pregnancy: maternal cardiac disease: the obstetrician's viewpoint." *CVR&R*, May: 40–45.

Lutter, L. D. 1982 "Running athlete in office practice." *Foot and Ankle* 3(1):53–59.

MacNeil-Lehrer Report. 1991 "Eat smart." September 16.

Manetta, A., and C. Fuchtner. 1992 "The role of B-carotene in cancer chemoprevention." *Drug Therapy,* July: 55–60.

Manson, J. E., J. E. Buring, S. Satterfield, and C. H. Hennekens. 1991 "Baseline characteristics of participants in the Physicians' Health Study: a randomized trial of aspirin and beta-carotene in U.S. physicians." *Am J Prev Med* 7(3):150–54.

Mantzioris, E., M. J. James, R. A. Gibson, and L. G. Cleland. 1994 "Dietary substitution with an alpha-linolenic acid-rich vegetable oil increases eicosapentaenoic acid concentrations in tissues." *Am J Clin Nutr* 59:1304–9.

1995 "Differences exist in the relationships between dietary linolenic and alpha-linolenic acids and their respective long-chain metabolites." *Am J Clin Nutr* 61:320–24.

Manzoli, U., E. Rossie, G. P. Littarry, et al. 1990 "Coenzyme Q_{10} in dilated cardiomyopathy." *Int J Tissue React* 12:173–78.

Maresh, C. M., B. G. Sheckley, G. J. Allen, D. N. Camaione, and S. T. Sinatra. "Middle-age male distance runners: physiological and psychological profiles." *J Sports Med Phys Fit* 31:461–69.

Marx, J. L. 1987 "Oxygen free radicals linked to many diseases." *Science* 235:529–31.

Matthew, K., et al. 1994 "Influence of the perimenopause on cardiovascular risk factors and symptoms of healthy middle-aged women." *Arch Intern Med* 154:2349–55.

Mauer, I., A. Bernhard, and S. Zierz. 1990 "Coenzyme Q_{10} and respiratory chain enzyme activities in hypertrophied human left ventricles with aortic valve stenosis." *Am J of Cardiology* 66:504–5.

Maxwell, S., A. Cruikshank, and D. Thorpe. 1994 "Red wine and antioxidant activity in serum." *The Lancet* 344:193–94.

Mayo Clinic Nutrition Letter. 1990 "Psyllium and rice bran: more obscure than oat bran—but they lower cholesterol, too." *Mayo Clinic Nutrition Letter* 3(7):1–2.

McBarron, J. 1991 "Bariatrics." *The Bariatrician: American Journal of Bariatric Medicine,* spring: 9–16.

McCord, J. M. 1985 "Oxygen-derived free radicals in postischemic tissue injury." *New England Journal of Medicine* 312:159–63.

McCully, K. S. 1969 "Vascular pathology of homocysteinemia: implications for the pathogenesis of arteriosclerosis." *Am J Pathol* 56:111–28.

McKeigue, P. 1995 "Trans-fatty acids and coronary heart disease: weighing the evidence against hardened fat." *The Lancet* 345:269–70.

The Medical Letter. 1991 "Fish oil." *The Medical Letter,* January 11: 4.

Mehta, J., B. Yang, and W. Nichols. 1993 "Free radicals, antioxidants, and coronary heart disease." *J Myocardial Ischemia* 5(8):31–41.

Metropolitan Life Insurance Company. 1939 "Girth and Death." New York: Metropolitan Life Insurance Company.

Metz, R. 1987 "Obesity: an eclectic review." *Hosp Pract* 22(2):152.

Millane, T. A., D. E. Ward, and A. J. Camm. 1992 "Is hypomagnesemia arrhythmogenic?" *Clinical Cardiology* 15:103–8.

Mittleman, M. A., M. Maclure, G. H. Tofler, et al. 1993 "Triggering of acute myocardial infarction by heavy physical exertion." *New England Journal of Medicine* 329:1677–83.

Montano, C. B. 1994 "Recognition and treatment of depression in a primary care setting." *J Clin Psych* 55:19–34.

Morisco, C., C. Timarco, and M. Condroelli. 1993 "Effect of coenzyme Q_{10} therapy in patients with congestive heart failure: a long-term multicenter randomized study." *Clin Invest* 71:S134–S136.

Morris, D. L., et al. 1994 "Serum carotenoids and coronary heart disease." *Journal of the American Medical Association* 272:1439–41.

Morris, J. N., J. A. Heady, P.A.B. Raffle, et al. 1953 "Coronary heart disease and physical activity of work." *The Lancet* 2:1053.

Morris, J. N., A. Kogan, D. C. Patterson, et al. 1966 "Incidence and prediction of ischemic heart disease in London busmen." *The Lancet* 463(2):553–59.

Myers, M. I., R. Bolli, R. Lekich, et al. 1985 "Enhancement of recovery of myocardial infarction by oxygen free radical scavengers after reversible regional ischemia." *Circulation* 72:915–21.

National Heart, Lung, and Blood Institute. 1991 "National cholesterol education program: report of the expert panel in population strategies for blood cholesterol reduction: executive summary." *Arch Int Med* 151:1071–84.

Nerem, R. M., M. J. Levesque, J. F. Cornhill, et al. 1980 "Social environment as a factor in diet-induced atherosclerosis." *Science* 208:1475.

New England Journal of Medicine. 1994 "The alpha-tocopherol, beta-carotene cancer prevention study group: the effect of vitamin E and beta-carotene on the incidence of lung cancer and other cancers in male smokers." *New England Journal of Medicine* 330:1029–35.

Ornish, D., et al. 1990 "Can lifestyle changes reverse coronary heart disease? The lifestyle heart trial." *The Lancet* 336:129–33.

Pomare, E. W., and K. W. Heaton. 1973 "Alteration of bile salt metabolism by dietary fiber (bran)." *BMJ* Nov 3; 4(887):262–64.

Prescott, L. 1991 "Symposium: magnesium in clinical medicine and therapeutic: wide range of diseases linked to low magnesium levels." *Internal Medicine World Report,* June 15–30: 7.

Proctor, P. H., and E. S. Reynolds. 1984 "Free radicals and disease in man." *Physiol Chem Phys* 16:175.

Quintanilha, A. T. 1984 "Effects of physical exercise and/or vitamin E on tissue oxidative metabolism." *Biochem Soc Trans* 12:403–4.

Ravussin, E., S. Lillioja, W. C. Knowler, et al. 1988 "Reduced rate of energy expenditure as a risk factor for body-weight gain." *New England Journal of Medicine* 318:467–72.

Rayssiguier, Y., E. Gueux, I. Bussiere, et al. 1993 "Dietary magnesium affects susceptibility of lipoproteins in tissues to peroxidation in rats." *J Am Col N* 12:133–37.

Renaud, S., and M. de Lorgeril. 1992 "Wine, alcohol, platelets, and the French paradox for coronary heart disease." *The Lancet* 339:1523–26.

Rimm, E. B., et al. 1993 "Vitamin E consumption and the risk of coronary disease in men." *New England Journal of Medicine* 328:1450–56.

1996 "Vegetable, fruit and cereal fiber intake and risk of coronary heart disease among men." *Journal of the American Medical Association* 275(6):447–51.

Risch, H., et al. 1994 "Dietary fat intake and risk of epithelian ovarian cancer." *J of the Natl Canc Inst* 86(18):1409–15.

Roberts, S. B., J. Savage, W. A. Coward, et al. 1988 "Energy expenditure and intake in infants born to lean and overweight mothers." *New England Journal of Medicine* 318:461–66.

Roberts, T. L., et al. 1995 "Trans isomers of oleic and linoleic acids in adipose tissue and sudden death." *The Lancet* 345:278–82.

Salonen, J. T., K. Nyyssonen, and R. Salonen. 1995 Letter. "Fish intake and the risk of coronary disease." *New England Journal of Medicine* 333(14):937; discussion 938.

Salonen, J. T., K. Nyyssonen, T. P. Tuomainen, et al. 1992 "High stored iron levels are associated with excess risk of myocardial infarction in Eastern Finnish men." *Circulation* 86(3):803–11.

1995 "Increased risk of non-insulin dependent diabetes mellitus at low plasma vitamin E concentrations: a four-year follow-up study in men." *BMJ* Oct 28; 311(7013):1124–27.

Sastre, J., et al. 1992 "Exhaustive physical exercise causes oxidation of gluta-thione status in blood: prevention by antioxidant administration." *Am J Physiol* R992–R995.

Scragg, R., I. Holdaway, R. Jackson, and T. Lim. 1992 "Plasma 25-hydroxy-vitamin D3 and its relation to physical activity and other heart disease risk factors in the general population." *Ann Epidemiol* 2(5):697–703.

Seddon, J. M., et al. 1994 "Dietary carotenoids, vitamins A, C, and E, and advanced age-related macular degeneration." *Journal of the American Medical Association* 272:1413–20.

Shapiro, B. 1992 "Personal observations." Paper presented at the International Bioenergetic Conference, Miami.

Sheffy, B. E., and R. D. Schultz. 1979 "Influence of vitamin E and selenium on immune response mechanisms." *Fed Proc* 38:2139–43.

Shimomura, Y., et al. 1991 "Protective effect of coenzyme Q_{10} on exercise-induced muscular injury." *Biochem Biophys Res Comm* 176:349–55.

Shirlow, M. J., et al. 1985 "A study of caffeine consumption and symptoms: indigestion, palpitations, tremor, headache, and insomnia." *Int J Epid* 14(2):239–48.

Siegel, A. J. 1988 "New insights about obesity and exercise." *Your Patient and Fitness* 2(6):6–13.

Simon, J. A., J. Fong, J. T. Bernert Jr., et al. 1995 "Dietary alpha-linolenic acid lowers the risk of stroke." *Modern Medicine* 63:45.

Simon-Schnass, I., and H. Pabst. 1988 "Influence of vitamin E on physical performance." *Int J Vitam Nutr Res* 58:49–54.

Sinatra, S. T. 1984 "Stress and the heart: a cardiologist's point of view." *Postgraduate Medicine* 76:231–34.

1984 "Stress and the heart: behavioral interaction and plan for strategy." *CT Med* 48:81–86.

Sinatra, S. T., et al. 1990 "Effects of continuous passive motion, walking, and a placebo intervention on physical and psychological well-being." *J Cardiopul Rehab* 10(8):279–86.

Sinatra, S. T., and S. Chawla. 1986 "Aortic dissection associated with anger, suppressed rage, and acute emotional stress." *J Cardiopul Rehab* 6(5): 197–99.

Sinatra, S. T., and J. DeMarco. 1995 "Free radicals, oxidative stress, oxidized low-density lipoprotein (LDL), and the heart: antioxidants and other strategies to limit cardiovascular damage." *Connecticut Medicine* 59:579–88.

Sinatra, S. T., and L. A. Feitell. 1985 "The heart and mental stress, real and imagined." *The Lancet* 222–223.

Sinatra, S. T., and H. Hatch. 1987 "Physiological and psychological profiles of participants in a six-day Healing the Heart seminar." Unpublished.

Sinatra, S. T., and A. Lowen. 1987 "Heartbreak and heart disease: the origin and essence of coronary-prone behavior." *British Hol Med* 2:169–71.

Sirtori, C. R., et al. 1986 "Controlled evaluation of fat intake in the Mediterranean diet: comparative activities of olive oil and corn oil on plasma lipids and platelets in high-risk patients." *Am J Clin Nutr* 44:635–42.

Siscovick, D. S., T. E. Raghunathan, et al. 1995 "Dietary intake and cell membrane levels of long-chain n-3 polyunsaturated fatty acids and the risk of primary cardiac arrest." *Journal of the American Medical Association* 274:1363–67.

Sismann, G., et al. 1988 "Focus on diet and exercise." *Lipid Digest* 1(2):1–6.

Smith, J. B., C. M. Ingerman, and M. J. Silver. 1976 "Malondialdehyde formation as an indicator of prostaglandin production by human platelets." *J Lab Clin Med* 88(1)167–72.

Soma, M. R., and R. Peoletti. 1995 "Lipids and menopause." *CVR&R,* May: 10–11.

Southorn, P. A. 1988 "Free radicals in medicine. 1. Chemical nature and biologic reactions." *Mayo Clin Proc* 63:381–89.

Sperduto, R. 1993 "Macular degeneration." *Arch Ophth* 111:104–9.

Spiller, G. A., and J. E. Gates. 1989 "Effect of diets high in monounsaturated fats, plant proteins, and complex carbohydrates on serum lipoproteins in hypercholesterolemic humans." Paper presented at the International Symposium on Drugs Affecting Lipid Metabolism, November 8–11.

Stampfer, M. J., et al. 1993 "Vitamin E consumption and the risk of coronary disease in women." *New England Journal of Medicine* 328:1444–49.

Stampfer, M. J., M. R. Malinow, W. C. Willett, et al. 1992 "A prospective study of plasma homocysteine and risk of myocardial infarction in U.S. physicians." *Journal of the American Medical Association* 268:87–91.

Stanford, J. L., et al. 1995 "Combined estrogen and progestin hormone replacement therapy in relation to risk of breast cancer in middle-aged women." *Journal of the American Medical Association* 274:137–42.

Starkebaum, G., and J. M. Harlan. 1986 "Endothelial cell injury due to copper-catalyzed hydrogen peroxide generation from homocysteine." *J Clin Invest* 77:1370–76.

Steen, S. N., R. A. Oppliger, and K. D. Brownell. 1988 "Metabolic effects of repeated weight loss and regain in adolescent wrestlers." *Journal of the American Medical Association* 260:47–50.

Steinberg, D., et al. 1989 "Mechanisms of disease beyond cholesterol modifications of low-density lipoprotein that increases its atherogenicity." *New England Journal of Medicine* 320:915–24.

Stephens, N. G., et al. 1996 "Randomized controlled trial of vitamin E in patients with coronary artery disease: Cambridge Heart Study." *The Lancet* 347(9004):781–86.

Swain, J. F., I. L. Rouse, C. B. Curley, and F. M. Sacks. 1990 "Comparison of the effects of oat bran and low-fiber wheat on serum lipoprotein levels and blood pressure." *New England Journal of Medicine* 322:147–52.

Tanaka, J., R. Tominaga, M. Yoshitoshi, et al. 1982 "Coenzyme Q_{10}: the prophylactic effect on low cardiac output following cardiac valve replacement." *Annals of Thoracic Surgery* 33:145–51.

Teas, J. 1981 "The consumption of seaweed as a protective factor in the etiology of breast cancer." *Med Hypotheses* 7(5):601–13.

Thompson, P. D., E. J. Funk, R. A. Carleton, et al. 1982 "Incidence of death during jogging in Rhode Island from 1975–1980." *Journal of the American Medical Association* 247:2535–38.

Ubbink, J. B., W. J. H. Vermaak, A. van der Merwe, P. J. Becker. 1993 "Vitamin B-12, vitamin B-6, and folate nutritional status in men with hyperhomocysteinemia." *Amer J Clin Nutr* 57:47–53.

Ulbricht, T. L. 1991 "Coronary heart disease: seven dietary factors." *The Lancet* 338:985–92.

Vallance, S. 1977 "Relationship between ascorbic acid and serum proteins of the immune system." *BMJ* 2:437–38.

Van Camp, S. 1987 "The hazards of exercise." *Your Patient and Fitness* 1(4):18–21.

Verlangieri, A. J., and M. J. Bush. 1992 "Effects of d-a-tocopherol supplementation on experimentally induced primate atherosclerosis." *J Am Coll Nutr* 11:131–38.

Verschuren, W.M.M., D. R. Jacobs, B.P.M. Bloemberg, et al. 1995 "Serum cholesterol and long-term coronary heart disease mortality in different cultures." *Journal of the American Medical Association* 274:131–36.

Virtmo, J., E. Valkesia, G. Alfthan, et al. 1985 "Serum selenium and the risk of coronary disease and stroke." *Am J Epidemiol* 122:276–82.

Wald, N. J., S. G. Thompson, J. W. Densen, et al. 1985 "Corpus and cervical cancer: a nutritional comparison." *Am J Obstet & Gyn* 153:775–79.

Walker, A.R.P., and D. P. Burkitt. 1976 "Colonic cancer: hypotheses of causation, dietary prophylaxis, and future research." *Am J Dig Dis* 21(10):910–17.

Warshafsky, S., et al. 1993 "Effects of garlic on total serum cholesterol: a metanalysis." *Annals of Internal Medicine* 119(7), part I: 599–605.

Weiner, M. A. 1986 "Cholesterol in foods rich in omega-3 fatty acids." *New England Journal of Medicine* 315(13):833.

Weisburger, J. H. 1991 "Nutritional approach to cancer prevention with emphasis on vitamins, antioxidants, and carotenoids." *Am J Clin Nutr* 53:226S–237S.

Weiss, S. J., and A. F. LoBuglio. 1982 "Phagocyte generated oxygen metabolite and cellular injury." *Lab Invest* 47:5–18.

Whang, R. 1987 "Magnesium deficiency: pathogenesis, relevance, and clinical implications." *Am J of Med* 82:24–29.

Wilber, J. F. 1991 "Neuropeptides, appetite regulation, and human obesity." *Journal of the American Medical Association* 266:257–58.

Willett, W. C., J. E. Manson, M. J. Stampfer, et al. 1995 "Weight, weight change, and coronary heart disease in women: risk within the 'normal' weight range." *Journal of the American Medical Association* 273(6):461–65.

Witztum, J. L., and D. Steinberg. 1991 "Role of oxidized low-density lipoprotein in atherogenesis." *J Clin Invest* 88:1785–92.

Wynder, E. L., and T. Shigematsu. 1967 "Environmental factors of cancer of the colon and rectum." *Cancer* 20:1520.

Wyshak, G., and R. E. Frisch. 1994 "Carbonated beverage, dietary calcium, the dietary calcium/phosphorus ratio, and bone fractures in girls and boys." *Journal of Adolescent Health* 15:210–15.

INDEX

Achterberg, Jeanne, xxv
acidophilus, 135, 288–89
aerobic exercise, 173–74, 176–77
aging, xxix, 60, 82, 247–61
    albumin levels and, 249, 251–52
    DHEA and, 249–50
    DMAE and, 255–56
    free radicals and, 85, 252–54
    L-arginine and, 254
    L-deprenyl and, 256
    longevity and, 216, 248
    melatonin and, 216, 255, 257, 259
    prevention of, 258–59
    proanthocyanidins and, 256–57
    process of, 252–54
    recommendations for health, healing,
        and longevity, 259–61
    running and, 170
    stress and, 250–51
    symptoms of, 248–49
airplanes, 85
albumin, 249, 251–52
alcohol, 73–74
    calories in, 25–26
    wine, 74–75
allergies, 251
allopathic medical model, xx–xxii, 264
almonds, 187, 194
aloe vera, 288

aluminum, 121
Alzheimer's disease, 251, 256
amino acids, 30, 31–32
anchovies, xxviii, 186
anger, 166, 179, 239, 242
antibodies, 251
antioxidants, 65, 67, 75, 81, 84, 86–87,
    253
    exercise and, 171, 172
    proanthocyanidins, 256–57
    selenium as, 123–24
    vitamin A as, 94
    vitamin C as, 99
    vitamin E as, 101
apple-cinnamon bran muffins, 228
apples, 37
arachidonic acid, 23, 59, 60, 61, 67
arteries:
    hardening of (atherosclerosis), 43–44, 59,
        254
    See also heart disease
arthritis, 211–13
artichokes, chicken with, 229
asparagus, xxviii, 67, 84, 186
    recipe for, 237
asthma, xxi–xxii, xxvii
astragalus, 133
atherosclerosis (hardening of the arteries),
    43–44, 59, 254

Atkins, Robert, 20–21, 22–23, 24

bacteria, friendly, 135, 288–89
balsamic-olive oil dressing, 236
barley, 188
bean(s), 189
    nutritional data on, 271
    soup, Antiguan black, 219
beef:
    low-fat exceptional hamburgers, 235
    nutritional data on, 281
    roast eye of round with rosemary and
        potatoes, 234
bee pollen, 195–96
beet salad with lemon and honey, 220
beta carotene, 89, 91–92, 94–95, 260, 285
    exercise and, 171, 172
betaine HCL, 288
beverages, calories and sodium in, 270
BHA and BHT, 9
bicycling, 171, 174, 181
bioenergetics, xviii, xix, xx
bioflavonoids, xxviii, 74, 75, 147
biotin, 99, 286
blood pressure:
    lowering of, 210–11
    salt and, 72, 73
blueberries, pancakes with, 227
blueberry-cinnamon bran muffins, 228
bluefish, marinated, 233–34
boron, 287
botanicals, 127–34
    astragalus, 133
    cayenne, 128, 148, 261
    chamomile, 133–34, 148
    echinacea, 132–33, 261
    fenugreek, 133, 134
    ginger, 127–28, 148, 260
    ginkgo, 132, 261
    ginseng, 129–30, 148, 260
    gotu kola, 128–29, 260
    hawthorn berry, 130–32, 261
    for menopause symptoms, 148–49
    myrrh gum, 133, 134
    wild yam extract, 130, 148, 250
bran, 39, 40
    muffins, blueberry or apple-cinnamon,
        228
breads, 187, 278–79
breakfast, 6–7, 27, 267
breast cancer, 23, 140, 143, 144, 145, 146,
    150
    toxins and, 10
breathing, xix–xx, 164
broccoli, xxviii, 186
bromelain, 260, 288

buckwheat, 188
    pancakes with blueberries, 7, 227
BUN (blood urea nitrogen), 30
butter, 48

cabbage, xxviii, 186, 191
caffeine, 5, 6, 33, 76–78
    content in selected items, 76–77
cakes, 275–76
calcium, 41, 78, 88, 89, 114–16, 144, 286–
    87
    foods high in, 117
    recommended daily dietary allowances
        for, 115
calories, 11, 20, 25–26, 33, 63
    in alcohol, 25–26
    in beverages, 270
    in carbohydrates, 25, 27, 29, 36
    daily needs for, 54–55
    in fats, 25, 27, 29, 36, 55, 271–84
    nutritional data tables, 271–84
    in protein, 25, 27, 29, 30
    reducing intake of, 48
    weight loss and, 20
cancer, xix, xxviii, 23, 75, 85, 90, 91, 150,
    254
    breast, 10, 23, 140, 143, 144, 145, 146,
        150
    chemotherapy for, xxiv, 213
    colon, 37–38, 40
    emotions and, xix, xxv
    fats and, 56
    lung, 85, 92–93
    nutritional treatment of, xxv–xxvi, 204–
        6
    ovarian, 150
    personality and, xix
    prostate, 23, 202
    radiation therapy for, xxiv, 213
    radon and, 85
    toxins and, 10
    uterine, 143, 144, 145, 146
cantaloupe, 186
capsicum (cayenne), 128, 148, 261
carbohydrates, 26, 32, 63
    balancing fats and proteins with, 27–28,
        61, 66, 67
    calories from, 25, 27, 29, 36
    complex, 32, 33–34, 35, 37, 38, 66
    glycemic index and, 27–28, 33, 66, 67
    insulin and, 5, 21, 22–24, 27–28, 33, 66,
        67
    simple, 32–33, 35
cardiovascular disease:
    stroke, 43, 65
    See also heart disease

carotenoids, xxviii, 87
carrots, 191
cataracts, 87, 91, 254
cauliflower, 186
cayenne (capsicum), 128, 148, 260
cereals, nutritional data on, 272
chamomile, 133–34, 148
cheeses, 115, 273
chemotherapy, xxiv, 213
cherries, 186
chicken, 50–51, 280, 281
    with artichokes, 229
    grilled, spinach salad with mango,
        raspberries and, 230–31
    with pea pods and zucchini, 228–29
    Santiago's, 230
children, 137–40, 151
chive and sour cream dressing, 236
chlorophyll, 191–92, 197–98, 261
cholesterol, 21, 43–52, 59, 67, 150
    Atkins diet and, 23
    dairy products and, 49
    defined, 43
    in eggs, 50, 67
    emotions and, 45–47
    fiber and, 37, 39, 40
    food labels and, 8
    in foods (tables), 271–84
    French Paradox and, 74–75
    guidelines for blood levels of, 47
    heart disease and, 43–44
    lowering of, 48–52, 55, 208–10
    in meats, 50–51
    saturated fats and, 57, 62
    in shellfish, 51–52
    women's levels of, 142–43, 145
    See also HDL; LDL
choline, 99, 288
chromium picolinate, 260, 287
chronic fatigue syndrome, 119
cigarette smoking, 45, 149
coenzyme Q₁₀, xxviii, 82, 89–90, 103–11,
        199, 260, 289
    doses of, 109
    exercise and, 171, 172
    function of, 107
    purchasing of, 110
    selenium and, 123–24
    sources of, 109
    weight loss and, 108
    women and, 150
coenzymes, 93, 119
coffee, 6, 76–78
collard greens, 186
colon cancer, 37–38, 40
constipation, 38, 72, 206–7

cookies, 275
copper, 88, 89, 114, 126
corn, 188–89
coronary artery disease. See heart disease
cortisol, 250–51
crisis, as opportunity, 13–15
crying, 166
cyanocobalamin (vitamin B-12), 88, 97–98,
        259, 286
cycling, 171, 174, 181

dairy products, 23, 55, 61
    cholesterol and, 49
    milk, 26, 49, 68, 70, 273–74
    nutritional data on, 273–74
dancing, 171, 173–74, 179
DDT, 10
denial of pleasure, 1–2, 26
depression, xxv, 200–201
desserts, nutritional data on, 275–76
DHEA, 130, 249–50, 251, 252
diabetes, 38, 103, 141–42, 149
diet, 26
    American, 44
    Mediterranean. See Mediterranean diet
    suggestions for, 267–68
diets, weight-loss, 17–18, 20–21
    emotional healing and, 153
    protein restriction in, 31
    self-denial in, 2, 26
    self-forgiveness and, 3
diet sodas, 7–8
dinners, suggestions for, 268
disease and illness, 82, 248
    aging as, 252
    albumin levels and, 249, 251–52
    crisis in, as opportunity, 13–15
    emotions and. See emotions
    fiber and, 35, 36
    free radicals and, 84–86
    holistic approach to, xxvi
    prevention of, 258–59
DMAE, xxviii, 255–56
dopamine, 256

echinacea, 132–33, 260
eggs, 50, 67, 187, 274–75
eicosanoids, 59, 60–61
electromagnetic contamination, 85, 87
emotional healing, 153–67
    breathing in, 164
    exercises in, 166–67, 179
    meditation in, 164–66, 251
    patience in, 157–58
    positive goals in, 158–59
    reframing in, 154, 157, 165

sexuality in, 160–63
emotional support, 3–4, 46, 239–40, 248
emotions, xvii, xviii, 248
  alcohol and, 74
  anger, 166, 179, 239, 242
  asthma and, xxi
  cancer and, xix, xxv
  cholesterol and, 45–47
  exercise and, 173
  food and, 154–55, 239
  immune system and, xxv
  love, 46, 155, 160, 245, 246
  overweight and, xxvii
  release of, 166–67, 179
  repressed, 155–56, 157, 163, 166–67, 239
  weight loss and, 239–46
  See also stress
energy, xxiii, 2
  caffeine and, 6
  metabolic rate and, 18–19
  sugar and, 6
environmental toxins. See toxins and pollutants
enzymes, 134–35, 259–60, 288–89
essential fatty acids (EFAs), 21, 59–61, 65, 148
  linoleic acid, 59, 60, 148
  linolenic acid, 59, 60–61, 65, 67, 148
  omega–3, 4–5, 23, 48, 51, 52, 59–60, 61, 65, 66
estrogen, 144, 145, 146
estrogen replacement therapy, 143–44, 145–47, 149
exercise, 11–12, 68, 144–45, 169–84, 248
  aerobic, 173–74, 176–77
  amount needed, 173
  benefits of, 173–74
  cardiovascular health and, 173–74
  cooldown in, 178
  cycling, 171, 174, 181
  dancing, 171, 173–74, 179
  duration of, 176–77
  emotional release and, 179
  enjoyment of, 174–75, 183–84
  frequency of, 177
  heart attack and, 170–71, 173
  intensity of, 177
  isometric, 174
  jogging, 169, 171
  leisure, 174
  nutrition and, 171–72
  progression in, 177
  pulse rate in, 183
  push-ups, 182–83

recommendations for quantity and quality of, 176–77
  rope jumping, 177, 183
  rowing, 181
  running, 169, 170
  sit-ups, 182
  skiing, 173, 174, 180–81
  support groups for, 181–82
  swimming, 174, 181
  treadmill, 181
  walking, 11–12, 171, 173–74, 177, 180
  warm-ups in, 175–76, 178
  weight lifting, 174, 182–83
  weight loss and, 19
  for women, 150
  workout phase in, 178
eyes, 86–87, 254, 259
  cataracts in, 87, 91, 254
  macular degeneration in, xxviii, 87

fast, 24-hour juice and veggie, 216
fat, body, 53–55, 63, 173
  brown, 20
  See also overweight and obesity
fatigue, 119, 200–201
fats, 26, 36, 53–63, 85
  animal, toxins in, 55–56
  in Atkins diet, 23
  balancing protein and carbohydrates with, 27–28, 61, 66, 67
  calories from, 25, 27, 29, 36, 55, 271–84
  cancer and, 56
  colon cancer and, 38
  commonly used, fat content of, 62–63
  daily intake allowed, 54–55
  essential fatty acids. See essential fatty acids
  in foods (tables), 271–84
  heart disease and, 23, 55, 57, 59
  in high-fiber healthy-fat foods, 64
  hydrogenated, 57, 60, 62
  monounsaturated, 48, 49, 57, 58, 62–63, 66, 254
  nutritional data on (table), 276
  oils. See oils
  omega–3, 4–5, 23, 48, 51, 52, 59–60, 61, 65, 66
  polyunsaturated, 48–49, 57, 58, 62–63, 254
  rancid, 85
  reducing intake of, 21, 28–30, 48, 63
  saturated, 4, 23, 47–48, 49, 56–57, 62–63
  types of, 56–57
  unsaturated, 4–5
  See also cholesterol

fennel, pasta with tuna and, 225
fenugreek, 133, 134
fiber, 4–5, 23, 33, 34, 35–42, 63, 66, 248
  cholesterol and, 37, 39, 40
  colon cancer and, 37–38, 40
  food labels and, 8
  in foods (tables), 271–84
  heart disease and, 39–40, 41
  in high-fiber healthy-fat foods, 64
  insoluble, 36–38, 40
  minerals and, 41, 114
  in quick and easy food combinations, 42
  recommended daily intake of, 38, 39
  soluble, 37, 38, 39
  sources of, 37
fish, xxviii, 51, 61, 65, 186
  breaded sole, flounder, or fluke, 232
  contamination of, 52, 124
  grilled halibut Mediterranean style with
    lemon-basil vinaigrette, 231–32
  grilled tuna or swordfish with spinach,
    233
  marinated bluefish, 233–34
  Mediterranean seafood sauce with
    Jerusalem artichoke pasta, 222
  nutritional data on, 276–77
  pasta with fennel and tuna, 225
  See also seafood
flaxseed oil, 61–62, 65, 68
flounder, breaded, 232
flour, white, 67, 187
fluke, breaded, 232
folic acid, xxviii, 67, 88, 98–99, 138, 150,
  260, 286
Folk Medicine (Jarvis), 195
Food and Drug Administration (FDA), 8
foods:
  additives in, 8–11
  to avoid, 237–38
  emotions and, 154–55, 239
  labels on, 8–10, 62, 72–73
  microwaving of, 83–84, 85
  nutritional values in. See nutritional
    values in foods
  organic, 11
  processed, 13, 33, 35, 57, 60, 72–73
  seeds, 187, 193–94
  substitution of, 238
foods, healing, 185–98, 259–60
  beans, 189
  fruits, xxviii, 67, 192–93
  garlic, 186, 196–97, 260
  natural sweeteners, 195–96
  nuts, 187, 193–94
  onions, xxvii, 29, 186, 196–97
  parsley, 197–98

sea vegetables, 185, 186, 189, 190
shiitake mushrooms, 194
soups, 194
vegetables, xxviii, 67, 191–92
whole grains, 67, 187–89
free radicals, 13, 60, 81, 84–86, 216, 252–
  53
  aging and, 85, 252–54
  antioxidants and. See antioxidants
  exercise and, 171, 172
French Paradox, 74–75
fruits, xxviii, 67, 192–93
  nutritional data on, 277–78
fungi, 67

garlic, 186, 196–97, 260
  pasta with mushrooms, parsley and, 223–
    24
ginger, 127–28, 148, 260
ginkgo, 132, 260
ginseng, 129–30, 148, 260
glossary, 285–89
glutathione, 171, 172
glycemic index, 27–28, 33, 66, 67
goldenseal, 260
gotu kola, 128–29, 260
grain products, nutritional data on, 278–79
grains, whole, 67, 187–89
grapefruit, 186

halibut, grilled, Mediterranean style with
  lemon-basil vinaigrette, 231–32
hamburgers, low-fat exceptional, 235
hawthorn berry, 130–32, 261
HDL (high-density lipoproteins), 28, 45,
  47, 48, 51, 55, 57, 58, 66, 173
  classification of levels of, 48
  women's levels of, 142–43, 145, 149
healing, xiv, xvi
  empowerment and, xxii–xxiii
  holistic, xxvi
  importance of multiple techniques of,
    xxiii–xxvii
  nutritional. See nutritional healing
  patient's responsibility for, xx–xxii, xxiii
  physician/patient collaboration in, xxii–
    xxiii
  recommendations for, 259–61
Healing the Heart workshops, 46, 166
health:
  optimum, 263–66
  recommendations for, 259–61
health care, xiii–xiv, 264
  allopathic model of, xx–xxii, 264
heart attack, xvi–xvii, 14, 15, 64, 91

exercise and, 170–71, 173
heart disease, xvi–xvii, xxviii, 23, 61, 85, 90, 91
  alcohol and, 73–74
  allopathic treatment for, xx
  breathing and, xix
  cholesterol and, 43–44
  coenzyme Q₁₀ and, 104–6, 107, 108, 109, 110
  exercise and, 173–74
  fats and, 23, 55, 57, 59
  fiber and, 39–40, 41
  French Paradox and, 74–75
  heart attack. *See* heart attack
  hormone replacement therapy and, 145
  insulin and, 28
  magnesium and, 118
  Mediterranean diet and, 64–65
  overweight and, xxvii, 17, 141, 142, 149
  patient's participation in healing of, xxii
  personality and, xvii, xviii
  protein restriction and, 31
  sodium and, 72, 73
  stress and, xviii
  vitamin C and, 100
  in women, 140–43, 145, 149, 150
Heartsense, xxix
herbs. *See* botanicals
high blood pressure, 72
  program for lowering, 210–11
Hirschmann, Jane R., 154
honey, 195
  -lemon dressing, 236
hormone replacement therapy (HRT), 143–44, 145–47, 149
  alternatives to, 147
human growth hormone, 257–58
hygiene, 251–52

illness. *See* disease and illness
immune system, xxv, 67, 81, 150, 248, 250
  albumin levels and, 251–52
  alcohol and, 73
  emotions and, xxv, 248
  free radicals and, 84
  vitamin E and, 103
impotence, 203
inositol, 99, 288
insulin, 5, 21, 22–24, 27–28, 33, 61, 66, 67, 68, 145
iodine, 88, 126, 287
iron, 41, 88, 89, 124–25, 126
  children and, 138–39
  foods high in, 125
isometric exercise, 174

Jarvis, D. C., 195
jogging, 169, 171
juice and veggie fast, 24-hour, 216

kale, 186
ketones, 21
kidney function, 30, 71, 72
kiwi, 186

L-arginine, 150–51, 254
L-carnitine, 288
L-deprenyl, 256
LDL (low-density lipoproteins), xxvii, 4, 37, 39, 45, 47, 51, 57, 58, 85–86
  classification of levels of, 48
  exercise and, 171
  lowering levels of, 47–48, 55, 62, 66
  saturated fats and, 47–48
  women's levels of, 142, 145
legumes, 66, 186
lemon-honey dressing, 236
lentils, 67, 186
lettuce, Boston, and watercress salad, 220–21
L-glutathione, 289
lighting, 258–59
linoleic acid, 59, 60, 148
linolenic acid, 59, 60–61, 65, 67, 148
lipotropic factors, 288
liver function, 71
longevity, 216, 248
  recommendations for, 259–61
  See also aging
love, 46, 155, 160, 246
  self-, 245, 246
Love, Medicine, and Miracles (Siegel), xix
Lowen, Alexander, xix, xx
LP(a), 57, 61
lunches, suggestions for, 267–68

macadamia nuts, 187
mackerel, xxviii, 186
magnesium, 78, 88, 114, 117–21, 260, 287
  cardiovascular consequences of deficiency in, 118
  causes of deficiency in, 120
  exercise and, 171, 172
  foods high in, 120
manganese, 114, 287
mango, spinach salad with grilled chicken, raspberries and, 230–31
MAO (monoamine oxidase), 256
maple syrup, 7
margarine, 62, 254
meats, 23, 31, 35–36, 51, 61
  cholesterol in, 50–51

low-fat exceptional hamburgers, 235
  nutritional data on, 273, 281
  roast eye of round with rosemary and
    potatoes, 234
meditation, 164–66, 251
Mediterranean diet, 58, 60, 64–65
  list of benefits of, 68
  modified, 24, 63, 64–70
  modified, guidelines for, 69–70
melatonin, 216, 255, 257, 259
memory, xxviii, 201–2, 251
menopause, 147, 148–49
  hormone replacement therapy and, 143–
    44, 145–47, 149
metabolism, 18–19, 55, 84
  free radicals and, 253–54
methionine, 288
microwaving, 83–84, 85
milk, 26, 49, 68, 70, 273–74
Miller, Alice, 155–56, 161
millet, 188
minerals, 12–13, 81, 82, 84, 113–26, 286–
    87
  antioxidant. See antioxidants
  balance of, 88
  boron, 287
  calcium. See calcium
  children and, 138–39
  chromium picolinate, 260, 287
  competition between, 114
  copper, 88, 89, 114, 126
  fiber and, 41, 114
  iodine, 88, 126, 287
  iron. See iron
  magnesium. See magnesium
  manganese, 114, 287
  phosphorus, 88, 286–87
  potassium, 78, 121–23, 287
  RDAs for, 87–88
  selenium, 89, 91, 123–24, 260, 287
  vanadium, 160, 287
  zinc, 41, 87, 88, 89, 114, 116, 138, 287
mineral supplements, xxviii, 12–13, 41,
    81–84, 87–93, 114, 126, 260
  advantages of, 90–91
  for children, 139, 140
  megadose hazards of, 88, 89
miso, 186, 189
  broth, 217
  -vegetable soup, 217–18
movement, 11–12, 19
  See also exercise
MSG (monosodium glutamate), 9
muffins, blueberry or apple-cinnamon, 228
Munter, Carol H., 154
mushrooms, 29

pasta with garlic, parsley and, 223–24
  shiitake, 194
myrrh gum, 133, 134

N-acetyl cysteine, 260
niacin (vitamin B–3), 88, 96, 286
Novil, Steven H., 67
nutrition, xxvii–xxviii, 25–34, 83–84
  exercise and, 171–72
  See also specific nutrients
nutritional healing, 199–213, 259–60
  for arthritis, 211–13
  for cancer, xxv–xxvi, 204–6
  for chemotherapy or radiation therapy
    patients, 213
  for cholesterol lowering, 208–10
  for constipation, 38, 72, 206–7
  for depression and fatigue, 200–201
  for high blood pressure, 210–11
  for impotence, 203–4
  for memory loss, 201–2
  for prostate health, 202–3
  for psoriasis, 83, 207–8
  See also foods, healing
nutritional supplements, 260
  chlorophyll, 191–92, 197–98, 261
  coenzyme Q$_{10}$. See coenzyme Q$_{10}$
  enzymes, 134–35, 260, 288–89
  L-glutathione, 289
  quercetin, xxvii, 74, 75, 260, 289
  See also botanicals; mineral supplements;
    vitamin supplements
nutritional values in foods (tables), 270–84
  beans/nuts/seeds, 271
  beverages, 270
  cereals, 272
  dairy products, 273–74
  desserts, 275–76
  eggs, 274–75
  fats/vegetable oils, 276
  fish/shellfish, 276–77
  fruits, 277–78
  grain products: breads/pasta/rice, 278–79
  meats, 273, 281
  miscellaneous, 279
  poultry, 280–81
  soups, 282
  vegetables, 283–84
nuts, 187, 193–94
  nutritional data on, 271

oils, 48, 49, 56, 57, 58, 60
  canola, 58
  commonly used, fat content of, 62–63
  nutritional data on (table), 276
  olive. See olive oil

See also fats
olive oil, 57, 58, 60, 61, 66, 215–16, 254
  –balsamic dressing, 236
omega oils, 60–61
  omega-3, 4–5, 23, 48, 51, 52, 59–60,
    61, 65, 66
onions, xxvii, 29, 186, 196–97
OPC (oligomeric proanthocyanidin), 256
organic foods, 11
osteoporosis, 101, 114, 143, 144, 149
Overcoming Overeating (Hirschmann and
  Munter), 154–55
overweight and obesity, 17–24, 48
  diets and, 2, 3, 17–18, 20–21
  emotions and, xxvii
  exercise and, 19
  genes and, 24
  heart disease and, xxvii, 17, 141, 142,
    149
  insulin and, 5, 21, 22–24, 27–28
  parents and, 3, 155–57, 161–62
  sexuality and, 160–63, 241–42
  See also weight loss
oxidation, 84, 85–86, 252
  See also free radicals; antioxidants

PABA, 99
pancakes, buckwheat, with blueberries, 7,
  227
pantothenic acid (vitamin B–5), 88, 96–97,
  260, 286
papain, 288
parents, 3, 155–57
  sexual boundaries and, 161–62
parsley, 197–98
  pasta with garlic, mushrooms and, 223–
    24
pasta, 66–67, 279
  à la Sinatra, 223
  easy Italian-style tomato sauce for, 221–
    22
  with fennel and tuna, 225
  with garlic, mushrooms, and parsley,
    223–24
  insulin resistance and, 66
  Jerusalem artichoke, Mediterranean
    seafood sauce with, 222
  Jerusalem artichoke, with fresh tomato
    sauce, 224
  low-glycemic, 67
  rye, with spinach, 224–25
PCBs, 10, 52
peaches, 186
peanuts and peanut butter, 193–94
pea pods, chicken with zucchini and, 228–
  29

pesticides, 10, 23, 52, 55–56, 82
phosphorus, 88, 286–87
phytoestrogens, 147
phytonutrients, 40, 66
pies, 275
plants. *See* botanicals
pollutants. *See* toxins and pollutants
potassium, 78, 121–22, 287
  foods high in, 122–23
potato chips, 29
potatoes, 191
  roast eye of round with rosemary and,
    234
poultry:
  nutritional data on, 280–81
  turkey, 50–51, 280–81
  See also chicken
premenstrual syndrome (PMS), 119, 147,
  148, 149
proanthocyanidins, 256–57
prostate, 202–3
  cancer of, 23, 202
protein, 26, 63
  amino acids in, 31
  balancing fats and carbohydrates with,
    27–28, 61, 66, 67
  breakdown of, 30
  calories from, 25, 27, 29, 30
  complete, 31–32
  excessive consumption of, 26–27, 30
  functions of, 30–31
  requirements for, 26–27
  sources of, 31–32, 67
psoriasis, 83, 207–8
puddings, 275
pumpkin seeds, 187
Pycnogenol, 256–57
pyridoxine (vitamin B-6), 89, 97, 260, 286

quercetin, xxvii, 74, 75, 260, 289

radiation, 85, 86
radiation therapy for cancer, xxiv
  nutritional healing and, 213
radon, 85
raspberries, 186
  spinach salad with grilled chicken,
    mango and, 230–31
recipes, 215–37
  beef, 234–35
  chicken, 228–31
  fish, 231–34
  muffins, 228
  pancakes, 227
  pasta, 221–25
  rice, 226–27

salad dressings, 236
salads, 220–21, 230–31
soups, 217–19
tofu, 235
vegetables, 221, 237
Reich, Wilhelm, xviii–xix
riboflavin (vitamin B-2), 88, 95–96, 286
rice, 279
rice, brown, 188, 279
fried, 226–27
with steamed vegetables, 226
Rolfing, xx
running, 169, 170

Saint-John's-wort, 261
salad dressings, 236
salads:
beet, with lemon and honey, 220
Boston lettuce and watercress, 220–21
Dad's Italian-style tomatoes, 221
spinach, with grilled chicken, mango,
and raspberries, 230–31
salmon, xxviii, 186
salt. See sodium
sardines, xxviii, 186
Scarsdale Diet, 21
seafood:
contamination of, 52
sauce, Mediterranean, with Jerusalem
artichoke pasta, 222
shellfish, 51–52, 65, 276–77
See also fish
Sears, Barry, 26–27, 28, 60, 61
sea vegetable(s), 185, 186, 189, 190
soup, 218–19
seeds, 187, 193–94
nutritional data on, 271
selenium, 89, 91, 123–24, 260, 287
self-denial, 1–2, 26
self-esteem, 240
self-forgiveness, 3
self-love, 245, 246
sesame seeds, 187, 194
tofu with, 235
sexual abuse, 161–63
sexuality, 160–63, 241–42
impotence and, 203–4
shellfish, 51–52, 65
nutritional data on, 276–77
shiitake mushrooms, 194
Siegel, Bernie, xix
skiing, 173, 174, 180–81
sodas, 7–8, 270
sodium (salt), 5, 7–8, 36, 72–73
in beverages, 270
sole, breaded, 232

soups, 194
Antiguan black bean, 219
canned and condensed, nutritional data
on, 282
miso broth, 217
miso-vegetable, 217–18
sea vegetable, 218–19
sour cream and chive dressing, 236
soybeans and soy products, 41, 68, 147,
186, 189
spinach, xxviii, 186
grilled tuna or swordfish with, 233
rye pasta with, 224–25
salad with grilled chicken, mango, and
raspberries, 230–31
steamed, 237
spirituality, xvii, 155, 265–66
squash, summer, 186
chicken with pea pods and zucchini,
228–29
pasta à la Sinatra, 223
strawberries, 186
stress, 68, 250–51
cholesterol and, 45–46
DHEA and, 250
exercise and, 173
heart disease and, xviii
illness and, xviii–xx
vitamin C and, 100
See also emotions
stroke, 43, 65
sugar, 5–6, 32–33, 35
alternatives to, 195–96
support, emotional, 3–4, 46, 239–40, 248
sweeteners, natural, 195–96
swimming, 174, 181
swordfish, grilled, with spinach, 233

thiamine (vitamin B-1), 88, 95, 286
tofu, 186, 189
with sesame seeds, 235
tomatoes, Dad's Italian-style, 221
tomato sauce:
easy Italian-style, 221–22
fresh, Jerusalem artichoke pasta with,
224
toxins and pollutants, 10, 13, 81, 84–85,
87, 258
aluminum, 121
in animal fats, 55–56
cancer and, 10
in fish, 52, 124
pesticides, 10, 23, 52, 55–56, 82
selenium and, 124
in water, 79, 84–85, 258
triglycerides, 28, 48, 141, 142, 149

tuna:
  grilled, with spinach, 233
  Mediterranean seafood sauce with
    Jerusalem artichoke pasta, 222
  pasta with fennel and, 225
turkey, 50–51, 280–81

uterine cancer, 143, 144, 145, 146

vanadium, 160, 287
vegetable recipes:
  asparagus, 237
  Dad's Italian-style tomatoes, 221
  miso-vegetable soup, 217–18
  rice with steamed vegetables, 226
  steamed spinach, 237
vegetables, xxviii, 67, 68, 191–92
  nutritional data on, 283–84
vitamins, 12–13, 81, 82, 84, 93–103, 285–
    86
  A, 86–87, 88, 89, 91, 94–95, 285
  antioxidant. See antioxidants
  B, 84, 94, 99
  B-1 (thiamine), 88, 95, 286
  B-2 (riboflavin), 88, 95–96, 286
  B-3 (niacin), 88, 96, 286
  B-5 (pantothenic acid), 88, 96–97, 260,
    286
  B-6 (pyridoxine), 89, 97, 260, 286
  B-12 (cyanocobalamin), 88, 97–98, 260,
    286
  balance of, 88
  beta carotene, 89, 91–92, 94–95, 171,
    172, 260, 285
  biotin, 99, 286
  C, 87, 88, 89, 90–91, 94, 99–100, 171,
    172, 260, 285–86
  children and, 138–39
  D, 88, 89, 94, 101, 144, 285
  E, 87, 88, 89, 91, 94, 101–3, 123, 148,
    171, 172, 260, 285
  fat-soluble, 94
  folic acid, xxviii, 67, 88, 98–99, 138,
    150, 260, 286
  RDAs for, 87–88
  water-soluble, 94
vitamin supplements, xxviii, 12–13, 41,
    81–84, 87–93, 172, 260
  advantages of, 90–91
  for children, 139, 140
  megadose hazards of, 88, 89, 94

walking, 11–12, 171, 173–74, 177, 180

  on treadmills, 181
walnuts, 187, 194
water, 5, 7, 8, 71, 72
  contamination of, 79, 84–85, 258
watercress and Boston lettuce salad, 220–21
weight:
  gain, causes of, 20, 27, 33
  ideal, finding, 268–69
weight lifting, 174, 182–83
weight loss:
  behavior change and, 242–43
  calories and, 20
  coenzyme Q10 and, 108
  diets for. See diets, weight-loss
  emotional repercussions of, 239–46
  emotional support and, 3–4, 239–40
  exercise and, 19
  fat intake and, 28–30, 63
  fiber and, 4–5
  friends' intrusions and, 246
  goals in, 158–59
  and HDL and LDL levels, 48
  healthy fats and, 4–5
  holistic approach to, 153–54
  parents and, 155–57, 161–62
  people's reactions to, 240–41
  reframing attitude toward, 154, 157
  relationships and, 242
  self-denial and, 2, 26
  sexuality and, 160–63, 241–42
  water and, 71–72
wheat, 189
Whitaker, Julian, 22, 23, 24
wild yam extract, 130, 148, 250
wine, 74–75
women:
  health strategies for, 149–51
  heart disease and, 140–43, 145, 149, 150
  hormone replacement therapy for, 143–
    44, 145–47, 149
  menopause in, 147, 148–49
  premenstrual syndrome in, 119, 147,
    148, 149

yam extract, 130, 148, 250
yams, 186

zinc, 41, 87, 88, 89, 114, 116, 138, 287
Zone, The (Sears), 26–27, 28, 60
zucchini, chicken with pea pods and, 228–
    29

ABOUT THE AUTHOR

STEPHEN T. SINATRA, M.D., F.A.C.C., is board certified in internal medicine and cardiology. He has special expertise in utilizing behavior modification and emotional release as tools for healthy living. Trained in Gestalt and bioenergetic psychotherapy, he is a certified bioenergetic analyst. Editor of the monthly Phillips' *HeartSense* newsletter, Dr. Sinatra is a much-sought-after speaker for medical conventions and anti-aging conferences.